VOLUME THIRTY NINE

INTERNATIONAL REVIEW OF RESEARCH IN MENTAL RETARDATION

VOLUME THIRTY NINE

INTERNATIONAL REVIEW OF RESEARCH IN MENTAL RETARDATION

Health Issues among Persons with Down Syndrome

Edited by

Richard Charles Urbano
Vanderbilt Kennedy Center for Research on Human Development and Department of Pediatrics
Vanderbilt University
Nashville, TN

ELSEVIER

AMSTERDAM • BOSTON • HEIDELBERG • LONDON
NEW YORK • OXFORD • PARIS • SAN DIEGO
SAN FRANCISCO • SINGAPORE • SYDNEY • TOKYO
Academic Press is an imprint of Elsevier

Academic Press is an imprint of Elsevier
525 B Street, Suite 1900, San Diego, CA 92101-4495, USA
30 Corporate Drive, Suite 400, Burlington, MA 01803, USA
84 Theobald's Road, London WC1X 8RR, UK
Radarweg 29, PO Box 211, 1000 AE Amsterdam, The Netherlands

First edition 2010

British Library Cataloguing in Publication Data
A catalogue record for this book is available from the British Library

Library of Congress Cataloging-in-Publication Data
A catalog record for this book is available from the Library of Congress

ISBN: 978-0-12-374477-7
ISSN: 0074-7750

Printed and bound in the United States of America
08 09 10   10 9 8 7 6 5 4 3 2 1

Contents

Contributors

Numbers in parentheses indicate the pages on which the authors' contributions begin.

Katherine Bathgate (67)
Telethon Institute for Child Health Research, Centre for Child Health Research, The University of Western Australia, Perth, Western Australia

Catia M. Bilardo (165)
Department of Obstetrics and Gynaecology, Fetal Medicine Unit Academic Medical Centre, Amsterdam, The Netherlands

Nico A Blom (165)
Department of Paediatric Cardiology, Leiden University Medical Center, Leiden, The Netherlands

Berto J. Bouma (165)
Department of Cardiology, Academic Medical Centre, Amsterdam, The Netherlands

Jenny Bourke (67)
Telethon Institute for Child Health Research, Centre for Child Health Research, The University of Western Australia, Perth, Western Australia

Susan J. Buckley (297)
Department of Psychology, Down Syndrome Education International, University of Portsmouth, UK

Shoumitro Deb (221)
Consultant Psychiatrist & Clinical Professor of Neuropsychiatry & Intellectual Disability, The Barberry-National Centre for Mental Health, Birmingham, University of Birmingham, UK

Aditya Deshpande (67)
Telethon Institute for Child Health Research, Centre for Child Health Research, The University of Western Australia, Perth, Western Australia

Klaartje van Engelen (165)
Department of Cardiology, Academic Medical Centre, Amsterdam, The Netherlands; Interuniversity Cardiology Institute of the Netherlands, Utrecht, The Netherlands; Department of Clinical Genetics Academic Medical Centre, Amsterdam, The Netherlands

Anna J. Esbensen (107)
Cincinnati Children's Hospital Medical Center, Division of Developmental and Behavioral Pediatrics, Cincinnati, OH, USA

Stephanie Fehr (67)
Telethon Institute for Child Health Research, Centre for Child Health Research, The University of Western Australia, Perth, Western Australia

Sonya Girdler (67)
Department of Occupational Therapy, School of Exercise, Biomedical and Health Sciences, Edith Cowan University, Perth, Western Australia

Samantha E. Goldman (37)
Vanderbilt Kennedy Center, and Department of Special Education, Vanderbilt University, Nashville, Tennessee, USA

Scott D. Grosse (257)
National Center on Birth Defects and Developmental Disabilities, Centers for Disease Control and Prevention, Atlanta, Georgia, USA

Johann K. Hitzler (129)
Division of Hematology/Oncology, Clinician-Scientist, Developmental and Stem Cell Biology, The Hospital for Sick Children, Toronto, Ontario, Canada

Robert M. Hodapp (37)
Vanderbilt Kennedy Center and Department of Special Education, Vanderbilt University, Nashville, Tennessee, USA

Helen Leonard (67)
Telethon Institute for Child Health Research, Centre for Child Health Research, The University of Western Australia, Perth, Western Australia

Ryan McHugh (221)
Speciality Registrar in Psychiatry for People with Learning Disability, Coventry & Warwickshire Partnership Trust, Brooklands Hospital, Birmingham, UK

Nancy Miodrag (37)
Vanderbilt Kennedy Center, Vanderbilt University, Nashville, Tennessee, USA

Barbara J. M. Mulder (165)
Department of Cardiology, Academic Medical Centre, Amsterdam, The Netherlands; Interuniversity Cardiology Institute of the Netherlands, Utrecht, The Netherlands

Heather Porter (195)
Department of Hearing & Speech Sciences, Vanderbilt Bill Wilkerson Center, Vanderbilt University, Nashville, Tennessee, USA

Nancy J. Roizen (3)
Division of Developmental-Behavioral Pediatrics and Psychology, Case Western Reserve University, Cleveland, Ohio, USA

Anne Marie Tharpe (195)
Department of Hearing & Speech Sciences, Vanderbilt Bill Wilkerson Center, Vanderbilt University, Nashville, Tennessee, USA

Kelly Thomas (67)
Department of Occupational Therapy, School of Exercise, Biomedical and Health Sciences, Edith Cowan University and Telethon Institute for Child Health Research, Centre for Child Health Research, The University of Western Australia, Perth, Western Australia

Richard C. Urbano (37)
Vanderbilt Kennedy Center and Department of Pediatrics, General Pediatrics Division, Vanderbilt University, Nashville, Tennessee, USA

Jeroen C. Vis (165)
Department of Cardiology, Academic Medical Centre, Amsterdam, The Netherlands; Interuniversity Cardiology Institute of the Netherlands, Utrecht, The Netherlands

Reviewers

Jennifer Blackford, PhD
Assistant Professor, Dept of Psychiatry and Vanderbilt Kennedy Center, Vanderbilt University
Jenni.blackford@vanderbilt.edu

Derek Chapman, PhD
Assistant Professor, Dept of Epidemiology and Community Health, Virginia Commonwealth University
dachapman@vcu.edu

Deborah Carran, PhD
Professor, Dept of Teacher Development and Leadership, School of Education, Johns Hopkins University
dtcarran@jhu.edu

Deborah Fidler, PhD
Associate Professor, Human Development and Family Studies, School of Education and Department of Psychology, Colorado State University
deborah.fidler@colostate.edu

Shuvo Ghosh, MD
Assistant Professor, Pediatrics, General Pediatrics, McGill University Health Centre
Shuvo.ghosh@muhc.mcgill.ca

Russell S. Kirby, PhD
Professor, Community and Family Health, College of Public Health, University of South Florida
rkirby@health.usf.edu

Craig Mason, PhD
Professor of Education and Applied Quantitative Methods, University of Maine
Craig.mason@umit.maine.edu

Karen Rabin, MD
Assistant Professor, Hematology-Oncology, Department of Pediatrics, Baylor College of Medicine
Krrabin@txccc.org

S. Trent Rosenbloom, MD
Department of Biomedical Informatics, Vanderbilt University
Trent.rosenbloom@vanderbilt.edu

Julie Lounds Taylor, PhD
Assistant Professor, Department of Pediatrics, Special Education Department and Vanderbilt Kennedy Center, Vanderbilt University
Julie.l.taylor@Vanderbilt.edu

Shihfen Tu, PhD
Associate Professor of Education and Applied Quantitative Methods, University of Maine
Shihfen.tu@umit.maine.edu

Paul Yoder, PhD
Department of Special Education and Vanderbilt Kennedy Center, Vanderbilt University
Paul.yoder@Vanderbilt.edu

Preface

In 1866, J. Langdon Down published the results of his careful observations of the characteristics of a group of patients at his institution, providing us with the first description of Down syndrome. However, it was not until 1957 that Lejune identified the underlying genetic mechanism responsible for Down syndrome. Using the latest technological advances, Lejune demonstrated that an extra copy of chromosome 21 existed in these individuals. Today we know that the extra copy of chromosome 21 (trisomy 21) accounts for 95% of all cases of Down syndrome.

Over the last 144 years, we have learned much about Down syndrome's impact on biological systems and its manifestations in intellectual, physical, and social development. Only within the last half century, however, significant progress has been made in improving the length of life of individuals with Down syndrome. With this phenomenal improvement in life expectancy, to around 60 years from the latest estimates, Down syndrome has been transformed from an acute condition with early death to a chronic condition with near-normal life span. As a consequence, management of the syndrome's major health issues has become a significant concern.

In addition to increased life expectancy, how we treat individuals with Down syndrome has changed. Today parents are no longer advised to place their child with Down syndrome in an institution "before they become attached to them." In fact, most children with Down syndrome live at home and participate fully in family life. When they enter the school system, they can be successfully integrated into the general education program. In addition, options now exist for aggressive early intervention to foster development in cognition, speech and language, and physical and social skills. Starting well before 3 years, interventions can be started to correct cardiac anomalies and to lessen speech, language, and motoric delays. Further, widespread infant hearing screening makes it possible to intervene with hearing loss and reduce its impact on speech and language.

Despite progress in understanding and treating health conditions associated with Down syndrome, much is left to learn. As the chapters in this volume illustrate, we often possess the big picture on health conditions, but the details are often missing. For example, it is well understood that individuals with Down syndrome are at risk of developing leukemia early in life (see Chapter 6). At the same time, however, we do not understood how identifiable characteristics of early leukemia are risk factors for or predictors of that condition's life course.

The authors in this volume provide an in-depth view of the conditions that affect individuals with Down syndrome and their families.

In Chapter 1 Nancy Roizen begins our in-depth coverage of the major health conditions affecting individuals with Down syndrome. She sets our concern with the health of individuals with Down syndrome in context when she says, "To enable children and adults with Down syndrome to be healthy and able to function well and live life fully, we need to be knowledgeable about the plethora of medical problems that are possible." She goes on to cover the medical problems and organ system anomalies potentially affecting individuals with Down syndrome: endocrine/metabolic/immune system disorders, cardiovascular disorders, gastrointestinal disorders, vision and hearing problems, cancer, motor/skeletal system disorders, neurological disorders, renal and urologic diseases, and obstructive sleep apnea and pulmonary problems. She emphasizes that individuals with Down syndrome are living longer, healthier lives and that Down syndrome should now be considered a chronic condition to be managed over the life span.

The next three chapters focus on the health outcomes most prominent in three distinct periods of life: infants and toddlers (Chapter 2), school-aged children (Chapter 3), adult and end of life (Chapter 4).

In Chapter 2, Robert Hodapp, Nancy Miodrag, Samantha Goldman, and I present the challenges facing individuals with Down syndrome from birth through early childhood. Although significant progress has been made in identifying and treating the health conditions affecting young children with Down syndrome, challenges still remain. The findings from large-scale population-based studies show that the prevalence of adverse birth outcomes, in-patient hospitalizations, and infant mortality are significantly higher for young children with Down syndrome. Hodapp et al. conclude their chapter by identify four areas needing additional emphasis in order to achieve better heath in young children with Down syndrome: (1) the interaction effects of health with such contextual factors as family characteristics, amount and quality of health services, and residential environment; (2) increased breadth and depth of population-level data; (3) freely available, flexible, and easy-to-use record linkage software; and (4) improved anticipatory guidance for parents and providers.

Progressing along the life span, Helen Leonard and her colleagues next cover health issues for school-aged children with Down syndrome. Many children in this age group have additional birth defects and health-related problems. They are at increased risk of cardiac, respiratory, gastrointestinal, ophthalmologic, ear and hearing, musculoskeletal, leukemia, thyroid, immune system, and dental problems. Repeating a theme from almost every chapter, Leonard et al. lament that there are so few studies of health issues in Down syndrome.

Anna Esbensen rounds out the series of age-related chapters with coverage of adult and aging issues. The increased life expectancy for individuals with Down syndrome has made it possible to study medical conditions common among adults, to show changes with age, and to examine the relationship of these conditions to mortality. In Chapter 4, Anna Esbensen reports that adults with Down syndrome are at increased risk of skin and hair changes, early onset menopause, visual and hearing impairments, adult-onset seizure disorder, thyroid dysfunction, diabetes, obesity, sleep apnea, and musculoskeletal problems. Care providers and families need to be on the alert beginning in early adulthood for changes in these age-related conditions, as they occur earlier in individuals with Down syndrome.

Thus far, the emphasis has been on age-related changes in health conditions. In the next five chapters, the focus switches to specific conditions that affect a large proportion of individuals with Down syndrome and their families: cancer (Chapter 5), cardiovascular disorders (Chapter 6), hearing loss (Chapter 7), dementia (Chapter 8), and sociodemographic and economic factors (Chapter 9).

While the overall incidence of cancer in children and adults with Down syndrome appears to be the same as that in the general population, the distribution of tumor types is markedly different. In Chapter 5, Johann Hitzler presents the current state of knowledge on tumors in children and adults with Down syndrome. He notes that leukemia is the most common childhood cancer in Down syndrome, with an incidence 10–20 times greater than in the general population. By contrast, solid tumors are markedly less frequent among these children and adults. Leukemia in children with Down syndrome is usually transient and does not convert into acute myeloid or acute lymphoblastic leukemia. However, 20% of the cases with transient childhood leukemia do convert to acute myeloid leukemia (AML) later in life. Finally, he reviews the intriguing evidence that two genes, CRLF2 and JAK2, may be associated with acute lymphoblastic leukemia (ALL) in Down syndrome.

At birth, almost half of the children with Down syndrome have some type of cardiac anomaly. In Chapter 6, Barbara Mulder and Jeroen Vis provide a comprehensive description of the anatomy of the heart, emphasizing the anatomical anomalies observed in Down syndrome. They review prenatal screening, intrauterine interventions, and the management of congenital heart defects in early childhood. They also cover pulmonary arterial hypertension and cardiac surgery during adulthood.

Another serious condition affecting half of the individuals with Down syndrome is hearing loss. In Chapter 7, Heather Porter and Anne Marie Tharpe describe the structure of the auditory system and the features specific to Down syndrome. They describe the methods available for diagnosing hearing loss and interventions available to compensate for that loss. For both diagnosis and intervention, they describe the challenges presented when working with individuals with Down syndrome.

Management of hearing loss for individuals with Down syndrome is critical to helping them maximize their communicative and cognitive potential.

In the section's final chapter, Shoumitro Deb and Ryan McHugh (Chapter 8) cover the single most important condition that has come to prominence from the increased lifespan of individuals with Down syndrome. Dementia, most notably Alzheimer's disease, appears earlier in life for individuals with Down syndrome and at a more advanced stage when diagnosed. Deb and McHugh emphasize that early changes associated with adult-onset dementias are difficult to diagnose in individuals with Down syndrome. The tools available for diagnosis require a high degree of clinical skill, do not have established psychometric properties, or were not designed for individuals with intellectual and developmental disabilities. Even when these diagnostic tools can be used, baseline measures taken early in adulthood are not always available. Thus, it is unclear if low levels of performance are characteristic of the syndrome or true deterioration in performance.

In the last chapter in this section (Chapter 9), Scott Grosse views the health issues for individuals with Down syndrome from the perspective of the family. He addresses two questions. First, he asks, "Are families of individual with Down syndrome different than other families of children with and without intellectual and developmental disabilities?" Specifically, he asks if there is a "Down syndrome advantage." Second, he asks, "What are the economic consequences of having a child with Down syndrome?" He provides a comprehensive review of the literature relating to both topics. Although a number of relevant studies relate to his first question, the literature on the economic impact of having a child with Down syndrome is severely limited. He extrapolates the findings from the intellectual and developmental disabilities literature to Down syndrome. More attention is need to this important question.

In the final chapter, Susan Buckley comments on the progress that has been in medical care and offers some cautions. From the perspective of a mother of a 40-year-old daughter with Down syndrome and a researcher and practitioner, she offers her insight on how information on health issues in Down syndrome should guide families. Further, she notes the diversity among individuals with Down syndrome and suggests that population-level findings should be followed-up with studies of individual differences and patterns of health outcomes.

Progress in health care provided to children and adults with Down syndrome has changed their lives. These individuals are now living longer, healthier, and more fulfilling lives. This special issue highlights the progress that has been made and points the way to even greater gains in health care. It is particularly important, at this time, to have easily accessible, solid, scientific work to inform the public policy debate on how to best improve the services for individuals with Down syndrome.

Dr. Langdon Downs would be amazed at the progress we have made in the last 140-plus years. He would be in awe as are we with the realization of how much there is left to be learned. It is critical to continue our search for an even fuller knowledge base regarding every facet of Down syndrome. Additional research funding is also necessary to expand our knowledge base, make significant strides forward in health care, and discover additional ways we can help individuals with Down syndrome and their families have an optimal quality of life.

Richard C. Urbano

Series Preface

In this special issue, Dr. Richard C. Urbano assembles the leading experts to provide a state-of-the-art overview on the health of individuals with Down syndrome. As several contributors note, although life expectancy is increasing rapidly for these individuals, many health problems remain. Compared to the general population, persons with Down syndrome display much higher rates of congenital heart defects, respiratory problems, hearing–speech difficulties, leukemia, dementia, and other health problems.

As illustrated by this special issue, such problems can be approached from two viewpoints: the age of the individual and the person's specific medical condition. After a strong opening chapter by Dr. Nancy Roizen, the first section focuses on the early childhood, school age, and adult years, while the second focuses on cancer, heart defects, and other specific conditions. Both age- and condition-related perspectives are critical to appreciating health-related problems in individuals with Down syndrome.

Such problems also highlight the need for future policy initiatives. As noted by Madeline Will in her Afterword, the National Down Syndrome Society and National Down Syndrome Congress are working to increase U.S. federal support for coordinated health care and for further studies of the health problems of children and adults with the syndrome. The National Institutes of Health (NIH) and the Centers for Disease Control and Prevention (CDC) have hosted conferences and produced plans for future work and, under Madeline Will's leadership, policymakers are being made aware that such health problems require sustained clinical and research attention.

Rarely, it seems, has there been such a confluence of content and opportunity. As a result of a 100-plus year history, we currently know at least the basics about the syndrome's age- and condition-related health problems, with each sub-area featuring a small—albeit inadequate—research base. Now seems the perfect moment to highlight such issues, with opportunities (and benefits) imminent for policymakers, physicians, parents, and individuals with Down syndrome.

Last but in no way least, Rick Urbano is the perfect editor for this special issue. As a long-time researcher in developmental epidemiology, Rick has for the past 5 years focused on the health of young children with Down syndrome (see Chapter 2). As the database "guru" for the Vanderbilt Kennedy Center, Rick works with researchers (through our Eunice Kennedy Shriver-Intellectual and Developmental Research Center, or

IDDRC) and with parents, service providers, and disability policymakers (through our University Center for Excellence in Developmental Disabilities, or UCEDD). He appreciates research, service, and policy needs.

Finally, as series editor of the *International Review* and Rick's colleague and friend, I greatly appreciate his leadership of this volume. Rick's enthusiasm has been infectious, all the way from proposing the volume; to recruiting, encouraging, and editing contributions from a stellar cast of international researchers; to working with Elsevier's editorial, promotional, and production teams; to recruiting Madeline Will to write the Afterword. Rick sensed a major need for this type of one-stop resource. *Health Issues among Persons with Down Syndrome* is a testament to Rick's vision, perseverance, and hard work.

Robert M. Hodapp
Series Editor

Glossary of Terms*

Richard C. Urbano and S. Trent Rosenbloom

accommodation	The process by which the eye's lens increases optical power to produce a clear image on an object when it draws near the eye.
activating mutation	A mutation that results in increased activity of the affected gene.
acute lymphoblastic leukemia (ALL)	A type of leukemia that affects the white blood cells, the cells that normally fight infections.
acute megakaryoblastic leukemia (AMKL)	A type of leukemia related to acute myeloid leukemia, in which the leukemic cells have a platelet precursor phenotype.
acute myeloid leukemia (AML)	A type of leukemia, in which the leukemic cells (called blasts) display lineage features of myeloid white blood cells.
adenoidectomy	The surgical removal of the adenoids, which are lymph nodes located in the back of the throat behind the nose and below the tonsils.
AGA IgG	A type of antibodies called "anti-gliadin," which are antibodies produced against gliadin, a prolamin found in wheat, frequently found in patients with celiac disease and in relationship with tTG.
alopecia	Hair loss.
alopecia areata	Hair loss resulting from the immune system attacking the hair follicle.
amblyopia	A condition in which vision does not develop properly in each eye, often called "lazy eye."
amyloid plaque	A small disk-shaped growth or plaque, consisting of tangles of amyloid proteins, typically found in nervous tissue.
angiogenesis	Growth of new blood vessels from existing blood vessels.

* Definitions provided by Hitzler, Leonard et al., Mulder, and Vis and drawn from http://medical-dictionary.thefreedictionary.com/

antithyroid antibodies test	Test for antibodies that attack the thyroid.
aortic coarctation	A narrowing of the aorta, commonly found just distal to the origin of the left subclavian artery.
aphakia	Absence of the lens of the eye.
APOE	Apolipoprotein E.
apoptosis	Programmed cell death.
APP	Amyloid precursor protein.
arthrodesis	Joint fusion surgery.
ascites	Abnormal fluid accumulation in the abdominal cavity.
astigmatism	A vision condition that causes blurred vision due to either an irregular shape of the cornea or the curvature of the lens inside the eye.
atherosclerosis	A process of hardening and narrowing of the arteries. It is caused by inflammation and the slow accumulation of fatty deposits (plaque) on the inside of walls of the arteries.
atlantoaxial instability	A condition in which the two bones at the top of the spinal cord are unstable and provide inadequate support for the skull. Because people with Down syndrome can have more lax ligaments, the two bones at the top of the neck (called C1 and C2) may be prone to excessive movement.
atlantoaxial subluxation	When one or more of the bones of the cervical spine move out of position and create pressure on or irritate spinal nerves.
atresia	Congenital absence or closure of a normal body opening or tubular structure.
atrial septal defect (ASD)	A congenital heart defect in the muscle wall (i.e., septum) between the right and left atrium that enables blood flow between the left and right atria.
atrial septostomy	A procedure in which a small hole is created between the heart's right and left atria, the upper two chambers of the heart.
atrioventricular septal defect (AVSD)	A congenital heart defect characterized by a lack of separation between the right atrium and the left ventricle, creating communication between the two sides of the heart.

azoospermia A condition in which no sperm are produced, or do not appear in the semen.

B precursor acute lymphoblastic leukemia The most common form of childhood leukemia, defined by leukemic cells that show features normally found in precursor cells of B lymphocytes.

B-lymphocytes The precursors of antibody-forming plasma cells; these cells carry immunoglobulin and class II MHC (major histocompatibility complex) antigens on their surfaces.

balloon valvuloplasty A procedure in which a narrowed valve is dilated by expanding a balloon inside the valve.

blast An acute leukemic cell as defined by microscopy.

blast lineage Leukemic cells do not complete normal differentiation into mature blood cells but frequently display features found in normal blood cell lineages (e.g., lymphoid, myeloid). Diagnosis of leukemia includes the characterization of the blast lineage.

blepharitis Inflammation of the eyelids.

bone marrow aspirate The material obtained from a procedure to collect bone marrow cells (typically obtained from the hip bone) as part of the diagnosis of leukemia.

calcaneal valgus Club foot.

cardiomyopathy A condition of abnormal heart function.

cavopulmonary shunt A surgically created connection between the vena cava (inferior and superior) and the pulmonary arteries. This is a palliative procedure in patients with a univentricular circulation.

cerumen Ear wax.

chemotaxis The process in which cells migrate in response to the presence of certain trigger molecules in their environment.

chest radiography Also called a chest X-ray, is a projection radiograph of the chest used to diagnose conditions affecting the chest, its contents, and nearby structures.

chromosomal See chromosome.

chromosomal rearrangement The process by which abnormally structured chromosomes are created by rearranging their material with other adjacent chromosomes, e.g., in leukemic cells; see also chromosomal translocation.

chromosomal translocation	A form of a chromosomal rearrangement in which parts of one chromosome are moved (translocated) to another chromosome; translocations are a common mechanism underlying abnormal gene activity in leukemic cells.
chromosome	An organized structure of DNA molecules and protein found in the cell nucleus. Each chromosome contains hundreds or thousands of the genes that form our hereditary blueprint. The number of chromosomes in the normal human cell is 46 (23 pairs).
clonal	Derived from a single cell.
coarctation	Malformation or narrowing of one or more structures of the heart or blood vessels.
coding region	Part of a gene that determines the amino acid sequence of the encoded protein.
collagen VI	A microfibrillar component of many extracellular matrices, acting as a bridge between cell surfaces and the surrounding extracellular matrix.
congenital	Present at birth, either due to genetic or developmental causes.
conjugated hyperbilirubinemia	Accumulation in the blood of a bile pigment normally secreted by the liver.
constitutional trisomy	Trisomy present in all cells of the body.
cryptorchidism	A condition in which the male testes do not descend normally into the scrotal sacks, and occasionally associated with an increased lifetime risk of testicular cancer.
cyanosis	Physical sign where the skin appears bluish, caused by an excess concentration of deoxygenated hemoglobin in the bloodstream. In congenital heart disease, cyanosis is generally due to right-to-left shunting through the cardiac defect, bypassing the lungs.
cyanotic	The condition of having cyanosis.
cysteine rich with EGF domains 1 (CRELD1) gene	Gene encoding a cell surface protein that likely functions as a cell adhesion molecule.

cytogenetics Diagnostic discipline focused on the analysis of numerical and structural chromosomal abnormalities, e.g., in leukemic cells (blasts).

cytokine Type of secreted cellular signaling molecule, often involved in the inflammatory process.

dacryocutaneous Involving the nasolacrimal duct.

deletion A chromosomal change in which part of the DNA is lost.

DNA methylation An epigenetic process involving the addition of a methyl group to a DNA molecule, inducing a change in DNA structure in this case with the specific effect of reducing gene expression.

Down syndrome cell adhesion molecule (DSCAM) A cell adhesion molecule involved in the development of the nervous system, but which is also highly expressed in the heart during cardiac development.

Down syndrome CHD critical region The minimal region on chromosome 21 that needs to be triplicated to cause the congenital heart defects in Down syndrome.

Down syndrome critical region (DSCR) The minimal region on chromosome 21 that needs to be triplicated to cause the Down syndrome phenotype.

Down syndrome critical region 1 gene (DSCR1) Gene encoding an inhibitor of the calcineurin/NFAT signaling, expressed in many tissues including the heart. The gene is also named Regulator of Calcineurin 1, RCAN1.

dual-energy X-ray absorptiometry (DEXA) An enhanced form of X-ray technology that is used to measure bone density.

dual-specificity tyrosine-(Y)-phosphorylation-regulated kinase 1A (DYRK1A) gene Gene encoding a nuclear kinase that regulates several transcription factors, including NFAT transcription factors.

ductus arteriosus In the developing fetus, the ductus arteriosus, also called the ductus Botalli, is a normal vascular connection between the aorta and pulmonary artery that typically closes shortly after birth under the influence of increased oxygen in the bloodstream occurring as soon as air breathing begins.

duodenal	Relates to the duodenum, the first section of the small intestine.
duodenum	First part of the small intestine.
dysgammaglobulinemia	Immunodeficiency due to the reduction of certain types of antibodies.
dyslipidemia	Disorders in the lipoprotein metabolism. There is an excess of lipids (such as cholesterol) in the blood.
dysmorphic	An alteration in the normal form or appearance.
ECMO	Extracorporeal membrane oxygenation.
ectasia	A general term used to describe dilation or abnormal growth of a body structure.
effusion	An abnormal collection of fluid in a body cavity.
Eisenmenger syndrome	A syndrome resulting from longstanding pulmonary arterial hypertension as a consequence of preexisting systemic-to-pulmonary shunting that results in increased pulmonary vascular resistance leading to a reversed (right-to-left) shunt.
emmetropia	It is the ideal state of the eye in which no refractive error is present.
endocarditis	An infection of the endocardium (the membrane that lines the inner surfaces of the heart) or the heart valves.
endomysium	The fine connective tissue sheath surrounding a muscle fiber.
enteropathy	A disease of the intestinal tract.
epicanthic folds	A skin fold of the upper eyelid.
epigenetics	The study of heritable changes in gene function that occur without a change in the DNA sequence.
epiphora	Excessive tear production.
esodeviation	Term referring to either esophoria or esotropia, meaning convergent strabismus.
Eustachian tube	The narrow channel connecting the middle ear and the posterior nasopharynx.
euthyroid	A normal thyroid hormone status.

exodeviation Turning out.

facies Face or exterior aspect of a body part or organ.

failure to thrive A condition to describe a delay in a child's growth or development.

fibrillin A major component of elastin-associated microfibrils.

fistula An abnormal connection between an organ, vessel, or intestine and another structure.

flow cytometry Automated laboratory method to characterize the expression of specific markers on the surface and within cells; leukemic cells, for example, are first labeled with specific antibodies bound to fluorescing dyes; if the antigen or marker of interest is present on the leukemic cell, a fluorescence signal is detected as the cell flows through a detection unit.

folliculitis Inflammation or infection of one or more hair follicles.

foot pronation A rotational movement of the foot.

foramen ovale An opening in the fetal heart between the atria that allows blood to bypass the immature pulmonary circulation and to enter the left atrium from the right.

fusion gene Abnormal gene made up of parts derived from normally separate genes as a consequence of chromosomal translocation.

genomic Related to the entire collection of genes in an organism.

genomics Scientific discipline focused on the analysis of the collection of all genes in an organism (genome).

geographic tongue Benign migratory glossitis (inflammation of the tongue).

germ line Refers to cells and their genes in the absence of mutations.

glomerulonephritis A specific inflammatory disease of the kidneys.

glomerulosclerosis Hyaline deposits or scarring with the renal glomeruli.

Hashimoto's thyroiditis	A chronic autoimmune thyroiditis characterized by thyroid enlargement, reduced thyroid function, thyroid fibrosis, lymphatic infiltration of thyroid tissue, and the production of antibodies which attack the thyroid.
hearing loss (conductive, sensorineural)	Sensorineural, or nerve deafness; conductive, where sound is not transmitted into inner ear. "Mixed," is simply a combination of sensorineural and conductive hearing loss.
hemiplegia	Paralysis of one side of the body but not the other.
hepatosplenomegaly	Abnormal enlargement of liver and spleen.
Hirschsprung disease	Also known as congenital megacolon or aganglionic megacolon, is an abnormality in which certain nerve fibers are absent in segments of the bowel, resulting in severe bowel obstruction.
HLA	Human leukocyte antigen.
hydronephrosis	A swelling and dilation of the urine collecting system at the kidneys occurring when urine flow is obstructed.
hydroureter	The distention of the ureter with urine due to blockage of urine flow.
hypercholesterolemia	Higher than normal level of cholesterol in the blood, typically 240 mg/dL or above.
hyperdiploidy	Presence of an increased number of chromosomes in a cell.
hypergammaglobulinemia	The presence of an abnormally high amount of gamma globulins in the blood.
hyperglycemia	Abnormally elevated blood sugar level.
hyperkeratosis	Non-cancerous enlargement (hypertrophy) of the cornea or the horny layer of the skin.
hypermetropia	A defect of vision also called long-sightedness.
hypertelorism	Abnormally increased distance between the eyes.
hyperthyroidism	Overactivity of the thyroid gland characterized by weight loss, chest pain, cramps, diarrhea, and nervousness.
hypoplastic/dysplastic	Underdeveloped/abnormally developed.

hypospadias A condition in which the urinary meatus is abnormally developed and located low on the ventral penis.

hypothyroidism Deficiency of thyroid activity characterized by weight gain and decreased metabolism.

hypotonia Abnormally low muscular tone.

ichthyosis Skin disorder characterized by excessive amounts of dry surface scales.

IgA, Total The total serum level of Immunoglobulin A.

immunoglobulin A specific protein called an antibody, synthesized in response to the presence of a foreign substance (antigen).

insertion Mutation, in which there is an abnormal gain of DNA.

interproximal Area in between two teeth.

intracardiac Inside the heart.

intronic polymorphism Polymorphism of a segment of a gene situated between exons that are removed before transcription.

iritis Inflammation of the iris of the eye.

JAK Janus kinases belong to a family of proteins which participate in the transduction of cellular signals, e.g., the binding of growth factor or cytokine molecules to the cell surface, into altered gene activity in the cell nucleus.

karyotyping A test performed to analyze chromosomes by size and morphology to detect changes in chromosomal structure and arrangement.

keratoconus A deterioration of the structure of the cornea with gradual bulging from the normal round shape to a cone shape.

kinase Enzyme or enzymatic activity adding phosphate groups to a substrate.

lacrimal Located near or relating to the glands that produce tears.

lectins Antibody-sized glycoproteins—part carbohydrate, part protein.

leptin	A protein hormone with an important role in regulating body weight, metabolism, and reproductive functions.
lymphocyte	A type of T cell and B cell in the vertebrate immune system.
lymphoid	Associated with T or B lymphocytes and their cell lineages.
mandibular prognathism	Abnormal forward positioning of mandible (lower jaw) in relation to skeletal base beyond predetermined imaginary line in sagittal plane.
megakaryoblastic	Associated with an immature cell (megakaryoblast) within the platelet precursor lineage.
megakaryocytic	Associated with platelet precursors (megakaryocytes) and their blood cell lineage.
metatarsus primus	A condition in which the first metatarsal bone in the foot is rotated and angled away from the second metatarsal bone.
metatarsus primus varus	The part of the foot between the ankle and the toes.
micro-RNA	A type of non-coding RNA that binds to messenger RNA, thereby inhibiting translation of the messenger RNA to a protein. This is an epigenetic mechanism.
microcephaly	Abnormally small head or cranial capacity.
microcysts	A cyst only observable microscopically.
microdontia	A condition of having one or more disproportionately small teeth.
microphthalmos	Abnormal smallness in all dimensions of one or both eyes.
mitral valve	Heart valve, situated between the left atrium and the left ventricle; allows blood to pass from atrium to ventricle.
mitral valve prolapse	A heart problem in which the valve that separates the upper and lower chambers of the left side of the heart does not close properly.
mosaicism	The presence of a genetic change (e.g., trisomy 21) in some but not in all cells of the body, such as only in a proportion of cells and tissues.

moyamoya	From the Japanese, "a puff of smoke," a cerebrovascular disorder in which the main cerebral arteries at the base of the brain are replaced by a fine network of vessels.
mucositis	Inflammation and breakdown of mucosal membranes, e.g., as a side effect of chemotherapy.
multipotential hematopoietic progenitor cell	Precursor cell within the blood cell forming tissue, which is capable of giving rise to several types of mature blood cells, also called stem cells.
mutation	An abnormal alteration of the normal DNA sequence or resulting in an altered gene product or function.
myelodysplastic syndrome (MDS)	A blood cell disorder in which the normal maturation of blood cells is blocked; may develop into acute myeloid leukemia (AML).
myeloid	Associated with myeloid blood cells and their lineage (e.g., monocytic, granulocytic, erythroid, megakaryocyctic).
myelopathy	Disturbance or disease of the spinal cord.
myeloproliferative disorder	Hematological disorder characterized by the excessive production of blood cells, classified with hematological malignancies.
myoclonus	Shock-like contractions of a muscle or a group of muscles.
nasolacrimal duct	Tear duct between the inner canthus of the eye and the inside of the nose.
nasopharyngeal	Pertaining to the cavity of the nose and the nasal parts of the pharynx.
neurofibrillary tangles	Abnormal structures composed of twisted masses of protein fibers within nerve cells.
neutropenia	An abnormally low blood concentration of neutrophils, a subset of white blood cells, which plays an important role in the control of bacterial and fungal infections.
neutrophil	The most common type of white blood cell involved in immunity, a subset of white blood cells, which plays an important role in the control of bacterial and fungal infections.

nuchal translucency	Refers to the nuchal fluid accumulation visible in first trimester fetuses and measurable at ultrasound examination. A large nuchal translucency measurement at 11–14 weeks' pregnancy is a marker for Down syndrome and for cardiac defects.
nystagmus	A form of involuntary eye movement.
occipitoatlantal	Of or relating to the occipital bone of the skull and the atlas cervical vertebrae.
odontoid	Having the form of a tooth.
oligoarticular	Affecting a few joints.
oligoclonal	Derived from more than one cell line.
onychomycosis	A chronic fungal infection of the fingernails or toenails.
organomegaly	Abnormal enlargement of an organ, particularly an organ of the abdominal cavity.
oro-facial	Pertaining to mouth or face.
otolaryngology	The branch of medicine dealing with disease of the ear, nose, and throat.
palmoplantar	Of relating to or affecting both the palms of the hands and the soles of the feet.
palpebral	Pertaining to the eye.
partial anodontia	Congenital absence of one or more teeth.
partial trisomy 21	Only a part of chromosome 21 is triplicated, as opposed to full trisomy 21, in which the whole chromosome 21 is triplicated.
patent ductus arteriosus (PDA)	A heart condition occurring soon after birth in which the ductus arteriosus remains open, causing abnormal blood flow between two of the major arteries connected to the heart.
pericardial effusion	Abnormal fluid accumulation around the heart.
pes planus	Flat feet or fallen arches.
pharyngeal	Of relating to, located in, or coming from the pharynx.
phytohemagglutinin	PHA, a lectin found in plants that causes red blood cells to adhere together in the laboratory.

pleural effusion An abnormal fluid accumulation around the lungs.

pneumoeustachian (PE) tubes (Grommets) tiny tubes put in the eardrum to allow air to equalize between the middle ear and the atmosphere, and to allow abnormal ear fluid to drain.

point mutation Mutation in which a single DNA nucleotide is altered.

polyarticular Affecting many joints.

polysomnography A sleep study which monitors a person as they sleep, or try to sleep.

prenatal screening This currently consists of first (or second) trimester screening for Down syndrome and mid-trimester routine ultrasound investigation for the diagnosis of structural congenital defects, such as heart defects.

pronation Lowering or descending of the inner edge of the boot by turning the entire foot outward. Related to flat feet.

proteolytic Degradation of proteins by cellular enzymes.

PS-1 Presenilin-1.

ptosis An abnormally drooping upper eyelid.

pulmonary hypertension An abnormal elevation of the blood pressure present in the pulmonary arteries, occasionally associated with a syndrome of dyspnoea, fatigue, chest pain, and syncope caused by a progressive increase in mean pulmonary vascular resistance.

pulmonary vascular resistance The resistance that must be overcome to push blood through the pulmonary circulatory system.

pyloric stenosis A narrowing of the pylorus, which is the muscular sphincter at the passage between the stomach and the small intestine.

RCAN1 See Down syndrome critical region 1 gene (DSCR1).

reactive oxygen species (ROS) Chemically reactive products of oxygen within cells.

remission Stage following the initial treatment of cancer when cancer cells are no longer detectable.

rhinorrhea	An abnormal discharge from the nasal mucous membrane, especially if excessive.
seborrheic dermatitis	A common inflammatory disease of the skin characterized by oily and scaly lesions usually on the scalp, hairline, and face.
seminomas	A malignant tumor of the testis arising from sperm-forming tissue.
shunt	Movement of blood through a congenitally abnormal or surgically created connection or hole between two circuits. Cardiac shunts may be described as right-to-left, left-to-right, or bidirectional, or as systemic-to-pulmonary or pulmonary-to-systemic.
sinusitis	An abnormal inflammation of the sinuses, often caused by viral or bacterial infections.
solid tumor	Cancers not derived from blood cells and their precursors.
somatic mutation	Acquired mutation in a proportion of the cells of the body, e.g., leukemic cells, as opposed to a germ-line mutation, which is inherited and present in all cells of the body.
spermatogenic	Producing semen or spermatozoa.
stenosis	An abnormal narrowing in a blood vessel or other tubular organ or structure.
strabismus	A condition in which the eyes are not properly aligned with each other.
***Streptococcus mutans*-specific IgA**	Antibody produced in saliva against microorganism *Streptococcus mutans*.
subglottic stenosis	Abnormal narrowing below the glottis.
subluxation	An incomplete or partial dislocation.
T-lymphocyte	Lymphocyte cells which mature in the thymus and are involved in cell-mediated immunity.
T4, T3, or TSH	Tests for evaluating thyroid function and/or symptoms of hypothyroidism or hyperthyroidism include measures of thyroid-stimulating hormone (TSH). It is frequently ordered along with or preceding a T4 (thyroxine) test. Other thyroid tests that may be ordered include a T3 (tri-iodothyronine) test.

tachypnea Breathing faster rate than normal.

taurodontism Body of a tooth is enlarged at the expense of its root during development resulting in large tooth crown size.

teratomas A type of cancer that differentiates into different types of tissue, none of which is native to the area in which it occurs; usually found in the ovary or testis.

tetralogy of Fallot A syndrome of four congenital anatomic abnormalities of the heart: pulmonary artery stenosis, ventricular septal defect (VSD), deviation of the aortic origin to the right, and right ventricular hypertrophy.

thromboembolism The collective term for deep vein thrombosis and pulmonary embolism. A condition in which a blood clot (thrombus) forms in a vein, which in some cases then breaks free and enters the circulation as an embolus, finally lodging in and completely obstructing a blood vessel.

thymus A lymphoid organ that is located in the superior mediastinum and lower part of the neck and is necessary in early life for the normal development of immunological function.

thyrotoxicosis The presence of hyperthyroidism severe enough to cause abnormalities to other body systems, such as the cardiovascular system or the neurologic system.

tonic-clonic seizures A type of generalized seizure that affects the entire brain and is manifest as loss of consciousness and abnormal movements throughout the body, often called a grand mal seizure.

toxicity Adverse effects of therapeutic intervention, such as from chemotherapy for cancer.

transcript RNA generated from a gene.

transcription factor Protein able to bind to and regulate the activity (transcription) of a set of genes.

transglutaminase An enzyme, formed by cleavage and activation of protransglutaminase.

transposition of the great arteries	A congenital anatomic heart defect with a reversed connection of the great arteries and ventricles such that the pulmonary trunk arises from the left ventricle and the aorta arises from the right ventricle.
tricuspid valve	Heart valve, situated between the right atrium and the right ventricle; allows blood to pass from atrium to ventricle.
trisomy	Presence of three instead of the normal two copies of a specific chromosome.
tTG IgA	Anti-tissue transglutaminase immunoglobulin A. These are tissue transglutaminase-specific antibodies (IgA) produced during celiac disease.
tympanostomy tube (grommets)	See pneumoeustachian (PE) tubes.
uropathy	Any disease or other pathologic change in the urinary tract.
valgus	Characterized by an abnormal outward turning of a bone, especially of the hip, knee, or foot.
vasodilator	An agent that causes blood vessels to relax and dilate.
ventricular septal defect (VSD)	A congenital anatomic heart defect characterized by a hole in the muscular septum between the right and left ventricles of the heart.
vitiligo	An abnormal condition in which a loss of cells that give color to the skin (melanocytes) results in smooth, white patches in the midst of normally pigmented skin.
xerosis	Abnormal dryness, as of the eye, skin, or mouth.

INTRODUCTION

CHAPTER ONE

Overview of Health Issues among Persons with Down Syndrome

Nancy J. Roizen

Contents

Division of Developmental-Behavioral Pediatrics and Psychology, Case Western Reserve University, Cleveland, Ohio, USA

International Review of Research in Mental Retardation, Volume 39
ISSN 0074-7750, DOI 10.1016/S0074-7750(10)39001-X

Abstract

With increasingly effective medical interventions for congenital heart disease and leukemia, more individuals with Down syndrome (DS) are living into adulthood and old age. To enable children and adults with DS to be healthy and able to function well and live life fully, we need to be knowledgeable about the plethora of medical problems that are possible. In individuals with DS, each system has the potential of some or several types of medical problems that may require constant surveillance such as celiac disease or monitoring such as thyroid disease. These disorders may be more prevalent at different ages, such as arthropathy of DS, or constantly a potential issue, such as atlantoaxial subluxation. This chapter describes by system the multitude of potential medical problems that individuals with DS have an increased chance of developing at different ages.

1. Introduction

In the life of a person with Down syndrome (DS), he or she has the potential of having health issues in almost every system. Some health problems occur so commonly that every child needs evaluation including congenital heart defects and vision and hearing problems. Other problems such as thyroid disorders need monitoring; obesity and dental problems need prevention and management. Careful surveillance is indicated for gastrointestinal (GI) malformations, type 1 diabetes, seizures, atlantoaxial subluxation, leukemia, testicular cancer, arthritis, and obstructive sleep apnea. This chapter provides a detailed presentation of each of these systems.

2. Endocrine, Metabolic, and Immune System Disorders

2.1. Thyroid disorders

There has been long recognition of the association of thyroid disorders and DS (Forte et al., 1984), and consequently, routine monitoring is recommended. There are several types of thyroid disorders found in individuals with DS including congenital hypothyroidism, primary hypothyroidism, autoimmune (Hashimoto's) thyroiditis, compensated hypothyroidism (otherwise referred to as hyperthyrotropinemia or subclinical hypothyroidism), and hyperthyroidism. One in 141 newborns with DS has persistent primary congenital hypothyroidism, compared to 1 in 4000 in the general population (Forte et al., 1984). The cause of congenital hypothyroidism does not seem to be thyroid agenesis since most patients have normal thyroid scans (Kennedy, Jones, & Cuckle, 1992). Primary hypothyroidism develops after the newborn period with a high thyroid-stimulating hormone (TSH) and low T4 and is usually not associated with antithyroid antibodies. Karlsson, Gustafsson, Hedov, Ivarsson, and Anneren (1998) reported on a longitudinal study monitoring 85 children with DS for thyroid disorders up to 25 years of age. Hypothyroidism was found in 30 children and hyperthyroidism in 2 of the 85 children. Half of those with hypothyroidism acquired it before 8 years of age with only one displaying thyroid autoantibodies at diagnosis. This contrasted with the 15 children who were diagnosed after 8 years of age where 11 of the 13 tested were positive for thyroid autoantibodies indicating autoimmune thyroiditis. They documented slower growth before treatment in the 8 children with hypothyroidism who were younger than 8 years at diagnosis. In 7 of the 8 children, growth velocity increased with treatment.

Compensated hypothyroidism which is characterized by a mildly elevated TSH with normal or low normal free T4 is the type that is more controversial. The Turkish series of 320 children between 5 days and 10 years of age reported 1.8% of their children with hypothyroidism but an additional 23.3% with compensated hypothyroidism (Tuysuz & Beker, 2001). Gibson et al. (2005) from the United Kingdom reported that 25.3% of 122 children with DS screened for thyroid disorders had compensated hypothyroidism but only 30% of these children on retesting continued to have compensated hypothyroidism. Trostenburg, Vulsma, van Sante, Cheung, and Vijlder (2005) reported a randomized placebo-controlled trial of thyroxin from birth to 2 years in children with DS. At 24 months, the thyroxin-treated group had a 0.7-month smaller motor delay (seven motor developmental index points on the Bayley Scales of Infant Development II) and a greater gain in length (1.1 cm) and weight (378 g) but no differences in the mental developmental index compared to an untreated DS group.

As children with DS become adolescents, they have an increasing chance of developing hypothyroidism due to Hashimoto's thyroiditis. In a study of 200 school children, aged 4–19 years, with DS who were screened with TSH levels, 15 had a TSH greater than 10 mU/l, and all but one had evidence of Hashimoto's thyroiditis. Of the eight adolescents diagnosed with hypothyroidism, five were asymptomatic, and in the other three, symptoms included dry skin, lethargy, and cold intolerance (Noble et al., 2000). In a study by Rubello et al. (1995) of 10–20 year olds, 30%

had subclinical hypothyroidism. Nineteen percent of those tested positive for antithyroid antibodies. Two years later, 36% of the antithyroid antibody-positive group developed clinically evident thyroid disease compared to none of the antithyroid antibody-negative group.

In adults with DS, there are limited studies on thyroid disorders. But, in a 10-year follow-up study of adults, Prasher and Gomez (2007) found that compensated hypothyroidism was not found to be an early sign for definite hypothyroidism and recommend that routine screening in adults with DS who are euthyroid can be reduced to every 5 years instead of every 1–2 years.

Hyperthyroidism is less common than hypothyroidism in DS but more common than in the general population. In a retrospective chart review of 1832 medical records of children and adults with DS from a specialized medical center in Barcelona, 12 patients (6.5/1000) were diagnosed with hyperthyroidism at a mean age of 16.8 years (7 females). The most common presenting symptoms were decreased heat tolerance, sweating, increased irritability, and weight loss. All of the patients had diffuse goiter at physical examination and two presented with exophthalmos. Thyroid-stimulating immunoglobulin (Ig) levels were raised and imaging testing confirmed the diagnosis of Graves' disease (Goday-Arno et al., 2009).

2.2. Type I diabetes

Diabetes mellitus develops in an increased incidence in individuals with DS but is still uncommon and so surveillance is recommended. In a survey of 1453 people with DS in the United Kingdom, the risk ratio of type 1 diabetes mellitus was 2.8 compared to the general population (Goldacre, Wotton, Seagroatt, & Yeates, 2004). In a survey from Denmark (Bergholdt, Eising, Nerup, & Pociot, 2006), DS was 0.09% of the population and prevalence of DS in the population with type 1 diabetes was 0.38%, which is a 4.2-fold increased prevalence compared to the general population. The age of onset in DS was reported to be closer to 8 years of age compared to peak initiation rates in the general population at 14 years of age (Burch & Milunsky, 1969) and to exceed that in the general population by factors of 6.8 (0–9 year olds), 3.3 (10–14 year olds), and 3.0 (15–19 year olds) (Milunsky & Neurath, 1968).

2.3. Growth hormone

Growth retardation and microcephaly are characteristics of many children with DS and intervention has been explored in the past. Reports of low circulating levels of insulin-like growth factor I and diminished provoked and spontaneous secretion of growth hormone (GH) along with the availability of unlimited recombinant human GH in the early 1990s lead to investigations of treatment of children with DS with GH (Allen, Frasier, Foley, & Pescovitz, 1993). Anneren, Tuvemo, and Gustafsson (2000) reported on the results of treatment of 15 young children (mean age at start of treatment, 7.4 months) with DS with GH for 3 years. The mean height increased significantly from −1.8 to −0.8 SDS (Swedish standard) compared to the control group with DS whose mean height fell from −1.7 to −2.2 SDS. After cessation of treatment, growth velocity declined in the treated group and growth of the head did not increase during the GH treatment. There was no effect on mental or gross-motor development although there was some improvement in fine-motor development ($p < 0.01$). They did not recommend treatment of children with DS who do not have GH deficiency. In addition, there has been a question of whether treatment with GH is associated with an increased incidence of leukemia in children as individuals with DS already have an increased risk of developing leukemia (Allen, 1996).

2.4. Sexual development and function

Sexual development in females with DS is similar to the general population, but concerns of potential sexual abuse and hygiene issues make it an issue of concern for parents and caregivers. Goldstein (1988) reported that females with DS were similar to controls with an average age of menarche of 13.6 years, average duration of bleeding of 5.5 days, and the average length of cycle of 28.3 days. For families, menstrual hygiene, sexual abuse, pregnancy, and premenstrual syndrome can become concerns. To the family, sexual development brings the fear of sexual abuse. The fear is not unfounded, because sexual abuse occurs at a higher rate in the mentally handicapped population than in typical children (Elkins, 1987). Women with DS have reproductive capacity. Bovicelli, Orsini, Rizzo, Montacuti, and Baccetta (1982) reported on 30 pregnancies in women resulted in 10 offspring with DS, 18 who did not have any syndrome and 3 spontaneous abortions. The onset of menopause for women with DS is earlier (47.1 years) than for women with intellectual disability who do not have DS (49.3 years) or for women in the general population (51 years) (Schupf et al., 1997).

Reports on the sexual development in males with DS have been limited. Pueschel, Orson, Boylan, and Pezzullo (1985) reported that the patterns of sexual development of penile and testicular size as well as follicle-stimulating hormone, luteinizing hormone, and testosterone levels were similar to controls. But there have been other reports of small testes (Benda, 1969), decreased sperm counts, and small volumes of ejaculate in young men with DS (Stearns, Droulard, & Sahhar, 1960). Other factors that may contribute to a reduced capacity for reproduction could be a general unfitness of males with DS and reports of spermatogenic arrest causing azoospermia and sterility (Johannisson et al., 1983). Compared to females with DS, there have been only three reports of men with DS fathering a child (Sheridan et al., 1989; Zuhlke, Thies, Braulke, Reis, & Schirren, 1994; Pradhan, Dalal, Khan, & Agrawal, 2006).

2.5. Immune system

The combination of infections specifically pneumonias being a major cause of morbidity and mortality, the increased prevalence of autoimmune diseases such as thyroid disorders, type I diabetes, alopecia, and celiac disease and the increased prevalence of leukemias indicates that there are defects in the immune system in individuals with DS. An overview of the multiple studies of the immune system in the last 40 years (Kusters, Verstegan, Geman, & de Vries, 2009) reveals that there are inconsistent findings in relation to increases and decreases in lymphocyte subpopulations and Igs and a consistently decreased response to some vaccinations (e.g., influenza, pertussis, polio, and tetanus) but a normal response to hepatitis A and a decreased or normal response to pneumococcal and hepatitis B vaccine. This is despite hepatitis B virus carrier state being much higher among children with DS. The role and the function of natural killer (NK) cells and whether they are higher or lower in numbers and whether they are part of the theorized early senescence of the immune system are unclear (Kusters et al., 2009).

The most consistent abnormalities have been identified in the T cell system. The thymus in newborns with DS is smaller and has an abnormal structure. The TCR excision circle T_{REC} counts in the estimation of recent thymic emigrants are low possibly consistent with the theory of early senescence, which is one theory to explain the multiple abnormal functions of the immune system. Although absolute numbers of T lymphocyte populations gradually approach those of normal children over time, it is doubtful that they have normal function over time (de Hingh et al., 2005). The *in vitro* proliferative response to phytohemagglutin (PHA) is markedly below normal in infants and adults with DS (Kusters et al., 2009).

In children with DS, there is a considerable hypergammaglobulinemia of IgG and IgA after the age of 5 years, with high levels of IgG_1 and IgG_3 and low levels of IgG_2 and IgG_4, with IgM levels decreasing in adolescence. IgD levels are high. Paradoxically, in infants there is a profound B lymphocytopenia deficit with an absence of the normal enormous expansion in the first year of life. These abnormalities could be due to an intrinsic B lymphocyte defect or, more likely, due to the consequence of deficient T helper lymphocyte function leading to inadequate control of B lymphocyte activation and proliferation (Kusters et al., 2009).

Although the theory of precocious aging may explain some of the aberrant findings in the immune system, it is more likely that there are intrinsic deficiencies from the beginning (Kusters et al., 2009).

3. Cardiovascular and Gastrointestinal Disorders

3.1. Congenital heart disease

Echocardiograms at birth for all newborns with DS are routie. Efforts to find a less expensive method with acceptable sensitivity and specificity have been unproductive. About half of children with DS are born with congenital heart disease (Abbag, 2006; Freeman et al., 2008; Jaiyesimi & Baichoo, 2007). In a recent review of 1469 cases of DS, 44% had a congenital heart defect with the most frequent lesions being atrioventricular septal defect (39%), atrial septal defect (42%), and ventricular septal defects (43%). Less frequently were isolated tetralogy of Fallot (6%), aortic coarctation (1%), and other lesions (3%) (Freemen et al., 2008).

3.2. Coronary artery disease and hypertension

Despite problems with obesity and poor lipid profiles, individuals with DS have a low prevalence of coronary artery disease (Draheilm, McCubbin, & Williams, 2002; Vis et al., 2009). In addition, after adjusting for age, cigarette smoking, and medication use, women with DS had lower fasting plasma glucose and lower systolic blood pressure than those of comparison women with intellectual disability (van de Louw, Vorstenbosch, Vinck, Penning, & Evenhuis, 2009). These findings are unexplained although perhaps it is partially explained by individuals with DS having fewer atherosclerotic risk factors.

3.3. Feeding, chewing, and swallowing

Studies show that as many as 80% of children with DS have problems with nutrition and feeding. These problems include (1) inappropriate, excessive, or low intakes of nutrients and energy; (2) poor eating habits with retention of infantile feeding habits, food refusals, and unacceptable behavior around food; and (3) inappropriate parental feeding practices and delays in self-feeding skills in children beyond an age they are developmentally ready to acquire the skill (Pipes & Holm, 1980). In a study of feeding difficulties in 14 children with DS compared to a control group and using standardized feeding and oral-motor instruments, the children with DS lag behind and follow an aberrant pathway in oral-motor function. In particular, specific aspects of tongue and jaw function were impaired together with problems initiating and maintaining a smooth sequence of feeding actions (Spender et al., 1996). Although the prevalence of breast-feeding was similar to non-DS populations and nutritional intakes were adequate, there was a significant delay at which the age of solid food was introduced (median age 12 months for children with DS vs. 8 months in the controls; $p < 0.01$). In a study by Frazier and Friedman (1996), oral hypersensitivity interferes with the oral stage of swallowing and acceptance of textured foods. In addition, they noted a disordered pharyngeal phase of swallowing in 16 of 19 children studied with aspiration in 10 of 19 but silent in 8. Chewing and swallowing problems can continue to be an issue even in adolescents and adults.

3.4. Dental

Children with DS have potential problems with serious gingivitis that can be prevented with rigorous hygiene and malocclusion that can be treated with orthodontic work if the child has the ability to tolerate the discomfort. The most serious dental problem is early-onset periodontal disease that can rapidly progress with gingivitis and regression of the jaw bone that anchors the teeth. Individuals with DS have less dental caries but more periodontal disease with both thought to be related to changes in oral bacteria related to the aberrations in immunity. In addition to periodontal disease, almost all children with DS have malocclusions and some type of dental anomalies such as fused teeth, microdontia, and missing teeth. The average age of the eruption of teeth both primary and permanent is later than in typical children (Hennequin, Faulks, Veyrune, & Bourdiol, 1999).

3.5. Congenital gastrointestinal defects

GI defects are second to heart defects among the common serious structural birth defects associated with DS and as with heart defects are most likely to be identified in the newborn period. The Atlanta and National Down Syndrome Project reviewed the presence of congenital GI defects in a population-based study conducted from 1989 to 2004 in six geographic areas in 1892 infants with DS. In this population, 126 (6.7%) infants were identified with the following GI malformations: duodenal stenosis/atresia (3.9%), anal stenosis/atresia (1.0%), Hirschsprung disease (0.8%), esophageal atresia/tracheoesophageal fistula (0.4%), and pyloric stenosis (0.3%) (Freeman et al., 2009).

3.6. Celiac disease

Celiac disease needs surveillance in the population of individuals with DS. It is an immune-mediated enteropathy caused by permanent sensitivity to gluten (the protein in wheat, barley, and rye) in genetically susceptible individuals. In Europe and the United States, it may occur in 0.5–1.0% of the general population. In the population of children with DS, studies find small intestine biopsy proven celiac disease in 3–10% of children studied (Book et al., 2001; Carnicer et al., 2001; Nisihara et al., 2005; Uibo et al., 2006). It is increased in certain populations including children with DS as well as those with diabetes mellitus type 1 and thyroiditis (Sood, 2007). Guidelines from the North American Society for Pediatric Gastroenterology Hematology and Nutrition (NASPGHAN, 2005) recommends screening of at-risk groups including children with DS at 3 years of age whether symptomatic or not but were vague on follow-up screening.

The clinical presentation of celiac disease in a toddler includes diarrhea or constipation, abdominal distention or pain, failure to thrive, and/or anemia. Children can also be emotionally withdrawn, irritable, and fretful and have refractory developmental problems. As we have been able to screen more children, new clinical patterns in the presentation are emerging. In one study of 143 patients with celiac disease, children less than 3 years of age presented with GI symptoms but the majority of those older than 3 years of age presented with non-GI symptoms such as anemia, having a risk factor such as DS or having short stature, mood disorders, or alopecia with 11.2% being overweight (Telega, Bennet, & Werlin, 2008). In a study from Spain, in 18 children 2–15 years of age with DS and with positive screens and biopsies, 15 had clinical manifestations (8 GI and 7 extra-intestinal) and 3 were silent (Carnicer et al., 2001). Evaluation begins with screening with antitissue transglutaminase IgA or antitissue endomysial antibody. A quantitative IgA level is needed to confirm the presence of serum IgA concentration to assure that there is no false-negative results in an IgA-deficient individual. Definitive diagnosis of celiac disease requires a small intestine biopsy with positive histological findings. Several studies have resulted in recommendations to identify children with DS who are at higher risk of celiac disease. Wouters et al. (2009) recommended buccal swabs in the first year of life for HLA-DQ2/8 typing and initiating serologic screening of children with DS in whom the test results are positive for HLA-DZ2 or DZ8 at 3 years of age and no screening in those children whose test results are negative. No uniform approach as to the who and the how of initial screening is generally agreed upon except to screen those who are symptomatic.

3.7. Obesity

Obesity is a disease to be prevented with early dietary intervention. The high incidence of obesity in children and adolescents with DS is well known and begins to develop in the preschool years. Compared with their siblings, children with DS are less active, spend more time indoors, and prefer indoor activities. Several reports have demonstrated a lower resting metabolic rate, at least in childhood, which also contributes to the development of obesity (Luke, Roizen, Sutton, & Schoeller, 1994).

A more recent article on resting metabolic rate indicated that it was not reduced in adults with DS (Fernhall et al., 2005). Increased leptin levels for percent body fat may also be a factor (Magge, O'Neill, Shults, Stallings, & Stettler, 2008).

4. Sensory Systems

4.1. Vision

Ophthalmic abnormalities and disorders are common in children and adults with DS affecting 46–100% in a review, by Creavin and Brown (2009), of reports from all over the world and require annual evaluation. Abnormalities that are part of the phenotype and gestalt of the DS facies but not affecting vision are frequent such as slanting fissures (63–80%), epicanthic folds (> 60%), Brushfield spots (0–81%), hypertelorism (2–34%), and microphthalmos (1–7%) (Creavin & Brown, 2009).

Studies of refractive errors are broadly comparable as the defined boundaries of emmetropia can vary from 1.00 diopters (D) to 3.25 D, and consequently the definitions of hyperopia, myopia, and astigmatism vary. In a review of 13 studies, hyperopia (4–59%) was more common than myopia (8–41%) in 8 of the studies and in general astigmatism was recorded to be between 20 and 30%. Deficits in visual acuity were relatively common (30–62%) with amblyopia in 20% (Creavin & Brown, 2009). In a report of refractive errors in a population of 2–28 year olds from Macedonia with the diagnosis of DS made clinically, they report that 47.4% with myopia had a correction of less than or equal to −6.00 D and those with hyperopia had a correction of greater than or equal to +6.00 D in 38.1% (Antonelo & Vladimir, 2009).

Disorders of eye movements such as strabismus or squint are found in 20–60% and nystagmus generally 10–20%. When strabismus is divided by directions of deviation, esodeviation (15–52%) is more common than exodeviation (0–11%).

Lacrimal disease can be lacrimal obstruction (17–36%), congenital dacryocutaneous fistulae (1%), and epiphora (15–32%). The most common palpebral or eyelid abnormality is blepharitis, which is reported in less than 10% up to 50%. Another abnormality that is common is ptosis, which is reported to be from 3 to 7% and should be monitored for clinical significance as it can lead to amblyopia if the eyelid covers the eye too much.

Other disorders found in DS can be of low frequency but high impact such as cataracts, which are congenital in less than or equal to 5% and need to be identified in the first few weeks of life to prevent amblyopia or blindness. In the second decade of life and beyond, lens opacities can develop and need monitoring and sometimes require intervention (Creavin & Brown, 2009;

Roizen, Mets, & Blondis, 1994). Corneal abnormalities include keratoconus (0–12%), which is a bilateral noninflammatory corneal ectasia with an incidence of 1 per 2000 in the general population. Keratoconus generally comes on after puberty and can progress quickly and then go into a stage of quiescence (Rabinowitz, 1998). The association with DS is thought to be related to eye rubbing caused in part by blepharitis (Rabinowitz, 1998).

Glaucoma is another serious ophthalmological disorder that occurs with increased frequency in DS and can be congenital or of later onset. The frequency is inconsistent from study to study with it being less than or equal to 1% in some studies and 5–7% in others (Creavin & Brown, 2009). In one study of adults with a mean age of 35.1 years, 11.5% had glaucoma compared to 1.1% in the control population (Yokoyama, Tamura, Tsukamoto, Yamane, & Mishima, 2006).

In an institutionalized population of 97 adults with DS in the Netherlands, visual impairment was identified in only 4.5% of individuals with DS younger than 50 years of age with mild to moderate intellectual disability but much higher (74%) in those with severe or profound intellectual disability. In individuals older than 50 years of age with DS, in the group with mild to moderate intellectual disability the prevalence increased from 4.5 to 31%, which was thought to be related to early age-related cataracts and insufficiently corrected refractive errors. In the group with severe to profound intellectual disability, prevalences did not increase with age (Evenhuis, Theunissen, Denders, Verschuure, & Kemme, 2001).

5. Hearing

Hearing problems can develop at any time of life in a person with DS. Therefore, an annual evaluation of the hearing status of an individual with DS is indicated. At this time, children with DS as other children in their community are screened for hearing at birth and referred for evaluation if they fail the initial screen. In a cross-sectional study of auditory brainstem response testing done prior to the initiation of newborn hearing screening in unselected children aged 2 months to 3½ years with DS, 34% had normal hearing, 28% had unilateral loss, and 38% had bilateral loss. The type of loss was conductive in 19 ears, mixed in 14, and sensorineural in 16. The degree of loss was mild in 33 ears, moderate in 13, and severe to profound in 3 (Roizen, Wolters, Nicol, & Blondis, 1993). In a more recent study from China in school children 6.4–23 years of age (mean age 12.1 years) using tympanometric, transient evoked otoacoustic emission (TEOAE) and pure tone audiometric examinations revealed a high prevalence of mainly a mild to moderate loss in 78% of the ears and 90% of the participants (McPherson, Lai, Leung, & Ng, 2007). In a recent longitudinal study by Shott, Joseph, and

Heithaus (2001) children with DS and normal hearing were enrolled by 2 years of age and seen every 6 months or every 3 months if they had stenotic ear canals. By the end of a year, 98% of the children had normal hearing but 83% of these children required pressure equalization tube placement due to chronic ear infections and/or persistent middle ear effusions and 55% required two or more sets of tubes. Multiple pressure equalization tube placements may be required as Selikowitz (1993) reported that after placement there continued to be hearing loss in 40% of children with DS compared to less in control children. There are many factors that could possibly contribute to chronic otitis media such as increased upper respiratory infections possibly due to the immune dysfunction, and mid-face hypoplasia.

Although hearing loss is less common in adolescence than in childhood, up to one-half of adolescents with DS have a hearing impairment. The hearing loss most frequently seen is sensorineural (22%); with conductive (19%) and mixed (17%) hearing less common (Widen, Folsom, Thompson, & Wilson, 1987). Mild (15–25dB) losses due to impacted cerumen are common. Some audiologists believe that more individuals with DS can profit from hearing aids than have them (Balkany, Downs, Jafek, & Krajicek, 1979). In adults Evenhuis, van Zanten, Brocaar, and Roerdinkholder (1992) found hearing loss in 56 of 59 ears tested in a group of 35 institutionalized adults 35–62 years of age. Hearing loss can contribute to social and mental deterioration and should be monitored.

6. Cancer

6.1. Standardized Incidence Ratio (SIR)

Childhood leukemia is the most frequently observed cancer in individuals with DS. Despite having a similar overall incidence of cancers as that of the general population, individuals with DS have a different tumor profile. In general, large national cancer surveys refer to SIRs, which are defined as the ratios of observed number of cancer cases to those expected from the national cancer incidence rates by age and sex. The overall cancer risk in DS is equal to that of the general population (Patja, Pukkala, Sund, Iivanainen, & Kaski, 2006) or slightly increased with an SIR of 1.2 in the Danish study by Hasle, Clemmensen, and Mikkelsen (2000). In survey reports from multiple countries, there was an increased SIR for acute lymphocytic leukemia (SIR, 10.5–24.2), acute nonlymphocytic leukemia (SIR, 28.2) (Hill et al., 2003), and testicular cancer (SIR, 3.7–4.8) (Hill et al., 2003; Patja et al., 2006). By contrast there is a decreased SIR for solid tumors such as breast cancer. In the Hasle et al. (2000) study, there were only 24 solid tumors seen with 47.8 expected (SIR, 0.50) and no cases of breast cancer.

6.2. Leukemia

Leukemia constitutes about 60% of the cases of cancer overall in the Hasle et al. study (2000) and 97% of the cancer cases in children. The SIR for leukemia varied with age, being 56 at age 0–4 years and 10 at 5–29 years. No cases of leukemia were seen after the age of 29 years. The SIR for acute myeloid leukemia was 3.8 times higher than that for acute lymphoblastic leukemia in children aged 0–4 years. The cumulative risk of leukemia by the age of 5 years was 2.1% and that by 30 years was 2.7% (Hasle et al., 2000).

Leukemia in individuals with DS includes distinctive disease entities—transient myeloproliferative disorder (TMD), acute megakaryoblastic leukemia (AMKL), and acute lymphoblastic leukemia (ALL). The search for epidemiologic environmental risk factors has thus far been unsuccessful. However, it is believed that environmental factors along with genetic factors and altered folate metabolism play a significant role (Rabin & Witlock, 2009).

The frequency of TMD is unknown as newborns with DS are not routinely screened for leukocytosis. But, it has been estimated that between 4 and 10% of infants with DS are born with TMD with immature megakaryocytes in the peripheral blood (Pine et al., 2007; Zipursky, 2003). A major breakthrough has been made in the understanding of the connection between the seemingly mainly benign TMD and the development in the next few years of AMKL. In a subset of children with TMD, Wechsler et al. (2002) discovered that mutations of the *GATA1* gene are specific to those individuals who transition from TMD to AMKL. The *GATA1* gene is found on the X chromosome and is the hematopoietic transcription factor (Mundschau et al., 2003). To determine whether this mutation was present at birth in the population of children with DS, Pine et al. (2007) examined DNA from Guthrie cards of 590 infants with DS and reported that *GATA1* mutations were detected in 3.8% of the infants. In infants with DS, TMD is most frequently an asymptomatic leukocytosis but, less frequently, it can be a clinical picture resembling leukemia with massive organomegaly and fatal liver/and or respiratory failure or stillbirth.

The majority of cases of AML in DS are megakaryoblastic phenotype (AMKL). In patients with DS, AMKL almost exclusively occurs in children younger than 5 years of age and is distinguished by an unusually favorable clinical prognosis with a current event-free survival (EFS) rate at about 80% compared to 15–20% in patients with non-DS AMKL. The few AML cases in children with DS who are 5 years and older show no significant survival advantage compared with the general population (Gamis, Woods, & Alonzo, 2003).

DS ALL is similar to non-DS ALL in many ways: the incidence of DS ALL follows about the same age peak and range as non-DS ALL except that almost no cases occur in infants younger than 1 year of age in children with DS (Rabin & Witlock, 2009). Overall survival has been 10–20% lower in

DS ALL patients than in non-DS ALL patients in most protocols worldwide. But, if favorable risk patients who are underrepresented in the DS group are excluded from the analysis, the outcomes for DS and non-DS groups are comparable (Rabin & Witlock, 2009).

6.3. Testicular cancer

The increased incidence of testicular cancer is thought to be related in part to the increased prevalence of cryptorchidism in DS, which is a predisposing factor for seminomas testicular cancer. In a report of nine patients with DS identified with testicular cancer, two had bilateral tumors and four had cryptorchidism. Their ages ranged from 21 to 50 years of age. Of the 11 tumors identified, nine were seminomas and two were malignant teratomas undifferentiated. Five of the nine patients relapsed within 30 months, which is a high relapse rate (Hafeez, Sharma, Huddart, Dearnaley, & Horwich, 2007). There is one report of testicular cancer in a 2-year-old male with DS who also had cryptorchism (Dada, Kumar, & Kucheria, 2006).

6.4. Breast cancer

It is notable that females with DS are less likely to develop breast cancer than other females. This may be related to a life style characterized by less alcohol and cigarette use, earlier menopause, shortened life expectance, and possibly biological factors such as a protective cell microenvironment (Benard, Beron-Gaillard, & Satge, 2005).

7. Motor/Skeletal System

7.1. Ligamentous laxity

Orthopedic disorders are commonly seen in DS. Hypotonia, ligamentous laxity, and hyperflexibility of the joints contribute to the development of a variety of orthopedic disorders which are likely aggravated by the lack of physical activity and obesity. Examples include metatarsus primus varus with or without hallux abducto valgus, subluxation or dislocation of the patella, severe pes planus, atlantoaxial instability, genu valgum, and acetabular dysplasia with or without subluxing hips.

7.2. Atlantoaxial subluxation (ATL)

All of these disorders have the potential of leading to some degree of debilitation over time and therefore require surveillance to prevent problems with function. The identification and treatment of asymptomatic and symptomatic ATL is controversial, complicated, and perplexing. Depending on the age and method of radiologic screening [e.g., plain radiographs, computed tomography (CT), or magnetic resonance imaging (MRI)] and definition of ATL, 10–30% of patients with DS have atlantoaxial instability and 1–2% of these have symptomatic instability (Tredwell, Newman, & Lockitch, 1990; Pueschel et al., 1987). Many agree that ligamentous laxity of the posterior transverse ligament is likely to be a common cause of ATL in DS and is one of the factors that contributes to instability of vertebral movement at the atlantoaxial junction (Merrick et al., 2000) but not all (Ferguson, Putney, & Allen, 1997). Additionally, C-1 hypoplasia and occult spinal canal stenosis have been associated to an increased risk of compressive myelopathy (Matsunaga et al., 2007).

In the recent past, there has been a movement away from screening for subluxation with radiographs as screening is not cost-effective or specific and can either give parents a false sense of security or alarm them needlessly (Cohen, 2006). However, screening radiographs are required for participation in the Special Olympics and suggested for those undergoing anesthesia with tracheal intubation where neck extension is likely (Brockmeyer, 1999). Central to the effective identification of atlantoaxial subluxation is a careful history and physical examination on a regular basis and immediately in the symptomatic child (Brockmeyer, 1999). Patients with history positive for motor symptoms such as neck pain, radicular pain, gait difficulties with limping or dragging a leg, weakness with loss of motor skills such as climbing the stairs, change in bowel or bladder function, or head tilt require an immediate physical examination. Physical findings of weakness, head tilt, spasticity, sensory deficits, and hyperreflexia require further evaluation. Brockmeyer (1999) carefully reviewed the topic and made the following points: (1) When screening for atlantoaxial subluxation with the cervical spine series with flexion and extension views, the atlantodens interval (ADI) is an indirect measurement of instability and should be used with the better direct measure of the neural canal width (NCW) to determine consideration of an MRI which is indicated in those with a NCW width of less than 14 mm or an ADI of greater than 4.5 mm. (2) A special high-risk group that should be studied carefully is patients with biomechanically significantly bony anomalies at the atlantoaxial junction or the occipitoatlantal junction (e.g., os odontoideum). (3) Those with positive screens or who are symptomatic with either a negative or positive screen should have an MRI. If the MRI is positive, then surgical intervention should be considered.

Fortunately, there have been advances in surgery. A series of studies describing surgical intervention with posterior arthrodesis with or without internal fixation reported major complications in 21 of 25 children (Doyle, Lauerman, Wood, & Krause, 1996; Segal, Drummond, Zanotti, Ecker, & Mubarak, 1991). Other studies using occiput to C2 fusion and atlantoaxial fusion report bony union report a minimum of complications (Menezes & Ryken, 1992). In addition, parents should be counseled that participation in activities that may result in hyperextension, radical flexion, or direct pressure on the neck such as diving, high jumps, trampoline use, and contact sports such as soccer and football places them at increased risk of spinal cord injury (Pizzutillo and Herman, 2005).

7.3. Podiatric

The typical gait of the patient with DS has been described as Chaplinesque with external rotation of the hips, knees inflexion and valgus, and both tibias rotated. Individuals with DS in part related to hypotonia and ligamentous laxity have increased podiatric anomalies that can result in these postural alterations. In a study of 50 children with DS 4–10 years of age, compared to a control group, they were significantly more likely to have flat feet (60%), calcaneal valgus (24%), knee valgus (22%), and rigid flat foot (16%) with 16% having an anomaly known as a "pronated flat foot" (Concolino, Pasquizzi, Capalbo, Sinopoli, & Strisciuglio, 2006).

In adolescence and into adulthood, the foot problems associated with ligamentous laxity and excessive pronation begin to manifest themselves. Examples include severe hallux valgus and hammertoe deformities as well as plantar fasciitis, fatigue, and early onset of pedal arthritis associated with severe flat foot (Caselli, Cohen-Sobel, & Thompson, 1991). Early detection and management can reduce the need for subsequent surgical intervention (Prasher, Robinson, Krishnan, & Chung, 1995).

7.4. Arthritis

Another condition that requires surveillance in young children is "arthropathy of Down syndrome," which is a type of juvenile idiopathic arthritis (JIA). In a recent review, Juj and Emery (2009) reported on the children from University of Washington in addition to previous reported series (Olson, Bender, Levinson, Oestreich, & Lovell, 1990; Padmakumar, Evans, & Sills, 2002; Yancey, Zmijewski, Athreya, & Rosenberg, 1984) and cases in the literature (Herring, 1982; Sherk, Pasquariello, & Watters, 1982) for a total of 30 patients. In this group, age of onset varied from 20 months to 12 years with most being symptomatic before 8 years of age and with boys and girls equally affected. Seventy-two percent (18/25) of those reported had histories of morning stiffness, which is a helpful symptom. At diagnosis, 57% had polyarticular disease and 43% had oligoarticular disease of which 54% went on to develop polyarticular arthritis. Only 2 had positive inflammatory markers, but 72% (21/29 reported) had elevated erythrocyte sedimentation rate (ESR) at the time of diagnosis. Therapeutically, only 32% (8/25) responded to first-line therapies alone. Almost half of the individual with

JIA developed subluxation of the involved joints. Unlike JIA, no child developed iritis or other frequent ocular complications. Children with DS have an increased prevalence of arthropathy of DS (8.7/1000), which is almost 6 times that of 1.4/1000 for JIA in the general population (Miller & Cassidy, 2004). Providers need a high index of suspicion as the combination of delayed development, a challenging physical diagnosis, and hypermobile joints makes it difficult to appreciate limitations in range of motion on physical examination. A history of morning stiffness can be helpful. Juj and Emery (2009) reported an average delay from symptom onset to diagnosis of 2 years, which is an improvement from the 1990 report of Olson et al., of a mean time to diagnosis as 3.3 years.

7.5. Osteoporosis

Osteoporosis is generally an adult disease, but the roots lie in childhood and the peak bone mass that is achieved in early adulthood sets the level from which an adult looses bone mass starting in the third decade of life at a rate of about 1% annually (Steelman & Zeitler, 2001). Studies indicate that individuals with DS appear to achieve lower peak bone mass densities than other individuals with and without intellectual disability (Tyler, Snyder, & Zyzanski, 2000). In addition to the usual risk factors for osteoporosis, children with DS are more likely to have other disorders that are associated with osteoporosis such as JIA, acute lymphocytic leukemia and the chemotherapy treatment (Hawli, Nasrallah, & Fuleihan, 2009), anticonvulsant use, celiac disease, and hyperthyroidism. Life style characteristics such as low levels of physical activity and low calcium intake (Luke, Sutton, Schoeller, & Roizen, 1996) are also increased in DS. All of these risk factors are likely to contribute to the outcome of increased osteoporosis and osteopenia in adults with DS (Hawli et al., 2009; Tyler et al., 2000) that is reported to start with lower bone mineral density in young adults after 20 years of age (Baptista, Varela, & Sardinha, 2005).

8. Other Systems and Problems

8.1. Neurological disorders

8.1.1. Seizures

Patients with DS are at risk of a variety of neurologic problems, including intellectual disability, seizures, and strokes. About 8% of children and adolescents with DS have seizures including febrile seizures, which is lower than in the population of people with intellectual disability but higher than in the general population. The age of onset is bimodal with 40% before 1 year of age and 40% in the third decade of life (Pueschel,

Louis, & McKnight, 1991). Children tend to develop infantile spasms and tonic-clonic seizures with myoclonus. About half of the children with infantile spasms achieve seizure remission without relapse and partial restoration of their development. This is in contrast with infantile spasms in the general population which are associated almost uniformly with long-term problems with seizure control and a poor developmental prognosis (Stafstrom & Konkol, 1994). Seizures with onset after 13 years of age most frequently result from head trauma or delayed sequelae of heart disease and are tonic-clonic in type (Stafstrom, Patxot, Gilmore, & Wisniewski, 1991).

Adults develop partial simple or complex seizures (Pueschel et al., 1991). Adults with DS over 45 years of age who develop seizures are significantly more likely to develop signs of Alzheimer disease. Compared to the typical population where myoclonic seizures tend to occur late in the course of Alzheimer disease, in adults with DS, the onset of partial or tonic-clonic seizures often herald the onset of cognitive decline (Puri, Ho, & Singh, 2001).

8.1.2. Strokes

Moyamoya syndrome is a chronic, occlusive cerebrovascular disease of unknown pathogenesis in which there is progressive stenosis of the supraclinoid portions of the internal carotid arteries and tortuous arterial collaterals at the base of the brain. Moyamora disease has a bimodal presentation with the first peak in the first decade of life with symptoms related to cerebral ischaemia and the second peak in the fourth decade with intracranial hemorrhage. This unusual vascular complication occurs with a higher frequency in children with DS. Children typically present with ischemic event with a fixed unilateral neurological deficit or alternating hemiplegia with one report of a child with DS with a presumed perinatal stroke (Pysden, Fallon, Moorthy, & Ganesan, 2010). Children with DS may also develop seizures or involuntary movements. The adult presentation is hemorrhagic (Gordon, 1995).

8.1.3. Disintegrative syndrome

It is reported that a minority of adolescents and young adults with DS can present with a regression of skills for no identified reason. Prasher (2002) reported from Ireland that in their West Midlands health study of 357 adults over a 10-year period a significant minority between the ages of 15 and 30 years with a peak age of 22 years presented with a specific regressive/disintegrative disorder. Usually, after a normal period of development for an individual with DS, there is a gradual but severe deterioration in function. There is a regression and loss of previously acquired skills in expressive and receptive language, mobility, cognition, adaptive skills, and social skills. Frequently there are associated changes in personality, behavior, and mood and the person may become mute, withdrawn, have decreased social interaction, decreased interests and activities, and have a mild to severe low mood. A careful history should include changes in life supports such as the death of a grandparent and acute or chronic emotional trauma such as bullying or sexual abuse. Evaluation frequently includes tests for thyroid dysfunction, sleep disorders, depression, anemia, or a seizure disorder. Treatment with antidepressants can sometimes improve mood and some of the individuals have thyroid dysfunction (Brodtmann, 2009) or sleep disorders. But, in general, this phenomenon has not had a unifying etiology identified, nor has there been much success in treatment.

8.1.4. Renal and urologic diseases

The spectrum of renal and urologic disease in DS includes kidney disease with glomerulonephritis and anomalies including renal agenesis and microcysts as well as ectopic kidney; urinary tract anomalies with hydronephrosis, hydroureter, posterior urethral valves and anterior urethral obstruction, and hypospadias. Glomerular nephritis is largely acquired in the second and third decades (Lo, Brown, Fivush, Neu, & Racusen,. 1998; Mercer et al., 2004). A report from the North American Pediatric Renal Transplant Cooperative Study identified 14 patients with DS who underwent renal replacement for obstructive uropathy (4), hypoplastic/dysplastic renal disease (2), focal segmental glomerulosclerosis (2), and chronic glomerulonephritis (2) and others. Five graphs failed which was similar to the rate for all transplants, and they concluded that renal replacement was a reasonable option for this population with chronic renal failure. The increased incidence of renal disease and urinary tract anomalies in DS is reported sometimes incidentally in the autopsy case literature (Lo et al., 1998; Mercer et al., 2004). But in a report of 124 cases of children and young adults with DS, Ariel, Wells, Landing, and Singer (1991) found renal hypoplasia in 21.4%, glomerular microcysts in 23.7%, and simple renal cysts in 5.6% compared to a pediatric incidence of 0.1%. The clinical significance of these cysts is unknown (Mercer et al., 2004).

Reports of patients with DS being disproportionately represented in series of cases of posterior urethral valves (4.17%) (Bielek, Carvajal-Busslinger, & Bianchetti, 1996) have raised concern about unrecognized obstructive disease. The New York State Congenital Malformation Registry (Kupferman, Druschel, & Kupchik, 2009) recently compared the prevalence of renal and urinary tract anomalies in 3832 individuals with DS compared to the non-DS population of 3.4 million. They reported an overall increased odds ratio of 4.5 for these anomalies in the population with DS with a prevalence of 3.2% compared to 0.7% in the New York state population. The rates of renal agenesis per 10,000 in this study (23.5 vs. 3.2–3.5) were higher than in other population-based studies while rates of any urinary tract obstructive defect were similar (180 vs. 146–183), as were hypospadias and epispadias (80.9 vs. 81.7–124). The morbidity related to renal and urinary tract anomalies may be significant, and this study suggests screening with an early renal ultrasound in the newborn with DS to reduce morbidity in the DS population.

9. Obstructive Sleep Apnea and Pulmonary Problems

9.1. Obstructive sleep apnea

There is an increased incidence of multiple otolaryngologic problems in children with DS, in part related to smaller airways and immune aberrations. They have increased potential for ear infections and hearing loss, airway problems with obstructive sleep apnea and subglottic stenosis, and chronic rhinorrhea and sinusitis as well as important anesthetic considerations (Shott, 2006). Studies of populations selected for referral to sleep clinics have reported a high incidence of sleep apnea with Fitzgerald, Paul, and Richmond (2007) reporting sleep apnea in 91% of 33 children with DS (mean age, 4.9 years) referred for sleep studies with snoring. Much of our evidence-based data is from a prospective longitudinal study by Shott et al. (2006) at the Cincinnati Children's Hospital on a group of 65 children with DS and normal hearing starting before 2 years of age. In this study, 56 children between 4 and 63 months of age (mean age, 42 months) completed polysomnograms. Abnormal results and evidence of obstructive sleep apnea syndrome were found in 57% of the children. The parents of 69% of the children reported no sleep problems, and in this group, 54% had abnormal results. Of the parents who reported sleep problems in their children, 36% had abnormal sleep study results. Shott et al. (2006) recommended that all children with DS at 3–4 years of age receive polysomnography due to the high incidence of obstructive sleep apnea and poor correlation between parental impressions and the results of testing.

9.2. Respiratory illnesses

Respiratory illnesses are also increased in children with DS who are frequently hospitalized early in life. In a study of 213 children with DS, 54% had congenital heart disease. Almost half of the children (49.8%) were hospitalized before the age of 3 years with respiratory illnesses as the principal diagnoses in 38.3% of those hospitalized and affecting 64.9% of all hospitalized children with congenital heart disease (So, Urbano, & Hodapp, 2007).

In a study of 15,964 infants treated with extracorporeal membrane oxygenation (ECMO), children with DS were overrepresented by a factor of 3.6–5.9. In the ECMO-treated group, they were overrepresented in the group with primary persistent pulmonary hypertension (47.3% vs. 13%). Although survival to discontinuation of ECMO was similar to the other infants, survival to discharge was decreased for the infants with DS (65.9% vs. 75.6%) because of increased post-ECMO mortality (Southgate, Annibale, Hulsey, & Purohit, 2001). Children with DS are also disproportionally represented in hospital admissions for respiratory syncytial virus (RSV)-induced lower respiratory tract infections (LRTIs) accounting for 9.9% of admissions in one study (Bloemers et al., 2007). Interestingly, in a cohort of children with DS with and without hospitalization for RSV-LRTI there was no difference in the physician-diagnosed wheeze up to 2 years of age (36% vs. 30%). Although in the group of non-DS children, those with RSV-LRTI were more likely to have a wheeze compared to healthy control children (31% vs. 8%, $p = 0.004$) (Bloemers et al., 2010).

10. Dermatology Problems

The majority of children with DS (87%) develop a skin disorder associated with the syndrome such as palmoplantar hyperkeratosis (40.8%), xerosis (9.8%), seborrheic dermatitis (30.9%), fissured tongue (20%), geographic tongue (11.2%), and cutis marmorata (12.6%) (Ercis, Balci, & Atakan, 1996). By adolescence, dermatological problems frequently cause difficulties, especially folliculitis, which develops in 50–60% of adolescents with DS (Pueschel, 1990). Over half of adolescents with DS will have one or more of the following skin disorders: atopic dermatitis, cheilitis, ichthyosis, onychomycosis, seborrheic dermatitis, or xerosis (Ercis et al., 1996). The autoimmune disorders vitiligo and alopecia both arise more frequently in individuals with DS than in the general population (Scherbenske, Benson, Rotchford, & James, 1990).

11. Summary

Multiple medical problems and organ system abnormalities potentially affecting individual with DS have been presented in great detail. In order to highlight the most salient features of the health profiles of individuals with DS, the data are summarized in two ways. First, a brief summary of each of the areas is presented below. Second, an organized approach to medical problems in DS is presented in Table 1.1.

Table 1 Evaluation, prevention, and surveillance timetable from newborn through adulthood for persons with Down syndrome

	Newborn	First year	2—12 years	Adolescence 13—21 years	Adulthood > 21years	Comments
Evaluation						
Cardiac	Echocardiogram					
Hearing	Newborn screen	6 and 12 months	Every 6 months to 4 years then annually	1–2 years	1–2 years	Hearing screen
Vision	Check cataracts	<6 months	Every 1–2 years	Every 1–2 years	Every 1–2 years	Ophthalmologist who treats children
Thyroid	Screen	Screen 6 and 12 months	Annual screen	Annual screen	Annual screen	Thyroid-stimulating hormone (TSH)
Prevention						
Dental		+	++	++	++	Hygiene—dentist 1–2/ years
Obesity			+++	+++	++	Diet and exercise
Osteopenia			++	+++	++	Calcium, vitamin D, exercise

Surveillance						
Alzheimer					++	
Arthritis			+++			Arthropathy of Down syndrome
Atlantoaxial	subluxation		+	++	+	+
Discuss risk with						anesthesiologist
Celiac disease		++	+++	++	++	
Diabetes type 1			+++	++	+	
	Gastrointestinal deficits	+++		Hirschsprung disease		
Leukemia	CBC[1]	+++	+++	+		
Mitralvalve prolapse				+	+	
Seizures		+++	+	+	+++	
Testicular cancer		+	+	+	++	Especially if has cryptorchidism
Urologic anomalies	++	+				

+ = intensity of surveillance
CBC[1] = complete blood count

The main points made in each system discussed are listed below:

Endocrine/metabolic/immune systems: The person with DS has an increased prevalence of thyroid disorders that continue to develop over a life time. Identification of type 1 diabetes requires surveillance especially in childhood. Women have a reproductive capacity, but males, however, have limited reproductive capacity. The immune system has multiple qualitative and quantitative deficiencies that account for some of the problems with infections.

Cardiovascular: Children with DS have around a 50% chance of being born with a congenital heart malformation that is likely to be corrected surgically in early childhood. Interestingly, despite problems with obesity and poor lipid profiles, individuals with DS have a low prevalence of coronary artery disease.

Gastrointestinal: Infants and toddlers with DS can have problems with chewing and swallowing and frequently have continued issues in adulthood. Dental problems include gingivitis and eventual tooth loss can be prevented with rigorous hygiene. GI malformations occur in 6.7% of infants and are usually identified in the newborn period and treated surgically. Celiac disease, which has been identified in at least 5% of children with DS, requires evaluation of children with GI symptoms as well as mood disorders and anemia. Obesity is to be prevented by careful monitoring of growth curves and trajectories and dietary interventions.

Vision: Individuals with DS have a wide spectrum of possible visual problems, the most frequent of which are refractive errors but include other serious disorders such as cataracts and glaucoma which can result in blindness if untreated.

Hearing: Children with DS are screened at birth for hearing and require continued monitoring all through life as they can develop both conductive and sensorineural hearing loss.

Cancer: Despite having an incidence of cancer that is similar to the general population, the types of cancer differ with leukemia constituting about 60% of the cases overall and 97% of childhood cancers. There are few solid tumors except for testicular cancer, which has an increased prevalence especially in males with cryptorchism.

Motor/Skeletal system: Lax ligaments contribute to the development of multiple orthopedic and podiatric problems, the most potentially serious of which is atlantoaxial subluxation. Arthropathy of DS is rare but also requires vigilance as the average time from symptom onset to diagnosis is now 2 years. Osteoporosis is an adult disease that is to be prevented by diet and exercise in childhood and during the adolescent growth spurt when peak bone mass densities are established.

Neurological: Seizures are more common in DS with infants having an increased incidence of infantile spasms, followed by another peak in the 20's, and then in adults over 45 years of age with Alzheimer disease. A rare disorder referred to as disintegrative syndrome usually occurs in adolescents and young adults and includes a gradual but severed loss of function seemingly for no reason.

Renal and urologic diseases: Recent recognition that the spectrum of renal and urologic diseases is increased in individuals with DS has raised the question as to whether or not all newborns with DS should have a renal ultrasound.

Obstructive sleep apnea and pulmonary problems: Documentation of obstructive sleep apnea in the majority of 3–4 year olds with parents reporting no sleep problems in most of these children has lead the adoption of sleep studies in individuals with DS of all ages. Lower respiratory tract illnesses are a frequent reason for hospitalization in children with DS especially those with congenital heart disease.

In summary, individuals with DS are living longer, healthier lives than they did only a few decades ago. DS should now be considered a chronic condition in which most individuals with DS have some, but not all, of these medical problems. More importantly, with appropriate treatment and management they can realize their full potential and experience rich, productive lives.

REFERENCES

Abbag, F. (2006). Congenital heart diseases and other major anomalies among Down syndrome patients and short-term survival rate. *Saudi Medical Journal*, *27*, 219–222.

Allen, D. B. (1996). Safety of human growth hormone therapy: Current topics. *The Journal of Pediatrics*, *128*, 8–13.

Allen, D. B., Frasier, S. D., Foley, T. P., & Pescovitz, O. H. (1993). Growth hormone for children with Down syndrome. *The Journal of Pediatrics*, *123*, 742–743.

Anneren, G., Tuvemo, T., & Gustafsson, J. (2000). Growth hormone therapy in young children with Down syndrome and a clinical comparison of Down and Prader-Willi syndromes. *Growth Hormone & Igf Research*, *10* Supplement B, S87–S91.

Antonela, L., & Vladimir, T. (2009). Refractive errors in children and young adults with Down's syndrome. *Acta Ophthalmologica*, PMID 19843014.

Ariel, I., Wells, T. R., Landing, B. H., & Singer, D. B. (1991). The urinary system in Down syndrome: A study of 124 autopsy cases. *Pediatric Pathology*, *11*, 897–888.

Balkany, R. J., Downs, M. P., Jafek, B. W., & Krajicek, M. J. (1979). Hearing loss in Down's syndrome. *Clinical Pediatrics*, *18*, 116–118.

Baptista, F., Varela, A., & Sardinha, L. B. (2005). Bone mineral mass in males and females with and without Down syndrome. *Osterporosis International*, *16*, 380–388.

Benard, J., Beron-Gaillard, N., & Satge, D. (2005). Down's syndrome protects against breast cancer: Is a constitutional cell microenvironment the key? *International Journal of Cancer*, *113*, 168–170.

Benda, C. E. (1969). *Down's syndrome: Mongolism and its management*. New York: Grune & Stratton, Inc.

Bergholdt, R., Eising, S., Nerup, J., & Pociot, F. (2006). Increased prevalence of Down's syndrome in individuals with type 1 diabetes in Denmark: A nationwide population-based study. *Diabetologia*, *49*, 1179–1182.

Bielek, J., Carvajal-Busslinger, M. I., & Bianchetti, M. G. (1996). Posterior urethral valves in trisomy 21. *Pediatric Nephrology, 10*, 143–146.

Bloemers, B. L., van Furth, A. M., Weijerman, M. E., Gemke, R. J., Broers, C. J., van den Ende, K., et al. (2007). Down syndrome: A novel risk factor for respiratory syncytial virus bronchiolitis-a prospective birth-cohort study. *Pediatrics, 120*, e1076–e1081.

Bloemers, B. L., van Furth, A. M., Weijerman, M. E., Gemke, R. J., Broers, C. J., Kimpen, J. L., et al. (2010). High incidence of recurrent wheeze in children with Down syndrome with and without previous respiratory syncytial virus lower respiratory tract infection. *Pediatric Infectious Disease, 29*, 39–42.

Book, L., Hart, A., Black, J., Feolo, M., Zone, J. J., & Neuharsen, S. L. (2001). Prevalence and clinical characteristics of celiac disease in Down syndrome in a U.S. study. *American Journal of Medical Genetics, 98*, 70–74.

Bovicelli, L., Orsini, L. F., Rizzo, N., Montacuti, V., & Baccetta, M. (1982). Reproduction in Down syndrome. *Obstetrics and Gynecology, 59*(6 Suppl), 13S–7S.

Brockmeyer, D. (1999). Down syndrome and craniovertebral instability. Topic review and treatment recommendations. *Pediatric Neurosurgery, 3*, 71–77.

Brodtmann, A. (2009). Hashimoto encephalopathy and Down syndrome. *Archives of Neurology, 66*, 663–666.

Burch, R. R. J. & Milunsky, A. (1969). Early-onset diabetes mellitus in the general and Down's syndrome populations genetics, aetiology, and pathogenesis. *The Lancet, 15*(7594), 554–558.

Carnicer, J., Farre, C., Varea, V., Vilar, P., Moreno, J., & Artiga, J. (2001). Prevalence of celiac disease in Down's syndrome. *European Journal of Gastroenterology and Hepatology, 123*, 263–267.

Caselli, M. A., Cohen-Sobel, E., & Thompson, J. (1991). Biomechanical management of children and adolescents with Down syndrome. *Journal of the American Podiatric Medical Association, 81*, 119–127.

Cohen, W. I. (2006). Current dilemmas in Down syndrome clinical care: Celiac disease, thyroid disorders, and atlanto-axial instability. *American Journal of Medical Genetics Part C (Seminars in Medical Genetics), 142C*, 141–148.

Concolino, D., Pasquizzi, A., Capalbo, G., Sinopoli, S., & Strisciuglio, P. (2006). Early detection of podiatric anomalies in children with Down syndrome. *Acta Paediatrica, 95*, 17–20.

Creavin, A. L. & Brown, R. D. (2009). Ophthalmic abnormalities in children with Down syndrome. *Journal of Pediatric Ophthalmology and Strabismus, 46*, 76–82.

Dada, R., Kumar, R., & Kucheria, K. (2006). A 2-year-old baby with Down's syndrome, cryptorchidism and testicular tumor. *European Journal of Medical Genetics, 49*, 265–268.

de Hingh, Y. C., van der Vossen, P. W., Gemen, E. F., Mulder, A. B., Hop, W. C., Brus, F. L., & de Vries, E. (2005) Intrinsic abnormalities of lymphocyte counts in children with down syndrome. *Journal of Pediatrics, 147*, 744–770.

Doyle, J. S., Lauerman, W. C., Wood, K. B., & Krause, D. R. (1996). Complications and long-term outcome of upper cervical spine arthrodesis in patients with Down syndrome. *Spine, 21*, 1223–1231.

Draheilm, C. C., McCubbin, J. A., & Williams, D. P. (2002). Differences in cardiovascular disease risk between nondiabetic adults with mental retardation with and without Down syndrome. *American Journal of Mental Retardation, 107*, 201–211.

Elkins, T. E. (1987). Reproductive health concerns of the person with Down syndrome. *Journal of Pediatric Neurosciences, 3*, 28–36.

Ercis, M., Balci, S., & Atakan, N. (1996). Dermatological manifestations of 71 Down syndrome children admitted to a clinical genetics unit. *Clinical Genetics, 50*, 317–320.

Evenhuis, H. M., Thunissen, M., Denkers, I., Verschuure, H., & Kemme, H. (2001). Prevalence of visual and hearing impairment in a Dutch institutionalized population with intellectual disability. *Journal of Intellectual Disability Research, 45*, 457–464.

Evenhuis, H. M., van Zanten, G. A., Brocaar, M. P., & Roerdinkholder, W. H. (1992). Hearing loss in middle-age persons with Down syndrome. *American Journal of Mental Retardation, 97*, 47–56.

Ferguson, R. L., Putney, M. E., & Allen, B. L., Jr. (1997). Comparison of neurologic deficits with atlanto-dens intervals in patients with Down syndrome. *Journal of Spinal Disorders, 10*, 246–252.

Fernhall, B., Figueroa, A., Collier, S., Goulopoulou, S., Giannopoulou, I., & Baynard, T. (2005). Resting metabolic rate is not reduced in obese adults with Down syndrome. *Mental Retardation, 43*, 391–400.

Fitzgerald, D. A., Paul, A., & Richmond, C. (2007). Severity of obstructive apnea in children with Down syndrome who snore. *Archives of Disease in Childhood, 92*, 423–425.

Forte, P., Lifshitz, F., Bellisario, R., Davis, J., Lanes, R., & Pugliese, M. (1984). Abnormalities of thyroid function in infants with Down syndrome. *The Journal of Pediatrics, 104*, 545–549.

Frazier, J. B. & Friedman, B. (1996). Swallow function in children with Down syndrome: A retrospective study. *Developmental Medicine and Child Neurology, 38*, 695–703.

Freeman, S. B., Bean, L.H, Allen, E. G., Tinker, S. W., Locke, A. E., Druschel, C., et al. (2008). Ethnicity, sex, and the incidence of congenital heart defects: A report for the National Down Syndrome Project. *Genetics in Medicine, 10*, 173–180.

Freeman, S. B., Torfs, C. P., Romitti, P. A., Royle, M. H., Druschel, C., Hobbs, S. A. et al. (2009). Congenital gastrointestinal defects in Down syndrome: A report from Atlanta and National Down syndrome Projects. *Clinical Genetics, 75*, 180–184.

Gamis, A. S., Woods, W. G., & Alonzo, T. A. (2003). Increased age at diagnosis has a significantly negative effect on outcome in children with Down syndrome and acute myeloid leukemia: A report from the Children's Cancer Group Study 2891. *Journal of Clinical Oncology, 21*, 3415–3422.

Gibson, P. A., Newton, R. W., Selby, K., Price, D. A., Leyland, K., & Addison, G. M. (2005). Longitudinal study of thyroid function in Down's syndrome in the first two decades. *Archives of Disease in Childhood, 90*, 547–578.

Goday-Arno, A., Cerda-Esteva, M., Flores-Le-Roux, J. A., Chillaron-Jordan, J. J., Corretger, J. M., & Cano-Perez, J. F. (2009). Hyperthyroidism in a population with Down syndrome (DS). *Clinical Endocrinology, 71*, 110–114.

Goldacre, M. J., Wotton, C. J., Seagroatt, V., & Yeates, D. (2004). Cancers and immune related diseases associated with Down's syndrome: A record linkage study. *Archives of Disease in Childhood, 89*, 1014–1017.

Goldstein, H. (1988). Menarche, menstruation, sexual relations and contraception of adolescent females with Down syndrome. *European Journal of Obstetrics and Gynecological Reproductive Biology, 27*, 343–349.

Gordon, N. (1995). Alternating hemiplegia of childhood. *Developmental Medicine and Child Neurology, 37*, 464–468.

Hafeez, S., Sharma, R. A., Huddart, R. A., Dearnaley, D. D., & Horwich, F. (2007). Challenges in treating patients with Down's syndrome and testicular cancer with chemotherapy and radiotherapy: The Royal Dadsden experience. *Clinical Oncology, 19*, 135–142.

Hasle, H., Clemmensen, I. H., & Mikkelsen, M. (2000). Risks of leukaemia and solid tumors in individuals with Down's syndrome. *The Lancet, 355*, 165–169.

Hawli, Y., Nasrallah, M., & Fuleihan, G.E.-H. (2009). Endocrine and musculoskeletal abnormalities in patients with Down syndrome. *Nature Reviews/Endocrinology, 5*, 327–334.

Hennequin, M., Faulks, D., Veyrune, J.L, & Bourdoil, P. (1999). Significance of oral health in persons with Down syndrome: A literature review. *Developmental Medicine and Child Neurology, 41*, 275–283.

Herring, J. A. (1982). Cervical instability in Down's syndrome and juvenile rheumatoid arthritis. *Journal of Pediatric Orthopedics, 2*, 205–207.

Hill, D. A., Gridley, G., Cnattingius, S., Mellemkjaer, L., Linet, M., Adami, H. O., et al. (2003). Mortality and cancer incidence among individuals with Down syndrome. *Archives of Internal Medicine, 163*, 705–711.

Jaiyesimi, O. & Baichoo, V. (2007). Cardiology in the Omani Arab children with Down's syndrome. *Cardiology in the Young, 17*, 166–171.

Johannisson, R., Gropp, A., Winking, H., Coerdt, W., Rehder, H., & Schwinger, E. (1983). Down's syndrome in the male. Reproductive pathology and neiotic studies. *Human Genetics, 63*, 132–138.

Juj, H. & Emery, H. (2009). The arthropathy of Down syndrome: An underdiagnosed and under-recognized condition. *Journal of Pediatrics, 154*, 234–238.

Karlsson, B., Gustafsson, J., Hedov, G., Ivarsson, S-A., & Anneren, G. (1998). Thyroid dysfunction in Down's syndrome: Relation to age and thyroid autoimmunity. *Archives of Diseases in Children, 79*, 242–245.

Kennedy, R. L., Jones, T. H., & Cuckle, H. S. (1992). Down's syndrome and the thyroid. *Clinical Endocrinology, 37*, 471–476.

Kupferman, J. C., Druschel, C. M., & Kupchik, G. S. (2009). Increased prevalence of renal and urinary tract anomalies in children with Down syndrome. *Pediatrics, 124*, e615–e621.

Kusters, M. A. A., Verstegen, R. H. J., Gemen, E. F. A., & de Vries, E. (2009). Intrinsic defect of the immune system in children with Down syndrome: A review. *Clinical and Experimental Immunology, 156*, 189–193.

Lo, A., Brown, H. G., Fivush, B. A., Neu, A. M., & Racusen, L. C. (1998). Renal disease in Down syndrome: Autopsy study with emphasis on glomerular lesions. *American Journal of Kidney Disease, 31*, 329–335.

Luke A., Roizen, N. J., Sutton, M., & Schoeller, D. A. (1994). Energy expenditure in children with Down syndrome correcting metabolic rate for movement. *Journal of Pediatrics, 125*, 825–839.

Luke, A., Sutton, M., Schoeller, D. A., & Roizen, N. J. (1996). Nutrient intake and obesity in prepubescent children with Down syndrome. *Journal of the American Dietetic Association, 96*, 1262–1267.

Magge, S. N., O'Neill, K. L., Shults, J., Stallings, V. A., & Stettler, N. (2008). Leptin levels among prepubertal children with Down syndrome compared to their siblings. *The Journal of Pediatrics, 152*, 321–326.

Matsunaga, S., Imakiire, T., Koga, H., Ishidou, Y., Sasaki, H., Taketomi, E., et al. (2007). Occult spinal canal stenosis due to C-1 hypoplasia in children with Down syndrome. *Journal of Neurosurgery (6 Supplement on Pediatrics), 107*, 457–489.

McPherson, B., Lai, S. P., Leung, K. K., & Ng, I. H. (2007). Hearing loss in Chinese school children with Down syndrome. *International Journal of Pediatric Otorhinolaryngology, 71*, 1905–1915.

Menezes, A. H., & Ryken, T. C. (1992). Craniovertebral abnormalities in Down's syndrome. *Pediatric Neurosurgery, 18*, 24–33.

Mercer, E. S., Broecker, B., Smith, E. A., Kirsch, A. J., Scherz, H. C., & Massad, C. A. (2004). Urological manifestations of Down syndrome. *The Journal of Urology, 171*, 1250–1253.

Merrick, J., Ezra, E., Josef, B., Hendel, D., Steinberg, D. M., & Weintroub, S. (2000). Musculoskeletal problems in Down Syndrome European Paediatric Orthopaedic Society Survey: The Israeli sample. *Journal of Pediatric Orthopedics, 9*, 185–192.

Miller, M. L., & Cassidy, J. T. (2004). Juvenile rheumatoid arthritis. In R. E. Behrman, R. M. Cliegman, & H. B. Jenson, (Eds.), *Nelson's textbook of pediatrics*. (17th ed.). Philadelphia: Saunders.

Milunsky, A., & Neurath, P. W. (1968). Diabetes mellitus in Down's syndrome. *Archives of Environmental Health, 17*, 372–376.

Mundschau, G., Gurbuxani, S., Gamis, A. S., Green, M. E., Arceci, R. J., & Crispino, J. D. (2003). Mutagenesis of GATA1 is an initiating event in Down syndrome leukemogenesis. *Blood, 101*, 4298–4300.

NASPGHAN (2005). Guidelines for the diagnosis and treatment of celiac disease in children: Recommendations of the North American Society for Pediatric Gastroenterology, Hepatology and Nutrition. *Journal of Pediatric Gastroenterology and Nutrition, 40*, 1–19.

Nisihara, R. M., Kotze, L. M., Utiyama, S. R., Oliverira, N. P., Fiedler, P. T., & Messias-Reason, I. T. (2005). Celiac disease in children and adolescents with Down syndrome. *Journal de Pediatria, 81*, 373–376.

Noble, S. E., Leyland, K., Findlay, C. A., Clark, C., Redfern, J., Mackenzie, J. et al. (2000). School-based screening for hypothyroidism in Down's syndrome by dried blood spot TSH measurement. *Archives of Disease in Childhood, 82*, 27–31.

Olson, J. C., Bender, J. C., Levinson, J. E., Oestreich, A., & Lovell, D. J. (1990). Arthropathy of Down syndrome. *Pediatrics, 86*, 931–936.

Padmakumar, L. G., Evans, J., & Sills, J. A. (2002). Is arthritis more common in children with Down syndrome? *Rheumatology, 41*, 1191–1193.

Patja, K., Pukkala, E., Sund, R., Iivanainen, M., & Kaski, M. (2006). Cancer incidence of persons with Down syndrome in Finland: A population-based study. *International Journal of Cancer, 118*, 1769–1772.

Pine, S. R., Guo, Q., Yin, C., Jayabose, S., Druschel, C. M., & Sandoval, C. (2007). Incidence and clinical implications of GATA1 mutations in newborns with Down syndrome. *Blood, 110*, 2128–2131.

Pipes, P. L., & Holm, V. A. (1980). Feeding children with Down's syndrome. *Journal of the American Dietetic Association, 77*, 277–282.

Pizzutillo, P., & Herman, M. (2005). Cervical spine issues in Down syndrome. *Journal of Pediatric Orthopedics, 25*, 253–259.

Pradhan, M., Dalal, A., Khan, F., Agrawal, S. (2006). Fertility in men with Down syndrome: a case report. *Fertility and Sterilization, 86*, 1765. e1–3.

Prasher, V. P. (2002). Disintegrative syndrome in young adults with Down syndrome. *Irish Journal of Psychological Medicine, 19*, 101–102.

Prasher, V., & Gomez, G. (2007). Natural history of thyroid function in adults with Down syndrome—10-year follow-up study. *Journal of Intellectual Disability Research, 51*, 312–317.

Prasher, V. P., Robinson, L., Krishnan, V. H. R., & Chung, M. C. (1995). Podiatric disorders among children with Down syndrome and learning disability. *Developmental Medicine and Child Neurology, 37*, 131–134.

Pueschel, S. M. (1990). Clinical aspects of Down syndrome from infancy to adulthood. *American Journal of Medical Genetics, 7*, 52–56.

Pueschel, S. M., Findley, T. W., Furia, J., Gallagher, P. L., Scola, F. H., & Pezzullo, J. C. (1987). Atlantoaxial instability in Down syndrome: Roentgenographic, neurologic, and somatosentory evoked potential studies. *The Journal of Pediatrics, 110*, 515–521.

Pueschel, S. M., Louis, S., & McKnight, P. (1991). Seizure disorders in Down syndrome. *Archives of Neurology, 48*, 318–320.

Pueschel, S. M., Orson, J. M., Boylan, J. M., & Pezzullo, J. C. (1985). Adolescent development in males with Down syndrome. *American Journal of Diseases of Children, 139*, 236–238.

Puri, B. K., Ho, K. W., & Singh, I. (2001). Age of seizure onset in adults with Down's syndrome. *International Journal of Clinical Practice, 55*, 442–444.

Pysden, K., Fallon, P., Moorthy, B., & Ganesan, V. (2010). Presumed perinatal stroke in a child with Down syndrome and moyamoya disease. *Developmental Medicine and Child Neurology, 52*, 212–214.

Rabin, K. R., & Witlock, J. A. (2009). Malignancy in children with trisomy 21. *The Oncologist, 14*, 164–173.

Rabinowitz, Y. S. (1998). Keratoconus. *Survey of Ophthalmology, 42*, 297–329.

Roizen, N. J., Mets, M. B., & Blondis, T. A. (1994). Ophthalmic disorders in children with Down syndrome. *Developmental Medicine and Child Neurology, 36*, 594–600.

Roizen, N. J., Wolters, C., Nicol, T., & Blondis, T. A. (1993). Hearing loss in children with Down syndrome. *The Journal of Pediatrics*, *12*, S9–S12.

Rubello D., Pozzan G. B., Casara D., Girelli M. E., Boccato S., Rigon, F., et al. (1995). Natural course of subclinical hypothyroidism in Down's syndrome: Prospective study results and therapeutic considerations. *Journal of Endocrinology Investigation*, *18*, 35–40.

Scherbenske, J. M., Benson, P. M., Rotchford, J. P., & James, W. D. (1990). Cutaneous and ocular manifestations of Down syndrome. *Journal of the American Academy of Dermatology*, *22*, 933–936.

Schupf, N., Zigman, W., Kapell, D., Lee, J. H., Klien, J., & Levin, B. (1997). Early menopause in women with Down syndrome. *Journal of Intellectual Disability Research*, *41*, 264–267.

Segal, L. S., Drummond, D. S., Zanotti, R. M., Ecker, M. L., & Mubarak, S. J. (1991). Complications of posterior arthrodesis of the cervical spine in patients who have Down syndrome. *Journal of Bone and Joint Surgery*, *73A*, 1547–1554.

Selikowitz, M. (1993). Short-term efficacy of tympanostomy tubes for secretory otitis media in children with Down syndrome. *Developmental Medicine & Child Neurology*, *35*, 511–515.

Sheridan, R., Llerena, J. Jr., Matkins, S., Debenham, P., Cawood, A., & Bobrow, M. (1989). Fertility in a male with trisomy 21. *Journal of Medical Genetics*, *26*, 294–298.

Sherk, H. H., Pasquariello, P. S., & Watters, W. C. (1982). Multiple dislocations of the cervical spine in a patient with juvenile arthritis and Down's syndrome. *Clinical Orthopedics and Relat Research*, *162*, 37–40.

Shott, S. R. (2006). Down syndrome: Common otolaryngologic manifestations. *American Journal of Medical Genetics Part C (Seminars in Medical Genetics) 142C*, 131–140.

Shott, S. R., Amin, R., Chini, B., Heubi, C., Hotze, S., & Akers, R. (2006). Obstructive sleep apnea should all children with Down syndrome be tested? *Archives of Otolaryngology, Head, and Neck Surgery*, *132*, 432–436.

Shott, S. R., Joseph, A., & Heithaus, D. (2001). Hearing loss in children with Down syndrome. *International Journal of Pediatric Otorhinolaryngology*, *61*, 199–205.

So, S. A., Urbano, R. C., & Hodapp, R. M. (2007). Hospitalizations of infants and young children with Down syndrome: Evidence from inpatient person-record from a statewide administrative database. *Journal of Intellectual Disability Research*, *51*, 1030–1038.

Sood, M. R. (2007). Disorders of malabsorption. In R. Kliegman, H. B. Jenson, R. E. Berhman & B. F. Stanton (Eds.), *Nelson textbook of pediatrics* (18th ed., pp. 1591–1593).

Southgate, W. M., Annibale, D. J., Hulsey, T. C., & Purohit, D. M. (2001). International experience with trisomy 21 infants placed on extracorporeal membrane oxygenation. *Pediatrics*, *107*, 548–552.

Spender, Q., Stein, A., Dennis, J., Reilly, S., Percy, E., & Cave, D. (1996). An exploration of feeding difficulties in children with Down syndrome. *Developmental Medicine and Child Neurology*, *38*, 681–694.

Stafstrom, C. E., & Konkol, R. J. (1994). Infantile spasms in children with Down syndrome. *Developmental Medicine and Child Neurology*, *36*, 576–585.

Stafstrom, C. E., Patxot, O. F., Gilmore, H. E., & Wisniewski, K. E. (1991). Seizures in children with Down syndrome: Etiology, characteristics and outcome. *Developmental Medicine and Child Neurology*, *33*, 191–200.

Stearns, P. E., Droulard, K. E., & Sahhar, F. H. (1960). Studies bearing on fertility of male and female mongoloids. *American Journal of Mental Deficiency*, *65*, 37–41.

Steelman, J., & Zeitler, P. (2001). Osteoporosis in pediatrics. *Pediatrics in Review*, *22*, 56–65.

Telega, G., Bennet, T. R., & Werlin, S. (2008). Emerging new clinical patterns in the presentation of celiac disease. *Archives of Pediatrics and Adolescent Medicine*, *162*, 164–168.

Tredwell, S. J., Newman, D. E., & Lockitch, G. (1990). Instability of the upper cervical spine in Down syndrome. *Journal of Pediatric Orthopedics*, *10*, 602–606.

Tuysuz, B., & Beker, D. B. (2001). Thyroid dysfunction in children with Down's syndrome. *Acta Paediatrics, 90*, 1389–1393.

Tyler, C. V., Snyder, C. W., & Zyzanski, S. (2000). Screening for osteoporosis in community-dwelling adults with mental retardation. *Mental Retardation, 38*, 316–321.

Uibo, O., Teesalu, K., Metskula, K., Reimand, T., Saat, R., Sillat, T. et al. (2006). Screening for celiac disease in Down syndrome patients in Estonia revealed cases of subtotal villous atrophy without typical for celiac disease HLA-DQ and tissue transglutaminase antibodies. *World Journal of Gastroenterology, 12*, 1430–1434.

van de Louw, J., Vorstenbosch, R., Vinck, L., Penning, C., & Evenhuis, H. (2009). Prevalence of hypertension in adults with intellectual disability in the Netherlands. *Journal of Intellectual Disability Research, 53*, 78–84.

van Trotsenburg, A. S., Vulsma, T., van Rozenburg-Marres, S. L., van Baar, A. L., Ridder, J. C., Heymans, H. S., et al. (2005). The effect of thyroxine treatment started in the neonatal period on development and growth of two-year-old Down syndrome children: a randomized clinical trial. *Journal of Clinical Endocrinology and Metabolism, 90*, 3304–3311.

Vis, J. C., Duffels, M. G., Winter, M. M., Weijerman, M. E., Cobben, J. M., Huisman, S. A., et al. (2009). Down syndrome: A cardiovascular perspective. *Journal of Intellectual Disability Research, 53*, 419–425.

Wechsler, J., Greene, M., McDevitt, M. A., Anastasi, J., Karp, J. E., Le Beau, M. M., et al. (2002). Acquired mutations in GATA1 in the megakaryoblastic leukemia of Down syndrome. *Nature Genetics, 32*, 148–152.

Widen, J. E., Folsom, F. R., Thompson, G., & Wilson, W. R. (1987). Auditory brainstem responses in young adults with Down syndrome. *American Journal of Mental Deficiency, 91*, 472–479.

Wouters, J., Weijerman, M. E., van Furth, M., Schreurs, J. W. J., Crusius, J. B. A., von Blomberg, B. M. E., et al. (2009). Prospective human leukocyte antigen, endomysial immunoglobulin A antibodies, and transglutaminase antibodies testing fro celiac disease in children with Down syndrome. *The Journal of Pediatrics, 154*, 239–242.

Yancey, C. L., Zmijewski, C., Athreya, B. H., & Rosenberg, J. S. (1984). Arthropathy of Down's syndrome. *Arthritis and Rheumatism, 27*, 929–934.

Yokoyama, T., Tamura, H., Tsukamoto, H., Yamane, K., & Mishima, H. K. (2006). Prevalence of glaucoma in adults with Down's syndrome. *Japanese Journal of Ophthalmology, 50*, 274–272.

Zipursky, A. (2003). Transient leukemia: A benign form of leukemia in newborn infants with trisomy 21. *Journal of Haematology, 120*, 930–938.

Zuhlke, C., Thies, U., Braulke, I., Reis, A., & Schirren, C. (1994). Down syndrome and male fertility; PCR-derived fingerprinting, serological and andrological investigations. *Clinical Genetics, 46*, 324–326.

Health over the Life Span

CHAPTER TWO

Health Outcomes of Infants and Toddlers with Down Syndrome

Robert M. Hodapp,[*,†] Nancy Miodrag,[*] Samantha E. Goldman,[*,†] *and* Richard C. Urbano[*,‡]

Contents

Abstract

Reviewing large-scale, population-based studies, this chapter summarizes three health outcomes for young children with Down syndrome: (1) adverse birth outcomes (e.g., prematurity, low birthweight); (2) in-patient hospitalizations; and (3) early mortality. Prematurity and low birthweight occur several times more often among newborns with (vs. without) Down syndrome, and account for 14–25% of all newborns with the syndrome. From 1/2 to 3/4 of these infants experience nonbirth hospitalizations within their first 3 years, most beginning during their first year. Those infants with congenital heart defects experience hospitalization more often, earlier, and for longer periods; respiratory problems constitute the main reason for hospitalizations among children with (and without) heart defects. Newborns with Down syndrome die before their first birthday

[*] Vanderbilt Kennedy Center, Vanderbilt University, Nashville, Tennessee, USA
[†] Department of Special Education, Vanderbilt University, Nashville, Tennessee, USA
[‡] Department of Pediatrics, General Pediatrics Division, Vanderbilt University, Nashville, Tennessee, USA

International Review of Research in Mental Retardation, Volume 39
ISSN 0074-7750, DOI 10.1016/S0074-7750(10)39002-1

from 4 to 24 times more often than other newborns; congenital heart defects, African American mothers, and prematurity are the major risk factors. Future studies need to identify child, parent, and family risk factors for early health outcomes, tie health outcomes to medical services, and determine the influence on early health of pollution and other environments. Better data and data-linkage are also needed. With an expanded research base, physicians will be able to provide more precise anticipatory guidance to parents, early interventionists, and others who care for young children with Down syndrome.

1. Introduction

Health in Down syndrome is a glass that is either half full or half empty. In one sense, advances have been unprecedented. Early in the twentieth century, Lionel Penrose (1949) estimated that the life expectancy of persons with Down syndrome was 9 years in 1929 and 12 in 1949. By 1973, the median age of death had risen to 30 years, and was 56 by 1991, with current estimates approximately 58–60 years (Bittles & Glasson, 2004). Yang, Rasmussen, and Friedman (2002) also showed a rise from 25 to 47 years during the period from 1983 to 1997. Though life expectancies have risen for both the general population (Arias, 2007) and persons with disabilities (Long & Kavarian, 2008), rarely have such increases been on the order of 25–30 years over a 40-year span.

Moreover, such health advances often directly benefit young children. Even compared to 40 years ago, congenital heart defects are increasingly correctable via surgery, and most infants now survive their earliest years. In contrast to Penrose's earlier conclusions about death during childhood (when many children never reached adulthood), advances in pediatric medicine have greatly aided young children with Down syndrome.

But looked at another way, most of these children may be surviving, yet they continue to experience both major health issues that often require hospitalization and minor health issues that affect everyday functioning. Thus, compared to a population rate of 8 per 1000 births (0.8%), congenital heart defects are found in 44–60% of infants with Down syndrome (Freeman et al., 1998). Increased rates are also noted for leukemia, respiratory problems, celiac disease, hypothyroidism, and vision and hearing problems (Van Riper & Cohen, 2001). As Roizen (2003) notes, "The majority of children with Down syndrome will be born with or develop some major medical problem" (p. 88). "Low grade" medical health issues that also require access to health services also occur more frequently than in the general population (Schieve, Boulet, Boyle, Rasmussen, & Schendel, 2009).

Beyond changing the focus from mortality to morbidity, it is also important to highlight how young children with Down syndrome fare on other health outcomes. Such outcomes include prematurity and other adverse birth outcomes and in-patient hospitalization. These health outcomes, in turn, are especially salient to parents, teachers, and other non-medical professionals. Such outcomes are also salient to pediatricians, who routinely offer to parents anticipatory guidance—a dynamic process in which pediatricians provide educational information, guidance, and instruction on how to promote the child's health and development (Barkin et al., 2005). Anticipatory guidance is especially important for children with Down syndrome, whose early health issues can be persistent, severe, and complex.

In considering early health outcomes, we adopt an approach that is simultaneously age-specific and illness-general. It is age-specific in that we limit our focus to health-related outcomes that occur during the birth-to-5-year period. At the same time, our focus is not on individual health conditions; we leave for others discussions of prevalence, clinical characteristics, course, correlates, or treatments of specific health conditions. Instead, we center more on global, albeit important, outcomes that relate to overall health and well-being during the early childhood years.

By limiting our discussion to adverse birth outcomes, infant mortality, and hospitalizations, we are discussing only a subset of all possible health-related issues. We do not address the amount, type, timing, or predictors of children's less severe illnesses; physician's visits for those illnesses; vaccinations or well-child check-ups; or emergency department visits. Similarly, we do not examine medications or the pediatrician's continuing need to evaluate, monitor, prevent, and be vigilant about health conditions often found in young children with Down syndrome (Roizen, 2003).

In this chapter, then, we focus on several major health outcomes. First, we evaluate this area's main research approach, the use of large-scale, population-based, and (often) records-based information. Next, we review studies of adverse birth outcomes in Down syndrome, including low birthweight and prematurity. We then examine in-patient hospitalizations during infancy and the preschool years, before discussing early childhood mortality. We end the chapter by exploring next steps for future research.

2. Benefits of Examining Health Issues Using Large-Scale Databases

Similar to research on other aspects of disability, most studies on the health of children with Down syndrome are based on small samples of participants, usually those who present to a particular clinic or hospital.

These so-called samples of convenience provide a preliminary sense of many health concerns in these children.

But as small-scale studies using convenience samples are prone to several biases, the field has increasingly moved to large-scale studies. These studies examine hundreds or thousands of participants. Although we later provide examples, suffice for now to note that such studies utilize nationally representative questionnaires; data on all individuals throughout the country from the US Census or Vital Statistics Databases; or tests, interviews, medical histories, school records, or administrative databases from a state, region, or multi-county area (Hodapp & Urbano, 2009).

Such databases present three main advantages, in that each:

1) *Allows for Larger-Scale and Less Biased Examinations*

When discussing health problems in Down syndrome, rates vary widely, and one major source of variance concerns the size of each study's sample. When examining small numbers of children, divergent percentages can often arise for a particular problem condition. A good example concerns hearing impairments, in which estimates among children with Down syndrome range from 38% to 78% (Shott, Joseph, & Heithaus, 2001). But given how small-scale studies operate, such divergent rates are expected. Along with the fact that studies differ in their diagnostic criteria (e.g., Porter & Tharpe, 2010), studies with small samples make it more difficult to determine prevalence rates of co-occurring medical conditions.

A related problem concerns nonrepresentative samples. Almost by definition, samples of convenience do not represent the larger population from which they are drawn. Participants often reside near the hospital or clinic, and, because a hospital might excel at treating a specific condition, that hospital's clientele may overrepresent a certain medical problem. For their part, families of children are more likely to receive treatment when parents are married, are of higher socioeconomic status (SES), are White (vs. African American or Hispanic), and are of higher educational levels (Elster, Jarosik, VanGeest, & Fleming, 2003; Garland et al., 2005; Thompson & May, 2006).

Population-based studies, by contrast, are both larger in scale and less prone to nonrepresentative samples. Most nationally based questionnaire studies survey from 40,000 to 200,000 respondents, from which one can examine several hundred or more children with Down syndrome and their families (e.g., Schieve et al., 2009). Similarly, Census studies make use of the United States' 4.3 million births and 2.4 million deaths per year (Centers for Disease Control and Preventions, 2010). Though smaller in scale, statewide vital statistics databases provide information on thousands of births, deaths, marriages, and divorces each year, and their datasets (which in part go into the federal vital statistics data) often include extra fields and information. In some states, one can also make use of data pertaining to educational outcomes or hospital visits. Information pertains to individuals from all of the study area's ethnic, racial, educational, SES, or other groups, some of whom are often missed in smaller-scale studies.

2) *Allows for Examinations of Real-World Outcomes*

In contrast to many medical studies—which often focus on a specific disease—most large-scale datasets focus on health outcomes. Large-scale questionnaires ask how often (over the past week or month) the child has been sick, gone to the doctor, or been hospitalized. For example, using a National Health Interview Survey examining health in 3–17 year old children with Down syndrome, Schieve et al. (2009) asked parents if their child had a impairment that impacted health and how often and what kinds of health care services they utilized (e.g., physiotherapy, hospital emergency). In addition to child-related information, some questionnaires ask whether mothers have needed to stay home or miss work. Similarly, hospitalization records can determine the timing, length, and reason for in-patient hospitalizations, or the timing, causes, and correlates of death.

This focus on real-world health outcomes has both strengths and limitations. The main limitation concerns its more general focus. Using hospital records or large-scale questionnaire data, we often cannot know specifics about the child's disease, and whether the child has one of several types of congenital heart defect, cancer, or respiratory problem. No information is provided as to why one versus another treatment option was chosen, or the thought processes undertaken by the physician or parents. Further, what is recorded or omitted is determined by the primary purpose of the data system.

Conversely, large-scale studies often provide a perspective closer to that of those who care for that child. By highlighting the amount, timing, length, and causes of hospitalization when a baby has Down syndrome, the chances that specific health outcomes might occur become clearer to parents, interventionists, genetic counselors, and others. Though rarely considered, this more "parent-centered" perspective seems critical. Indeed, in interviewing parents of children and young adults with three disability conditions, Minnes and Steiner (2009) found that parents highlighted the need for better interactions between their physicians and their children with disabilities (see also Muggli, Collins, & Marraffa, 2009). Similarly, the American Academy of Pediatrics Committee on Children with Disabilities (2001) encourages pediatricians to work with parents to attain appropriate medical and other services for children with all disability conditions. Yet even today, most physicians receive inadequate training in the care of children with disabilities

(Burge, Ouellette-Kuntz, McCreary, Bradley, & Leichner, 2002; Special Olympics, 2005).

3) *Provides Practical Information about Those Outcomes*

By focusing on large samples across entire populations, population-based studies also allow one to examine various characteristics of health outcomes. In their examinations of child psychiatric conditions, for example, Costello, Foley, and Angold (2006) note how it is important to go beyond prevalence rates, to focus as well on the age at which the child's condition is usually first seen; the course of the condition; the identification of co-morbid health problems; and the specification of characteristics of the child, parents, family, or neighborhood that make a condition more likely to appear. Such studies can also tell us the chances that a condition, once diagnosed, might reappear (and predictors of such reappearance).

Finally, in providing practical information about health outcomes of young children with Down syndrome, we also need to emphasize the advantages of linking information from multiple sources. In several of the studies described below, we link information on the same person or family, either within a single type of record or across record types (Urbano, 2007). In examining hospitalizations across the first 3 years of life, So, Urbano, and Hodapp (2007) linked information about multiple hospital visits of the same child. Goldman, Urbano, and Hodapp (2010) linked newborns' birth and death records. By linking an individual's records together, administrative databases become increasingly useful. By "following" each child over time, either in multiple instances of a single record (e.g., hospitalizations) or from one record type to another (e.g., Birth to Death), we are able to join together—for thousands of children—multiple types of information, multiple instances of a single event across time, and multiple children in the same family.

3. State of the Art Concerning Health Information on Young Children with Down Syndrome

Before beginning, it is instructive to examine current consensus health guidelines concerning young children with the syndrome. These guidelines arise from two sources. The first guide, entitled *Health Care Guidelines for Individuals with Down Syndrome: 1999 Revision* (Cohen, 1999), was produced by the Down Syndrome Medical Interest Group (DSMIG) of the National Down Syndrome Society (NDSS). These individuals, consisting of physicians and other interested medical professionals, often direct Down syndrome clinics and see in their practice many of these children and their families. Their *Guidelines* reflect best clinical practice in the United States (Van Riper & Cohen, 2001) and include a checklist of exams, labs and consults, developmental concerns, and recommendations for parents at each stage of the child's life, from neonatal stage to adulthood. The latter half of the document provides information about co-occurring medical issues in Down syndrome, including cardiac problems, dental care, hearing and vision problems, thyroid disease, feeding issues, leukemia, respiratory infections, orthopedic disorders, gastrointestinal disorders, speech and language problems, seizure disorders, and psychiatric disorders.

The second set of recommendations was produced by the Committee on Genetics from the American Academy of Pediatrics (AAP, 2001). Developed in 2001, *Health Supervision for Children with Down syndrome* was designed to help pediatricians who provide health care to these children. Similar to the DSMIG publication, the AAP guidelines outline the same medical considerations according to major milestones from birth through early adulthood. For newborns and infants, the medical emphasis revolves around feeding and constipation issues, strabismus and other vision problems, otitis media and other hearing problems, congenital heart defects, thyroid disease, respiratory tract infections, and childhood leukemia.

In neither case, then, is the focus on health outcomes per se. In addition, within each guide little attention is given to those factors that are associated with each health condition. We now turn to these issues, especially as they relate to adverse birth outcomes, in-patient hospitalization, and death.

4. Adverse Birth Outcomes among Newborns with Down Syndrome

In contrast to Penrose's day, most newborns with Down syndrome survive into adulthood, although several important health problems remain. Even at birth, the rates of prematurity, low birthweight, and small for gestational age are much higher than rates seen among infants without Down syndrome.

To date, only two published studies—examining three cohorts of newborns with Down syndrome—have examined these issues. In the first, Frid, Drott, Olausson, Sundelin, and Anneren (2004) examined the medical records of newborns that were born with Down syndrome. Frid et al. (2004) focused on two cohorts, those born in northern Sweden from 1973 to 1980 ($N = 219$), and those born from 1995 to 1998 ($N = 88$). Newborns were identified as having Down syndrome from three sources: from the Medical Birth Register (covering 99% of all Swedish births) and from both the Swedish Register of Congenital Malformations and the Hospital

Discharge Register (used to identify additional newborns with Down syndrome). Authors examined birth outcomes among newborns with Down syndrome in two ways: comparing earlier to later cohorts within the Down syndrome group and comparing rates of several birth outcomes in the two cohorts (1973–1980 and 1995–1998) to general population rates during these two time periods.

In a second, ongoing study, Hodapp, Urbano, and Rosenbloom (2010) compared the birth outcomes of 1043 newborns with Down syndrome born from 1990 to 2005 to the general Tennessee birth population (1.2 million). Infants were primarily identified via official Birth records, with extra infants identified as having the syndrome when they had—in one or more hospitalizations—a notation that they also had Down syndrome (i.e., an ICD-9 code of 758.0 was among the child's secondary diagnoses).

As Table 2.1 shows, findings across all three cohorts were remarkably similar. In Swedish cohorts from the 1970s and from the late 1990s—as well as in a large Tennessee group from 1990 to 2005—higher-than-population levels persist of newborns who are premature (<37 weeks), who are of low birthweight (<2500 g), and who are small for gestational age (<10% line of weight per gestational age, by gender). In addition, Frid et al. (2004) note higher rates of Caesarian sections and both studies reported lower APGAR scores.

Several additional issues also deserve mention. First, these adverse birth outcomes are very high compared to overall population rates and when considered as a percentage of all Down syndrome births. Compared to newborns in the general population, those with Down syndrome are born prematurely, at low birthweight, and small for gestational age several times more often. High percentages of Down syndrome births are affected: depending on cohort and outcome, adverse birth outcomes occur in from 1 in 7 (14%) to 1 in 4 (25%) of all newborns with Down syndrome.

A second issue concerns the cohorts themselves. Although only two studies exist, births occurred in two distinct populations (Sweden and Tennessee), with three separate cohorts, from 1970 to 2005. Yet despite this diversity of time and culture, consistent findings accrued. Even in the presence of divergent base rates—Tennessee shows much higher rates of such outcomes than does Sweden—newborns with Down syndrome consistently experience elevated rates of prematurity, low birthweight, and other adverse birth outcomes.

5. Early Hospitalization

Similar to adverse birth outcomes, the findings from large-scale studies converge on the conclusion that in-patient hospitalization is a fairly common occurrence among young children with Down syndrome. In our

Table 2.1 Preterm births, birthweight, small for gestational age, and APGAR scores in three birth cohorts

Study	Cohort, time period, sample size	Target group	Comparison group	Preterm birth (mean GA in weeks)	Birthweight (mean BW, gm)	Small-for-gestational-age (SGA)	APGAR 5 min
Hodapp et al. (2010)	Tennessee, USA, 1990–2005, $N = 1043$	Children with DS	Children in the GP	DS over 2 times more likely to be preterm than non-DS DS = 37.7; non-DS = 38.8	DS over 3 times more likely to be LBW than non-DS DS = 2891 g; non-DS = 3263 g	DS over 2 times more likely to be SGA than non-DS	DS = 8.33; non-DS = 8.86
Frid et al. (2004)	Northern Sweden, 1973–1980, $N = 219$	Children with DS	Children in the GP	DS = 38.3; GP = 39.7	DS = 3054 g; GP = 3492 g	DS = 13.4%; GP = 4.1%	DS = 8.6; GP = 9.3
Frid et al. (2004)	Northern Sweden, 1995–1998, $N = 88$	Children with DS	Children in the GP	DS = 38.4; GP = 39.3	DS = 3082 g; GP = 3550 g	DS = 13.5%; GP = 3.0%	DS = 8.9; GP = 9.6

DS, Down syndrome; GP, general population; GA, gestational age in weeks based on last menstrual period; g, grams; LBW, low birthweight.

own work, this conclusion arose early, when we noted the age of each patient from among 8325 in-patient stays at Tennessee hospitals over the years 1997–2002. Compared to older children and adults (and excluding all birth hospitalizations), 0–5 year old children with Down syndrome experienced hospitalization frequently. Frid, Anneren, Rasmussen, Sundelin, and Drott (2002) also noted that, compared to utilization during the 4–6, 7–10, and beyond-10 year periods, health care utilization among Swedish infants with Down syndrome was strikingly high during both the neonatal/post-neonatal and the 0–3 year periods.

5.1. Hospital stays during infancy

Three studies performed in-depth examinations of hospitalization among children with Down syndrome during the earliest years. These studies—by So et al. (2007), Boulet, Molinari, Grosse, Honein, and Correa-Villasenor (2008), and van Trotsenburg, Heymans, Tijssen, de Vijlder, and Vulsma (2006)—again converge on the idea that hospitalization occurs often, early, and for extended periods of time. In the sections below, we describe the studies themselves, then various aspects of such hospitalizations.

5.1.1. Study descriptions

In a first study, So et al. (2007) used Tennessee Hospital Discharge Records to "follow forward" infants with Down syndrome from birth until 3 years. Only infants born from 1997 to 1999 were chosen for study, as this was the period during which Tennessee's Hospital Discharge Data System was fully operational and the time period during which each child could be followed in the records from birth until their third birthday. To avoid over-sampling sicker infants, study participants included only those newborns identified as having Down syndrome in their birth hospitalization (and did not include children who were only identified as having Down syndrome through subsequent, nonbirth hospitalizations). The main outcome measure included the child's nonbirth hospitalization(s) over the first 3 years of life.

In a second study, Boulet et al. (2008) examined health insurance claims data for 420 children, aged 0–4 years of age, whose families were enrolled in a private health insurance plan. Although 5 years of data were used to identify children with Down syndrome, 1 year's data (2004) were used in analyses. The main comparisons were between children with and without Down syndrome, for each yearly age period, and comparisons focused on in-patient hospitalizations, outpatient visits, and drug claims, with cost analyses highlighted. In-patient birth hospitalizations of less than 4 days were excluded from in-patient admissions.

Finally, a third study by van Trotsenburg et al. (2006) examined hospital admission and medication use rates in 196 neonates with Down syndrome (of which 181 completed the trial), who were enrolled in a previously reported randomized clinical trial in the Netherlands. The researchers randomly assigned infants to two groups over the first 2 years of life—91 infants received a treatment of thyroxine and 90 infants received a placebo. Assessments included hospitalization before and during the trial, medication use during the trial, and the consequences of hospitalization and medication use rates in relation to children's early neurodevelopment (i.e., mental and motor development at 24 months).

5.1.2. Amount of in-patient hospitalization

Taking these three studies together, several findings stand out. First, extremely high percentages of children with Down syndrome are hospitalized within their first year of life. In So et al. (2007), the percentage of infants hospitalized was 49.8% (106/213), with 87.7% of all hospitalized children showing one or more nonbirth hospitalizations before their first birthday. Rates in Boulet et al. (2008) were even higher, with 75% (73/97) of children with Down syndrome hospitalized within their first year. For those infants who did not have Down syndrome, the hospitalization rate within the first year was 16%. van Trotsenburg et al. (2006) found that 83.2% (163/196) of neonates with Down syndrome were admitted to the hospital before trial entry, and 52.5% (95/181) visited the hospital during the trial.

5.1.3. Ties to congenital heart defects

In all three studies, clear ties were noted between increased in-patient hospitalization and the presence of congenital heart defects. Among the So et al. (2007) sample, 67.0% of all children with a congenital heart defect were hospitalized, compared to 29.6% of children without heart defects. In addition, all children who were hospitalized 5 or more times (5–9 times) had congenital heart defects. Although focused more on financial issues, Boulet et al. (2008) also noted wide discrepancies in health care costs between those children with Down syndrome with and without heart defects, with discrepancies especially striking during the first year. While van Trotsenburg et al. (2006) list several reasons for their hospitalizations, congenital heart disease had the second highest rates (following lung/airway diseases) from trial entry to age 1 (i.e., 36 children, 30% of the time) and from trial entry to age 2 (i.e., 38 children, 22.3% of the time).

5.1.4. Timing of hospitalizations

The timing of such hospitalizations was early. In So et al. (2007), most nonbirth hospitalizations occurred early on, with median survival time to first nonbirth hospitalization equaling 103 days. Of the 245 nonbirth hospital visits (by the 106 children who were hospitalized), 67.6% occurred in the first year, 25.7% in the second, and 5.7% in the third. Similarly, in van Trotsenburg et al. (2006), 66% of hospital admissions during the trial happened in the first year of life, whereas 89.6% of hospital admissions that occurred before entry to the clinical trial were within 24 hours of the birth.

In the So et al. (2007) study, timing of hospitalization also differed by whether the newborn had a congenital heart defect. Among those hospitalized children who had a heart defect, the estimated median time to first hospitalization was 96 days (95% CI = 78–114 days), compared to a median time to first hospitalization of 197 days (95% CI = 46–347) among those infants who did not have a heart defect.

5.1.5. Length of in-patient stays

Van Trotsenburg et al. (2006) noted that, of the 95 infants with Down syndrome who were hospitalized during the trial (52.5%), the average number of admission days was 19.75. Across all hospitalized children in So et al. (2007), those with congenital heart defects averaged 19.59 days in the hospital over their first 3 years of life, compared to an average of 6.86 days for hospitalized children without heart defects. Frid et al. (2004) noted a similar discrepancy in the total lengths of hospital stay over their first 3 years for newborns with heart defects (35.6 days) versus without such defects (8.5 days).

5.1.6. Reasons for hospital stays

Although some in-patient days were devoted to corrective surgery for children with heart defects, less than half (42.8%) of the So et al. (2007) children with heart defects had cardiac surgery, and such hospitalizations accounted for 19.3% of all hospitalizations for these children. Even for children with congenital heart defects, most hospitalizations and days spent in the hospital were not related to cardiac surgeries.

Instead, most hospitalizations had as their primary or secondary diagnoses pneumonia, bronchitis, or other respiratory conditions. Considering only primary diagnoses, respiratory conditions were the primary cause of hospitalization in 32.8% of all hospitalizations of children with congenital heart defects, and 56.2% of these children's hospitalizations listed respiratory problems as either a primary or secondary diagnosis. For children who did not have heart defects, a full 70.5% of all hospitalizations listed respiratory conditions as the primary diagnosis (diseases of the digestive system were next most common primary diagnosis, accounting for 11.4% of the hospitalizations of children without heart defects). In van Trotsenburg et al. (2006), reasons for hospital admissions included lung/airway disease, congenital heart disease, congenital gastrointestinal disease, urinary tract disease, central nervous system (e.g., infantile spasms), surgery (e.g., orthopedic), and other (e.g., apparent life-threatening event, skin infection).

5.2. Hospital stays during the 2–5 year period

Compared to the first 2 years of life, during the 2–5 year period hospitalizations are less common and less costly. As shown in Table 2.2, the few published studies of this issue show that, compared to the 0–1 year and 1–2 year periods, fewer children are hospitalized during this period. In Boulet et al. (2008), 21 children aged 3–4 years were hospitalized, compared to 73 and 50 during the 0–1 year and 1–2 year periods, respectively. Similarly, Frid et al.'s (2004) later period, covering the 4–6 year age-span, showed a marked decrease in the mean number of in-patient days compared to the 0–3 year period (24.9 days during the 0–3 year period; 3.6 during the 4–6 year period). Overall health care costs, though still high (especially for children with congenital heart defects), also decline during this period (Boulet et al., 2008).

Still, many 2–5 year old children with Down syndrome do experience in-patient hospital stays. To obtain a better sense of these hospitalizations, we recently examined our Tennessee in-patient data for this age period. Overall, 82 children were hospitalized during the 2–5 year period. Most children, 54.9% (45 of 82), experienced a single visit, whereas the remainder were hospitalized from 2 to 8 times. Four children were hospitalized for 17, 29, 36, and 45 days.

Again, most hospitalizations were related to respiratory problems. Table 2.3 delineates the primary diagnoses noted for the first hospitalization of these 82 children. Pneumonia, bronchitis, and asthma again accounted for most hospitalizations. As the table focuses solely on primary diagnoses, respiratory problems are minimized; respiratory problems will be more implicated in hospitalizations when one includes secondary conditions. Table 2.4 outlines "all other diagnoses" ($n = 32$), each identified once; it should be noticed that respiratory conditions of various kinds make up the majority.

Overall, young children with Down syndrome experience high levels of hospitalization. Such hospital stays most often begin during the first year of life, and frequently involve pneumonia, bronchitis, and other respiratory problems. Congenital heart defects are also implicated in hospitalizations, to some extent for heart surgeries, but more as a risk factor for subsequent respiratory problems. Hospitalizations during the 2–5 year period, though less common than during earlier years, nevertheless occur often. Throughout the first 5 years, respiratory concerns are often either primary or secondary diagnoses underlying such hospitalizations.

Table 2.2 Comparison of studies on early in-patient hospitalizations in children with Down syndrome

Authors and publication date	Sample, years of data collection and sample size	Study design	Percentage of admissions	Total number of admissions	Number of admissions	Length of stay	Sample with CHD	Hospitalized health conditions
Boulet et al. (2008)	Infants and children with DS from MarketScan database 2000–2004 $N=420$	Population-based retrospective study examining health care expenditures for children with DS	75% had at least 1 hospital admission	298 times	Average number of visits is 3 to 4 times higher for children with DS than without $n=73$ (0–1 years); 50 (1–2 years); 21 (3–4 years)	2.5 times greater than children without DS	~48%	CHD

So et al. (2007)	Infants and young children with DS from HDDS database 1997–2002 $N = 213$	Population-based retrospective study examining hospitalizations of children with DS	49.8% had at least 1 hospital admission	245 times	Median visits = 2	19.59 and 6.86 days[a]	54%	CHD, pneumonia, acute bronchitis/ bronchiolitis
van Trotsenburg et al. (2006)	Neonates with DS 1999–2003 $N = 196$ $n = 181$ who completed the trial	Single-center, randomized, double-blind, 24 months clinical trial comparing thyroxine administration with placebo	83.2% (before trial) 52.5% (during trial)	197 times	Mean visits = 2.07 (SD = 1.55); median visits = 2 (range 1–8)	19.75 days (SD = 22.68)	38 children	CHD and lung/ airway disease, gastrointestinal disease

[a]LOS reported for children with and without CHD, respectively.
DS, Down syndrome; HDDS, Tennessee's Hospital Discharge Data System; CHD, congenital heart disease/defects.

Table 2.3 Type, frequency, and percentage of primary diagnoses at first admission ($n = 82$)

Health condition	Frequency	Percentage
Acute bronchiolitis due to respiratory syncytial virus	2	2.4
Acute bronchiolitis (due to other infectious organism)	5	6.1
All other diagnoses[a]	32	38.4
Asthma, unspecified	3	3.7
Asthma, unspecified type, with status asthmaticus	2	2.4
Asthma, unspecified with (acute) exacerbation	3	3.7
Bronchopneumonia	2	2.4
Croup	3	3.7
Diabetes with other specific manifestations	2	2.4
Endocardial cushion defects/ atrioventricular septal defect	2	2.4
Missing	1	1.2
Other and unspecified noninfectious gastroenteritis	4	4.9
Patent ductus arteriosus	3	3.7
Pneumonia	14	17.1
Volume depletion disorder	4	4.9
Total	82	100

Note: [a] See Table 2.4 for each of the 32 additional diagnoses ($n = 32$).

Table 2.4 All other primary diagnoses at first admission (from Table 2.1, $n = 32$)

Health condition	Frequency	Percentage
Respiratory		
Acute bronchitis	1	1.2
Acute tracheitis without mention of obstruction	1	1.2
Chronic adenoiditis	1	1.2
Chronic tonsillitis and adenoiditis	1	1.2
Extrinsic asthma with acute exacerbation	1	1.2
Influenza with other respiratory manifestations	1	1.2

(*Continued*)

Table 2.4 (*Continued*)

Health condition	Frequency	Percentage
Mediastinitis	1	1.2
Other diseases of trachea and bronchus	1	1.2
Pneumonia due to Chlamydia	1	1.2
Stenosis of larynx	1	1.2
Respiratory subtotal	10	11.2
Digestive system		
Acute appendicitis with generalized peritonitis	1	1.2
Blood in stool	1	1.2
Digestive subtotal	2	2.4
Heart		
Ostium secundum type atrial septal defect	1	1.2
Ventricular septal defect	1	1.2
Heart Subtotal	2	2.4
Urinary system		
Bilateral small kidneys	1	1.2
Pyelitis or pyelonephritis	1	1.2
Urinary System Subtotal	2	2.4
Other		
Acute lymphoid leukemia	1	1.2
Acute nonsuppurative otitis media	1	1.2
Anorexia	1	1.2
Cellulitis and abscess of leg	1	1.2
Closed fracture of second cervical vertebra	1	1.2
Convulsions	1	1.2
Diarrhea	1	1.2
Disseminated candidiasis	1	1.2
Hemorrhage complications	1	1.2
Infection and inflammatory reaction due to virus	1	1.2
Intestinal infection	1	1.2
Mechanical complication of nervous system device	1	1.2
Neuromyelitis optica	1	1.2
Partial unilateral paralysis of vocal cords	1	1.2
Primary thrombocytopenia	1	1.2
Pyogenic arthritis involving lower leg	1	1.2
Other subtotal	16	19.2
Total	32	38.4

6. Early Mortality

In line with findings on adverse birth outcomes and early hospitalization, young children with Down syndrome also have higher-than-expected rates of mortality during infancy and early childhood. In a study using the surveillance records of the Metropolitan Atlanta Congenital Defects Program, Rasmussen, Wong, Correa, Gambrell, and Friedman (2006) found a survival rate of children with Down syndrome of 92.9% to 1 year and of 88.6% until 10 years. The best predictors of mortality were maternal race (with African American babies dying more often than Caucasian babies), presence of heart defects, low birthweight, and the interaction of maternal race and heart defects.

While Rasmussen et al. (2006) present the overall picture, a host of studies provide a more in-depth analysis of mortality during infancy. Summarized in Table 2.5, these studies have been performed in Tennessee and in the five-county region of the Metropolitan Atlanta Congenital Defects Program, as well as in the Netherlands, Western Australia, Italy, and Israel. Most studies utilized official registries, usually of birth but sometimes also involving neonatal and/or death registries. Participant numbers ranged from 322 (Weijerman et al., 2008) to 1332 (Bittles, Bower, Hussain, & Glasson, 2006), with the median study examining 668 newborns (Rasmussen et al., 2006; Sadetzki et al., 1999). Publication dates begin in the early 1990s (Mastroiacovo, Bertollini, & Corchia, 1992), and four of eight studies included some infants born since 2000.

Even given this diversity, studies converge on the conclusion that mortality rates among newborns with Down syndrome are extremely high. Depending on the study and on infant mortality rates in each reference group, odds ratios of infant mortality in Down syndrome range from 5.8 to 24.3 times those seen in the larger birth population. Compared to newborns without Down syndrome, then, the chances that these children will die before they reach their first birthday are highly elevated.

Beyond such high odds ratios, high percentages of newborns with Down syndrome are affected. Even acknowledging wide variations across studies, from 4.0%—or 1 in 25 newborns—to 24.5%—or almost 1 in 4 newborns—will die before they reach their first birthday. Even the median rate across these 8 studies—7.25%—translates into 1 per 14 deaths during infancy.

A few additional points deserve mention. First, in contrast to newborns who die among the general population, proportionately more deaths in Down syndrome occur after 1 month. In Sadetzki et al. (1999), 70% of all deaths within the first year occurred during this post-1-month period, compared to less than 27% of all infant deaths in the general population. Similarly, Shin, Kucik, and Correa (2007) and Goldman et al. (2010) found

Table 2.5 Comparison of studies on infant mortality rates (IMR) among infants with Down syndrome

Authors and publication date	Location and years of record	Databases used	Total *N*	Down syndrome IMR (%)	General population IMR (%)	Odds ratio
Bittles et al. (2006)	Western Australia, 1953–2000	Disability Services Commission of Western Australia Database, Western Australia Cancer and Death Registry, National Death Index	1332	6.5	0.5*	13.0
Goldman et al. (2010)	Tennessee, 1990–2006	Tennessee Department of Health Birth and Death Registry, Hospital Discharge Records	1305	7.4	0.89	8.3
Leonard, Bower, Patterson, and Leonard (2000)	Western Australia, 1980–1996	Birth Defects Registry, Maternal and Child Health Research Database	440	8.3	0.5*	16.6
Mastroiacovo et al. (1992)	Italy, 1978–1992	Italian Multicentric Registry of Birth Defects	620	20.2	1.4	14.4
Rasmussen et al. (2006)	5 counties of metropolitan Atlanta, 1979–1998	Metropolitan Atlanta Congenital Defects Program, State of Georgia Certificate of Live Birth, National Death Index	645	7.1	1.1	6.5

(*Continued*)

Table 2.5 (*Continued*)

Authors and publication date	Location and years of record	Databases used	Total *N*	Down syndrome IMR (%)	General population IMR (%)	Odds ratio
Sadetzki et al. (1999)	Israel, 1979–1983, 1987–1991	Israeli National DS Birth Registry, National Population Registry, National Central Bureau of Statistics	692	24.5	1.0	24.3
Shin et al. (2007)	5 counties of metropolitan Atlanta, 1979–2003	Metropolitan Atlanta Congenital Defects Program, Georgia vital records, National Death Index	922	6.4	1.1	5.8
Weijerman et al. (2008)	The Netherlands, 2003	Dutch Pediatric Surveillance Unit, Statistics Netherland, National Dutch Neonatal Registry, National Dutch Obstetric Registry	322	4.0	0.48	8.3

*General population mortality rate obtained from published sources.

that 66% and 56% of all deaths in the Down syndrome group occurred in the post-neonatal period (i.e., 28–364 days). In all three studies, the age distribution of mortality differs from that seen among those newborns that die in the general population.

Second, as most studies relied on Birth, Neonatal, and Death registries, it was not always possible to discern the exact causes of death. In Rasmussen et al. (2006), 16% of deaths to African American mothers noted "Down syndrome" as the sole cause of death, and Down syndrome was listed as the only available cause for 22% of all deaths in the work of Goldman et al. (2010). Any study using official death records as its data source is likely to have a similar problem.

7. Remaining Issues

We now discuss three unaddressed issues concerning health of young children with Down syndrome.

1) *Need to Add Context to Studies of Health of Young Children with Down Syndrome*

In considering health outcomes in young children with Down syndrome, we know a fair amount about the general picture, much less about the details. For adverse birth outcomes, early hospitalizations, and infant mortality, we know the basic rates in Down syndrome and comparisons to young children in the general population. We know some about the timing of early hospitalizations and death, and the reasons underlying each outcome. Beyond this more global information, however, details remain sketchy.

The most important details concern interactions between early health and the contexts in which these children develop. Specifically, few existing studies provide information about the influence on these children's health of parent or family characteristics; of the amount or quality of medical or other services (e.g., Schieve et al., 2009); or of how the child's health status interacts with relevant environments. The following characteristics seem especially important:

Parental race, socioeconomic status (SES), and education. In studies examining children in the general population, the mother's race, SES, and educational status have been tied to outcomes related to health (prematurity, infant mortality, lack of health care) and education (held back a grade, high school drop-out, not attending or graduating college). Although mechanisms underlying many of these outcomes remain unknown, mothers who are younger, less educated, from minority backgrounds, and unmarried are more likely to have children whose outcomes are less successful (Brooks-Gunn & Duncan, 1997).

When considering the health of children and adults with Down syndrome, the sole family characteristic that has been somewhat examined involves the race of the mother. Rasmussen et al. (2006) found that, compared to White mothers, African American mothers were more likely to have children who died and children with congenital heart defects and African American mothers were at especially high risk of early mortality. Similarly over the period from 1968 to 1987, Friedman (2001) found lower life expectancies in African American versus White individuals with Down syndrome.

Race may also tie to other personal characteristics. In comparing African American to White mothers of newborns with Down syndrome, we found that higher percentages of African American mothers were younger when they gave birth (Hodapp & Urbano, 2008). Indeed, 37.5% of African American and 22.8% of White mothers were 23 years or younger when they gave birth to their newborns with Down syndrome. In both racial groups, younger mothers were more likely to not have graduated high school and to be unmarried. From prior studies of health care utilization, mothers who were younger, less educated, and unmarried were least likely to know about, access, and receive health care for their children (Elster et al., 2003; Garland et al., 2005; Thompson & May, 2006).

Also connected to race are the twin issues of education and class. Above and beyond parenting an infant who is typically developing infant, mothers of infants with Down syndrome require information about the child's condition, caregiving, and locally available services. Most likely, mothers who are more educated and of higher SES will be better able to learn about Down syndrome, early intervention services, and how to obtain appropriate health care. Well-educated, middle- or upper-class mothers are also more likely to access parent groups such as the NDSS and the National Down Syndrome Congress (NDSC). These parent groups have been shown helpful in fostering mothers' personal growth and in providing education and support to many mothers of children with disabilities (Solomon, Pistrang, & Barker, 2001). To date, however, no studies have explored connections between the health status of young children with Down syndrome and parental education, class, or specific support.

Amount and quality of health services. Beyond parent and family characteristics, receiving health services relates to where one lives. As has been well-documented, medical specialists more often work in large teaching hospitals, which disproportionately exist within major metropolitan areas.

Beyond this divide between urban and nonurban areas, different localities also feature greater or fewer numbers of physicians of different specialties. In the United States, localities are divided into rational service areas, defined as "... individual counties, groups of counties, or communities that have displayed certain obvious primary, obstetrical, and pediatric care service patterns for residents of that county, community, and/or surrounding areas. Determining factors for delineating rational service areas include natural or artificial barriers (mountains, bad roads), migration patterns for care, the presence or absence of health manpower or facilities, patients' payment capabilities, etc" (State of Tennessee, 2005, p. 7).

Using these demarcations, areas are rated as to the numbers of physicians, pediatricians, obstetricians/gynecologists, and other specialists. In Tennessee, the availability of health services is judged in each of the state's grand divisions (West, Middle, and East Tennessee), rational service areas, and 95 counties. In each instance, areas are rated in terms of the ratio of the numbers of physicians, pediatricians, or obstetricians/gynecologists relative to the size of the local population, with underserved areas highlighted.

Although informative, this information has yet to be tied to medical care for young children with Down syndrome. Given that, during the 0–3 year period, most families are served by (state-provided) early intervention services, health service areas may or may not be most relevant for whether these children receive adequate health care. Indeed, the field knows little about the degree to which various services interconnect, the degree to which families who are well integrated into early intervention, school, or other services also receive consistent, adequate health care. Though Krahn, Hammond, and Turner (2006) discuss health disparities among persons with disabilities, studies that examine health services or outcomes for young children with Down syndrome are scant.

The child's residential environment. A final, related issue concerns the exact residential environment in which children reside. Although it may be difficult to identify which aspects of the environment most influence the health of children with Down syndrome, several clues derive from the types of problems most often experienced by these children. As noted above, early hospitalization and death most often relate to pneumonia, bronchitis, and other respiratory conditions. Such conditions are exacerbated by the environments in which children live.

What role might high levels of ambient air pollution play in the deaths or hospitalizations of young children with Down syndrome? We cannot say for certain, but there is a growing concern about the potential links between high levels of air pollution and increased incidence of birth defects in the United States (Croser & Seiter, 2004) and the world (van Kraayenoord, 2008; Weinhold, 2009). To date, few studies have focused on the effects of high levels of air pollution on the health of children with disabilities.

But among infants in the general population, several studies have linked infant mortality to high levels of air pollution. Ritz, Wilhelm, and Zhao (2006) examined infant deaths in southern California, assigning each deceased infant to the air monitoring station nearest the child's home and comparing that child to 10 control infants. In the early post-neonatal period (from 28 days to 3 months), the risk of respiratory death increased from

20% to 30% per 1-parts per million increase in carbon monoxide levels 2 weeks before death. Similarly, using exact residential information, Currie, Neidell, and Schmieder (2009) examined three types of pollution (CO; O_3; and PM_{10}) and found that increased exposure to carbon monoxide related both prenatally and post-natally to infant health.

In beginning collaborations with an expert in environmental studies and geographic information systems (GIS), we are currently examining the potential ties of air pollution levels to infant mortality and morbidity in Down syndrome. So far, our GIS expert has modeled the amount of air pollution exposure for infants born during several years between 1990 and 2005 (Pantaleoni, 2010). Such work combines pollution readings from the Environmental Protection Agency (EPA), from mobile stations (i.e., 5700 state Department of Transportation stations measuring amount of traffic each day), and from stations adjacent to landfills and other stationary sources of pollution. Measurements are then combined with measures of wind, weather, topography, and ground covering. Pollution levels are estimated for each child, for each week of life. We will then compare air pollution levels of "unaffected" children to those infants who died or were hospitalized for respiratory illnesses.

2) *Attaining Better Data and Achieving Better Linkage*

Across large-scale examinations of early health in Down syndrome, the field needs better data. In most current studies, there is a trade-off between breadth and depth, such that large-scale, population-based studies examine many people and do well at examining persons from different racial-ethnic, educational, marital, and other backgrounds (breadth), even as their data sources often do not ask important information (depth). To give an example, both Rasmussen et al. (2006) and Goldman et al. (2010), examining early death in Down syndrome, used official death records. In about 1/5 of cases "Down syndrome" was listed as the underlying (often the only) cause of death.

Beyond the need for physicians to fill out existing forms correctly, an additional issue concerns moving to include additional information on all existing vital statistics records. As currently operated in the United States, the National Center for Health Statistics (NCHS) establishes the format and content for vital statistics reporting to the federal government. These NCHS standards are stable over time, with major changes made once a decade at the time of the decennial US Census. For the most part, recent updates have included such things as moving from ICD-9 to ICD-10 codes in death records, or adding the subcategories of "suspected," "pending," or "confirmed" diagnoses of Down syndrome in birth records. In addition, NCHS closely monitors the quality of data submitted by the states. To improve the quality of these data, the NCHS reimburses states for records submitted based on the quality of the data.

Although these changes are useful and important, additional changes in future years might allow us to progress even more. Already, the field of epidemiology/public health has made great strides in asking—in increasingly simpler ways—about difficult issues. Consider maternal health and depression. Although mothers of children with disabilities are at increased risks of chronic health problems (Brehaut et al., 2009) and feel more depressed and physically burdened when their child has both disabilities and externalizing behavior problems (Lach et al., 2009), many aspects of health among mothers of children with disabilities remain unknown (Miodrag & Hodapp, 2010). Such information would be expanded greatly by adding a few questions to the child's birth or hospitalization records. For example, maternal depression might be briefly assessed using the CES-D (Radloff, 1977) or other short-form depression screener, and respondent health has been examined by using a single question ("How would you say that in general your health is?"—to which respondents answer 1-poor to 5-excellent). Such self-reported overall health ratings correlate fairly highly with both longer and more objective health measures (Idler & Benjamini, 1997).

Large-scale studies would also be aided by the development of better ways to link datasets. Currently, matching one record to another is performed using either deterministic—or exact—matches or probabilistic matching procedures (Tu, Mason, & Song, 2007), with the most common matching variables—the mother's social security number, name (first, last, maiden), and exact date of birth (month, day, year) (Urbano, 2007). But the process remains cumbersome, with many (often manual) steps to perform.

Recently, advances have been made in producing publicly available, automated software to perform these linkage tasks (Jurczyk, Xiong, Cragan, & Correa, 2008). The Vanderbilt Kennedy Center, a Eunice Kennedy Shriver Intellectual and Developmental Disabilities Research Center, has initiated a project to create an open-source, community-supported software package that provides researchers access to automated linkage technology. The project, named Coupler, targets researchers with computer skills in the "moderate" level (i.e., they can use SPSS and SAS scripting languages). A few of Coupler's advantages include that it (1) is easy to install and run (and does not require a systems administrator); (2) can be customized by the end-user; (3) is "platform-independent," in that it can be run using various computer operating systems (e.g., Windows, Mac, Linux); (4) supports multiple databases and file formats (i.e., any format supported by Java Database Connectivity, JDBC); (5) supports viewing, merging, and editing of linked databases; and (6) has available source code, documentation, tutorials, and sample datasets (Github, 2010; for current status of the project, see http://coupler.github.com).

3) *Improving Anticipatory Guidance*

As noted throughout this chapter, infants and toddlers with Down syndrome are at increased risk of adverse health outcomes. But how do health care professionals prepare caregivers for what to expect at a time when development is so precious and exposed? One such approach involves anticipatory guidance. Although beginning to be used in the field of early intervention (e.g., Fidler, Philofsky, & Hepburn, 2007), anticipatory guidance has always been "a cornerstone of primary care pediatrics" (Barkin et al., 2005, p. 372). First defined in the American Public Health Association's (1955) clinical manual in the mid-1950s, anticipatory guidance involves gathering and providing education and information to caregivers. The goal is to prepare caregivers psychologically to manage their child's health care needs and to anticipate health conditions and events. Many clinical strategies are used, with physician- or parent-initiated discussions most common, printed materials less so (Young & Boltri, 2005). Other anticipatory guidance techniques include verbal advice, videos, books, parenting classes, and most recently, the Internet (Schuster, Duan, Regalado, & Klein, 2000).

While seemingly easy to perform, providing anticipatory guidance has its challenges. In most instances, physicians have limited time to address parental concerns during health care visits (Schuster et al., 2000), and some physicians may not be adequately trained to discuss certain topics. Families also differ in their communication styles, family structures, and ability and openness to hear difficult information. Nonetheless, given the prevalence and severity of health conditions in young children with Down syndrome, it seems important that physicians provide such anticipatory guidance.

How might such anticipatory guidance look? In the case of a newborn with Down syndrome who requires heart surgery, anticipatory guidance might include a pediatric cardiologist discussing a pamphlet outlining the signs and symptoms of an atrioventricular septal defect, or a nurse showing parents the equipment to be used during surgery and outlining the preparatory measures needed for such a surgery. Or another medical professional might explain the child's increased risks of bronchitis, pneumonia, or other respiratory problems, explain the need to contact physicians quickly when respiratory problems first develop, and verbally counsel parents about their fears and concerns. Ultimately, the practice of anticipatory guidance must revolve around ways to manage these children's health conditions, thereby supporting parents during stressful times.

8. Conclusion

Over the past 40 years, great strides have been made in increasing life expectancy and performing surgery to correct the congenital heart defects of approximately half of these children. Yet at the same time, newborns with the syndrome continue to experience extremely high rates of such adverse birth outcomes as prematurity and low birthweight. During their first year of life, from 50% to 75% of infants experience in-patient hospitalizations (most often for respiratory conditions) and those with congenital heart defects are especially prone to early, lengthy, and repeated hospitalizations. Even rates of infant and early mortality, though much improved from 40 to 50 years ago, continue to occur from 4 to 24 times rates in the general population. It is now time to learn more about the causes of early health outcomes, to publicize their existence throughout the Down syndrome community, and to help physicians and parents care for the health needs of infants and young children with Down syndrome.

ACKNOWLEDGMENTS

We thank Craig Mason, PhD, and Shuvo Ghosh, MD, for their thoughtful editorial comments on earlier drafts of this paper.

This research was supported by a Greenfield Discovery Grant from the Vanderbilt Kennedy Center's Nicholas Hobbs Society and NICHD grants P30HD 15052 and RO3HD 050468.

Hospital discharge data from the Tennessee Hospital Discharge Data System, 1996–2005, and vital statistics datasets, 1990–2005, were provided by the Tennessee Department of Health, Office of Health Statistics, Nashville, Tennessee.

The contents of this study and the views expressed herein are solely the responsibility of the authors and do not necessarily represent the official views of any of the funding agencies or the Tennessee Department of Health.

REFERENCES

American Academy of Pediatrics Committee on Children with Disabilities (2001). Role of pediatrician in family centered early intervention services. *Pediatrics*, *107*, 1155–1157.

American Academy of Pediatrics Committee on Genetics (2001). Health supervision for children with Down syndrome. *Pediatrics*, *107*, 442–449.

American Public Health Association, Inc (1955). *Health supervision of young children*. New York: Author.

Arias, E. (2007). United States life tables, 2004. *National Vital Statistics Reports*, *56*(9), 1–40. Hyattsville, MD: National Center for Health Statistics.

Barkin, S. L., Scheindlin, B., Brown, C., Ip, E., Finch, S., & Wasserman, R. C. (2005). Anticipatory guidance topics: Are more better? *Ambulatory Pediatrics*, *5*, 372–376.

Bittles, A. H., Bower, C., Hussain, R., & Glasson, E. J. (2006). The four ages of Down syndrome. *European Journal of Public Health*, *17*, 221–215.

Bittles, A. H., & Glasson, E. J. (2004). Clinical, social, and ethical implications of changing life expectancy in Down syndrome. *Developmental Medicine and Child Neurology*, *46*, 282–286.

Boulet, S. L., Molinari, N.-A., Grosse, S. D., Honein, M. A., & Correa-Villasenor, A. (2008). Health care expenditures for infants and young children with Down syndrome in a privately insured population. *Journal of Pediatrics*, *153*, 241–246.

Brehaut, J. C., Kohen, D. E., Garner, R. E., Millar, A., Lach, L. M., Klassen, A. F., et al. (2009). Health among caregivers of children with health problems: Findings from a Canadian population-based study. *American Journal of Public Health*, *99*, 1254–1262.

Brooks-Gunn, J., & Duncan, G. (1997). The effects of poverty on children and youth. *Futures of Children*, *7*, 55–71.

Burge, P., Ouellette-Kuntz, H., McCreary, B., Bradley, E., & Leichner, P. (2002). Senior residents in psychiatry: Views on training in developmental disabilities. *Canadian Journal of Psychiatry*, *47*, 568–571.

Centers for Disease Control and Prevention (CDC). (2010). FASTATS: Birth and death statistics. Retrieved from http://www.cdc.gov/nchs/fastats/

Cohen, W. I. (1999). Health care guidelines for individuals with Down syndrome: 1999 Revision (Down syndrome preventive medical check list). *Down Syndrome Quarterly*, *4*, 1–16.

Costello, E. J., Foley, D. L., & Angold, A. (2006). The epidemiology of child and adolescent psychiatric disorders: II. Developmental epidemiology. *Journal of the American Academy of Child and Adolescent Psychiatry*, *45*, 8–25.

Croser, M. D., & Seiter, M. (2004). *Pollution, toxic chemicals, and mental retardation: Framing a national blueprint for health promotion and disability prevention*. Proceedings of a National Wingspread Summit. Washington, DC: American Association on Intellectual and Developmental Disabilities.

Currie, J., Neidell, M., & Schmieder, J. F. (2009). Air pollution and infant health: Lessons from New Jersey. *Journal of Health Economics*, *28*, 688–703.

Elster, A., Jarosik, J., VanGeest, J., & Fleming, M. (2003). Racial and ethnic disparities in health care for adolescents: A systematic review of the literature. *Archives of Pediatric and Adolescent Medicine*, *157*, 867–874.

Fidler, D. J., Philofsky, A., & Hepburn, S. L. (2007). Language phenotyping and intervention planning: Research and practice. *Mental Retardation and Developmental Disabilities Research Reviews*, *13*, 47–57.

Freeman, S. B., Taft, L. F., Dooley, K. J., Allran, K., Sherman, S. L., Hassold, T. J., et al. (1998). Population-based study of congenital heart defects in Down syndrome. *American Journal of Medical Genetics*, *80*, 213–217.

Frid, C., Anneren, G., Rasmussen, R., Sundelin, C., & Drott, P. (2002). Utilization of medical care among children with Down's syndrome. *Journal of Intellectual Disability Research*, *46*, 310–317.

Frid, C., Drott, P., Olausson, P. O., Sundelin, C., & Anneren, G. (2004). Maternal and neonatal factors and mortality in children with Down syndrome born in 1973–1980 and 1995–1998. *Acta Paediatrica*, *93*, 106–112.

Friedman, J. M. (2001). Racial disparities in median age at death of persons with Down syndrome—United States, 1968–1997. *Morbidity and Mortality Weekly Report*, *50*, 463–465.

Garland, A. F., Lau, A. S., Yeh, M., McCabe, K. M., Hough, R. L., & Landsverk, J. A. (2005). Racial and ethnic differences in utilization of mental health services among high-risk youths. *American Journal of Psychiatry*, *162*, 1336–1343.

Github. (2010). *Github social coding* Retrieved from http://github.com/

Goldman, S. E., Urbano, R. C., & Hodapp, R. M. (2010). *Determining the amount, timing, and causes of mortality among infants with Down syndrome*. Manuscript submitted for publication.

Hodapp, R. M., & Urbano, R. C. (2008). Demographics of African-American and European-American mothers of newborns with Down syndrome. *Journal of Policy and Practice in Intellectual Disabilities*, *5*, 187–193.

Hodapp, R. M., & Urbano, R. C. (2009). Using large-scale databases to examine families of children with intellectual and developmental disabilities. *International Review of Research in Mental Retardation*, *37*, 131–177.
Hodapp, R. M., Urbano, R. C., & Rosenbloom, S. T. (2010). *Down syndrome and adverse birth outcomes: Findings from a population-based study*. Manuscript submitted for publication.
Idler, E. L., & Benjamini, Y. (1997). Self-rated health and mortality: A review of twenty-seven community studies. *Journal of health and social behavior*, *38*, 21–37.
Jurczyk, P., Xiong, L., Cragan, J. D., & Correa, A. (2008). Fine-grained record integration and linkage tool. *Birth Defects Research. Part A. Clinical and Molecular Teratology*, *82*, 822–829.
Krahn, G. L., Hammond, L., & Turner, A. (2006). A cascade of disparities: Health and health care access for people with intellectual disabilities. *Mental Retardation and Developmental Disabilities Research Reviews*, *12*, 70–82.
Lach, L. M., Kohen, D. E., Garner, R. E., Brehaut, J. C., Miller, A. R., Klassen, A. F., et al. (2009). The health and psychosocial functioning of caregivers of children with neurodevelopmental disorders. *Disability and Rehabilitation*, *31*, 741–752.
Leonard, S., Bower, C., Patterson, B., & Leonard, H. (2000). Survival of infants born with Down's syndrome: 1980–96. *Paediatric and Perinatal Epidemiology*, *14*, 163–171.
Long, T., & Kavarian, S. (2008). Aging with developmental disabilities: An overview. *Topics in Geriatric Rehabilitation*, *24*, 2–11.
Mastroiacovo, P., Bertollini, R., & Corchia, C. (1992). Survival of children with Down syndrome in Italy. *American Journal of Medical Genetics*, *42*, 208–212.
Minnes, P., & Steiner, K. (2009). Parent views on enhancing the quality of health care for children with fragile X syndrome, autism, or Down syndrome. *Child: Care, health and development*, *35*, 250–256.
Miodrag, N., & Hodapp, R. M. (2010). Chronic stress and health among parents of children with intellectual and developmental disabilities. *Current Opinion in Psychiatry*, *23*(4).
Muggli, E. E., Collins, V. R., & Marraffa, C. (2009). Going down a different road: First support and information needs of families with a baby with Down syndrome. *Medical Journal of Australia*, *190*, 58–61.
Pantaleoni, E. (2010). *Toward a geospatial model that links air pollution to mortality among infants with Down syndrome*. Manuscript submitted for publication.
Penrose, L. S. (1949). The incidence of Mongolism in the general population. *Journal of Mental Science*, *95*, 685–688.
Porter, H., & Tharpe, A. M. (2010). Hearing loss and Down syndrome. *International Review of Research in Mental Retardation*, *39*, 195–220.
Radloff, L. S. (1977). The CES-D Scale: A self-report depression scale for research in the general population. *Applied Psychological Measurement*, *1*, 385–410.
Rasmussen, S. A., Wong, L. Y., Correa, A., Gambrell, D., & Friedman, J. S. (2006). Survival in infants with Down syndrome, metropolitan Atlanta, 1979–1998. *Journal of Pediatrics*, *148*, 806–812.
Ritz, B., Wilhelm, M., & Zhao, Y. (2006). Air pollution and infant death in southern California, 1989–2000. *Pediatrics*, *118*, 493–502.
Roizen, N. J. (2003). The early interventionist and the medical problems of the child with Down syndrome. *Infants and Young Children*, *16*, 89–95.
Sadetzki, S., Chetrit, A., Akstein, E., Luxenburg, O., Keinan, L., Litvak, I., et al. (1999). Risk factors for infant mortality in Down's syndrome: A nationwide study. *Pediatric and Perinatal Epidemiology*, *13*, 442–451.
Schieve, L. A., Boulet, S. L., Boyle, C., Rasmussen, S. A., & Schendel, D. (2009). Health of children 3 to 17 years of age with Down syndrome in the 1997–2005 National Health Interview Survey. *Pediatrics*, *123*, e253–e260.

Schuster, M. A., Duan, N., Regalado, M., & Klein, D. J. (2000). Anticipatory guidance: What information do parents receive? What information do they want? *Archives of Pediatrics and Adolescent Medicine, 154,* 1191–1198.

Shin, M., Kucik, J., & Correa, A. (2007). Causes of death and case fatality rates among infants with Down syndrome in metropolitan Atlanta. *Birth Defects Research. Part A. Clinical and Molecular Teratology, 79,* 775–780.

Shott, S. R., Joseph, A., & Heithaus, D. (2001). Hearing loss in children with Down syndrome. *International Journal of Pediatric Otorhinolaryngology, 61,* 199–205.

So, S. A., Urbano, R. C., & Hodapp, R. M. (2007). Hospitalizations of infants and young children with Down syndrome: Evidence from inpatient person-records from a statewide administrative database. *Journal of Intellectual Disability Research, 51,* 1030–1038.

Solomon, M., Pistrang, N., & Barker, C. (2001). The benefits of mutual support groups for parents of children with disabilities. *American Journal of Community Psychology, 29,* 113–132.

Special Olympics (2005). *Changing attitudes, changing the world: The health and health care of people with intellectual disabilities.* Washington, DC: Special Olympics.

State of Tennessee, Department of Health, Community Services Division, Community Services Section (2005). *Tennessee Health Access Plan, Update.* Nashville, TN: Author.

Thompson, R., & May, M. A. (2006). Caregivers' perceptions of child mental health needs and service utilization: An urban 8-year old sample. *Journal of Behavioral Health Sciences and Research, 33,* 474–482.

Tu, S., Mason, C. A., & Song, Q. (2007). Second-order linkage and family datasets. *International Review of Research in Mental Retardation, 33,* 53–78.

Urbano, R. C. (2007). Record linkage: A research strategy for developmental epidemiology. *International Review of Research in Mental Retardation, 33,* 27–52.

van Kraayenoord, C. (2008). Environmental pollution, environmental health, and disabilities. *International Journal of Disability, Development and Education, 55,* 1–4.

Van Riper, M., & Cohen, W. I. (2001). Caring for children with Down syndrome and their families. *Journal of Pediatric Health Care, 15,* 123–131.

van Trotsenburg, A. S. P., Heymans, H. S. A., Tijssen, J. G. P., de Vijlder, J. J. M., & Vulsma, T. (2006). Comorbidity, hospitalization, and medication use and their influence on mental and motor development of young infants with Down syndrome. *Pediatrics, 118,* 1633–1639.

Weinhold, B. (2009). Environmental factors in birth defects: What we need to know. *Environmental Health Perspectives, 117*(Oct), A442–A447.

Weijerman, M. E., Van Furth, A. M., Noordegraaf, A. V., Van Wouwe, J. P., Broers, C. J., & Gemke, R. J. (2008). Prevalence, neonatal characteristics, and first-year mortality of Down syndrome: A national study. *Journal of Pediatrics, 152,* 15–19.

Yang, Q., Rasmussen, S. A., & Friedman, J. M. (2002). Mortality associated with Down's syndrome in the USA from 1983 to 1997: A population-based study. *Lancet, 359,* 1019–1025.

Young, R., & Boltri, J. (2005). How do family physicians provide anticipatory guidance during well-child visits? *Journal of the American Board of Family Medicine, 18,* 440–444.

CHAPTER THREE

Overview of Health Issues in School-aged Children with Down Syndrome

Kelly Thomas,[*,†] Sonya Girdler,[*] Jenny Bourke,[†] Aditya Deshpande,[†] Katherine Bathgate,[†] Stephanie Fehr,[†] *and* Helen Leonard[†]

Contents

Abstract

Background: School-aged children with Down syndrome experience an array of medical conditions and health care problems. Although there have been vast improvements in the medical management of these conditions, they still significantly impact on quality of life for families and children with Down syndrome. However, despite the magnitude of this

[*] Department of Occupational Therapy, School of Exercise, Biomedical and Health Sciences, Edith Cowan University, Perth, Western Australia
[†] Telethon Institute for Child Health Research, Centre for Child Health Research, The University of Western Australia, Perth, Western Australia

International Review of Research in Mental Retardation, Volume 39
ISSN 0074-7750, DOI 10.1016/S0074-7750(10)39003-3

problem limited literature has described the overall health status of children with Down syndrome.
Aim: The purpose of this review was to describe the medical conditions commonly experienced by school-aged children with Down syndrome and to consider the clinical implications of this knowledge.
Methods: Electronic searches of Medline, CINAHL, and PsychINFO and manual searches of reference lists identified relevant articles from 1990 to 2009. Studies were included if the topic involved one or more medical comorbidity and participants were children aged 18 years or younger with a diagnosis of Down syndrome. Articles were excluded at the title or abstract level if they were not peer-reviewed, in a language other than English, or did not meet the inclusion criteria. A narrative review of this research was possible.
Results: Common medical conditions experienced by school-aged children with Down syndrome include: heart disease; respiratory problems; gastrointestinal disorders; obesity; ophthalmological, ear, and hearing problems; musculoskeletal problems; leukemia and thyroid conditions; frequent infections; and dental disease. Prevalence estimates for these conditions varied depending on the diagnostic criteria or study methodologies.

1. Introduction

Down syndrome is a chromosomal birth disorder and the single most common cause of intellectual disability in Western Australia (Bower, Leonard, & Petterson, 2000). The worldwide prevalence of Down syndrome varies and may be determined by accessibility to prenatal screening (Weijerman et al., 2008), socio-cultural attitudes, religious beliefs, and political legislation regarding termination of pregnancy (Bittles, Bower, Hussain, & Glasson, 2006). Surveillance of congenital anomalies through population-based registries in Europe (Eurocat, 2010) reports birth prevalences of Down syndrome varying from 4.57 in the Czech Republic to 22.67 per 10,000 livebirths in Southern Ireland for the period 2004–2008 (Table 3.1). Total birth prevalence, including livebirths, terminations, fetal deaths/stillbirths over 20 weeks also varies from 12.86 in the Ukraine to 41.4 per 10,000 births in Paris, France. A review of prevalence of Down syndrome livebirths in the published literature representing birth years from 1967 to 2003 is shown in Table 3.2. The prevalence varies from a low of 2.18/10,000 livebirths in Taiwan (1993–2001) to a high of 17.2/10,000 livebirths in Ireland (1980–1989). Although there is ethnic variation, no clear temporal trends were evident from these data over these time periods.

In Western Australia, since 1980 the number of children born with Down syndrome has remained relatively stable at approximately 1 per 1000 births; however, the overall cases of Down syndrome conceptions (livebirths, stillbirths, and terminations of pregnancy) has more than doubled, from 1.2 per 1000 conceptions in 1980–84 to 2.6 per 1000 in 2006 (Bower,

Table 3.1 Down syndrome (per 10,000 births) for selected EUROCAT registries from 2004 to 2008

Registry	Year range	Live births		All cases (live births, stillbirths/ fetal deaths and terminations)	
		N	Rate per 10,000 births	*N*	Rate per 10,000 births
Dublin (Ireland)	2004–2008	277	22.67	303	24.68
Norway	2004–2006	231	13.29	341	19.46
Wessex (UK)	2004–2008	173	12.38	397	28.29
Sweden	2007–2008	254	12.31	569	27.49
Northern England (UK)	2004–2008	198	12.26	373	22.98
Ukraine	2005–2008	131	11.52	147	12.86
Wales (UK)	2004–2008	185	10.97	378	22.3
Thames Valley (UK)	2004–2008	134	10.92	320	25.94
East Midlands & South Yorkshire (UK)	2004–2008	328	9.40	638	18.19
Paris (France)	2004–2008	101	7.65	553	41.40
Czech Republic	2004–2007	192	4.57	830	19.69

Source: EUROCAT Website Database: http://www.eurocat-network.eu (data uploaded 14/04/2010)

Table 3.2 Birth prevalence of Down syndrome-literature published between 1979 and 2008

References	Country, birth years	Method of case ascertainment	Prevalence per 10,000 live births	95% CI
(Weijerman et al., 2008)	Netherlands, 2003	Dutch Pediatric Surveillance Unit and National Dutch Neonatal and Obstetric registries and capture–recapture	16.0	14.37–17.93[a]
(Egan et al., 2004)	USA, 2001	National Centre for Health Statistics	4.5	4.27–4.68[a]
(Reimand et al., 2006)	Estonia, 1999–2003	Population-based	11.7	10.24–13.24[a]
(Besser et al., 2007)	Metro Atlanta, 1999–2003	Metropolitan Atlanta Congenital Defects Program	11.6	N/A
(Canfield et al., 2006)	USA, 1999–2001	National Birth Defects Prevention Network – Varies from state to state	12.4[a]	12.10–12.66[a]
(Hei-Jen et al., 2005)	Taiwan, 1993–2001	National Birth Defects Registration and Notification system	2.18	1.94–24.49[a]
(Lai, 2002)	Singapore, 1993–1998	National Birth Defects Registry	10.24	9.11–11.48[a]
(Siffel, Correa, Cragan, & Alverson, 2004)	Atlanta and Georgia USA, 1990–1999	Metropolitan Atlanta Congenital Defects Program	9.44*	8.52–10.42[a]

(Morris, Mutton, & Alberman, 2002)	UK, 1990–1998	National Down Syndrome Cytogenetic Register & reports from cytogenetics laboratories	9.5	9.27–9.76[a]
(Huang, 1998)	UK, 1990–1997	National Down Syndrome Cytogenetic Register	9.9	9.65–10.18[a]
(Wortelboer et al., 2000)	Netherlands, 1989–1996	Northern Netherlands (EUROCAT) and cytogenetics laboratories	11.5	9.94–13.15[a]
(Bishop, 1997)	California USA, 1989–1991	California Birth Defects Monitoring Program & California Health Services Genetic Disease Branch	11.3	10.64–12.06[a]
(Freeman et al., 1998)	Atlanta USA, 1989–1995	Metropolitan Atlanta Congenital Defects Program	9.60	8.46–10.92[a]
(Bell, Rankin, & Donaldson, 2003)	Northern England, 1985–1999	Northern Congenital Abnormality Survey	10.3	9.48–11.18[a]
(Olsen, Cross, Gensburg, & Hughes, 1996)	New York State USA, 1983–1992	New York State Congenital Malformations Registry	10.4	N/A
(Centre for Disease Control, 1994)	17 states USA, 1983–1990	Population-based birth defects registers	9.2	9.0–9.41[a]
(S. Leonard, Bower, Petterson, & Leonard, 2000)	Western Australia, 1980–1996	Western Australian Birth Defects Registry	11.1	0.99–1.16
(Binkert, 2002)	Eastern Switzerland 1980–1996	Cytogenetics labs	10.0	N/A

(*Continued*)

Table 3.2 (*Continued*)

References	Country, birth years	Method of case ascertainment	Prevalence per 10,000 live births	95% CI
(Hayes et al., 1997)	EHB Ireland, 1980–1989	Dublin Eurocat Registry	17.2	15.56–19.02[a]
(Stoll, Alembik, Dott, & Roth, 1998)	Strasbourg France, 1979–1987	North Eastern France Birth Defects Register & 11 maternity hospitals	9.6*	7.95–11.58[a]
(Mikkelsen, Fischer, Hansen, Pilgaard, & Nielsen, 1983)	Denmark, 1979–1980	Danish Cytogenetic Central Register	8.6	6.97–10.42[a]
(Wilson, Chan, & Herbert, 1992)	University of Southern California Medical Center, 1974–1988	Genetics division at medical centre–predominantly Latino	16	14.34–17.74[a]
(Frid, Anneren, Rasmussen, Sundelin, & Drott, 2002)	Northern Sweden, 1973–1980	Swedish Register of Congenital Malformations, Cytogenetic register, Medical Birth Register	11.9	10.39–13.56[a]
(Fryers, & Mackay, 1979)	Salford C.B UK, 1961–1975	Salford Mental Handicap Register	12.1	N/A

*Denominator includes stillbirths and/or spontaneous fetal deaths.
[a] Calculated using information provided in the paper.

Callaghan, Cosgrove, & Quick, 2007). This change in the epidemiology of Down syndrome has been largely the result of increasing maternal age (Melve et al., 2008) and the widespread utilization of early prenatal screening (Besser, Shin, Kucik, & Correa, 2007).

It is well documented that Down syndrome is strongly correlated with maternal age (Sherman, Allen, Bean, & Freeman, 2007). Due to the changing roles of women in westernized societies, major socio-demographic shifts have resulted in increasing maternal age. Within the Australian context, women's participation in the workforce has increased from 40% in 1979 to 55% in 2006 (Australian Bureau Statistics, 2006, 2009) and their educational attainment is now similar to that of men (Australian Bureau Statistics, 2007). As a result, the postponement of childbirth has contributed to the overall increase in Down syndrome conceptions (Bower et al., 2007).

The large increase in the reporting of Down syndrome conceptions is attributed to the accessibility and utilization of antenatal screening programs. In Australia, since 1999, the rate of women's participation in antenatal screening programs has increased 2.5-fold to 44% (O'Leary, Breheny, Reid, Charles, & Emery, 2006) and the proportion of Down syndrome cases diagnosed prenatally for women under 35 has increased from 3 to 60% (Collins, Muggli, Riley, Palma, & Halliday, 2008). As a result, fetuses which would usually have spontaneously miscarried, are now being detected, contributing to an increase in the reporting of Down syndrome conceptions (Collins et al., 2008; Leonard, 2005). However, a corresponding increase in terminations of Down syndrome pregnancies has resulted in a relatively stable prevalence of Down syndrome livebirths (Bittles & Glasson, 2004). Rates of terminations are however influenced by countries' differing legislation regarding termination of pregnancy and their societies' socio-cultural beliefs (Bittles et al., 2006).

Developed countries have seen dramatic improvements in infant survival and overall life expectancy for people with Down syndrome. In Australia over the past 40 years, the average life expectancy of people with Down syndrome has increased from 18 to 60 years of age (Bittles & Glasson, 2004). Of particular significance is the improvement in infant survival whereby 91% of infants are expected to survive to 1 year and 85% to 10 years (Leonard, Bower, Petterson, & Leonard, 2000). These rates are comparable to other developed countries (Rasmussen, Wong, Correa, Gambrell, & Friedman, 2006; Viola & Rosano, 2005). Internationally, there are ethnic disparities with a seven-fold increase in the risk of infant mortality shown to be associated with black maternal race in the US, but only among infants without cardiac defects (Rasmussen et al., 2006). Within Australia, survival of Aboriginal children with Down syndrome is also significantly reduced compared to non-Aboriginal children (Leonard et al., 2000).

Several factors have contributed to improvements in the survival rates for children with Down syndrome. The most important of these has been surgical advances in the management of congenital heart disease (Viola & Rosano, 2005). In addition, improved accessibility to antibiotics and vaccinations have contributed to a decline in morbidity and improved life expectancy of people with Down syndrome (Bittles & Glasson, 2004). Changes in community and health professionals' attitudes have also influenced health care accessibility and survival (Bittles & Glasson, 2004), whereby people with Down syndrome are now afforded a higher degree of equality in the health care system (Savulescu, 2001). Ethical debates still persist in relation to implementing policies of equality when accounting for limited resources (Savulescu, 2001). However, arguments for equality of access are supported by research which suggests that denying access of children with Down syndrome to surgical interventions such as cardiac surgery does not improve the efficiency of scarce health resources (Roussot, Lawrenson, Hewitson, Smart, & de Decker, 2006).

School-aged children with Down syndrome experience an array of medical conditions and health care problems. A summary of published prevalences of individual medical conditions in Down syndrome is presented in Table 3.3, showing, for example, a variation in the prevalence of congenital heart defects from 44 to 56% (46% in WA) and in hearing loss from 31 to 50% (10.5% in WA). Although there have been vast improvements in the medical management of these conditions leading to increased rates of infant and child survival (Leonard, 2005), these comorbidities still impact on quality of life for families and children. However, despite the magnitude of this problem only limited literature is available describing the overall health status of children with Down syndrome. Therefore, the objective of this narrative literature review is to describe the medical conditions commonly experienced by school-aged children with Down syndrome and to consider the clinical implications of this knowledge.

2. Methods

Databases Medline, CINAHL, and PsychINFO were electronically searched from 1990 to 2009 to identify relevant peer-reviewed English publications. Sample characteristics were restricted to those where the majority of subjects were children younger than 18 years. The main search terms were: Down syndrome, medical conditions, cardiac, gastrointestinal, respiratory, ophthalmic, ear, hearing, thyroid, diabetes, musculoskeletal, cancer and leukemia, and dental and oral health. These terms were truncated and exploded to include relevant disorders and terminology under these headings and adjusted to match the specific database being searched.

Table 3.3 Prevalence of individual medical conditions in Down syndrome

Medical Condition	Author, publication year	Prevalence of medical conditions (%)	Source of case ascertainment	Prevalence (%) of medical condition in WA [95% CI] (Leonard S. et al., 1999 and unpublished data)
Congenital heart defects	(Freeman et al., 2008; Freeman et al., 1998; Frid, Anneren, Rasmussen, Sundelin, & Drott, 2002; Halliday, Collins, Riley, Youssef, & Muggli, 2009; Nisli et al., 2008; So, Urbano, & Hodapp, 2007; Torfs, & Christianson, 1998; Yam, 2008)	44–56	Population-based; Tertiary/pediatric clinics	46% [26.42–39.48]
Gastrointestinal Disorders				
Congenital gastrointestinal defects	(Freeman et al., 2009; Frid, Anneren, Rasmussen, Sundelin, & Drott, 2002; Torfs, & Christianson, 1998)	6.7–10.9	Population-based; active surveillance registers	2.84% [1.05–6.09]

(*Continued*)

Table 3.3 (*Continued*)

Medical Condition	Author, publication year	Prevalence of medical conditions (%)	Source of case ascertainment	Prevalence (%) of medical condition in WA [95% CI] (Leonard S. et al., 1999 and unpublished data)
Celiac Disease	(Bonamico et al., 2001; Book et al., 2001a; Carlsson et al., 1998; Mackey et al., 2001; Zachor, Mroczek-Musulman, & Brown, 2000, Uibo et al., 2006)	4.6–13	Clinic case series	0.95% [0.11–3.38]
Constipation	N/A	-	-	18.4% [13.07–23.87]
Obesity	(Grammatikopoulou et al., 2008; Luke, Sutton, Schoeller, & Roizen, 1996)	50^{a}–67.6^{b}	Hospital/School and Down Syndrome Association	36.7% with BMI z-scores > 1 standard deviation above the mean for age in general population; 14.4% with BMI z-scores > 2 standard deviations
Ophthalmological Problems				
Refractive errors	(Fimiani et al., 2007)	96	Clinic-based	43.60% [36.81–50.57]
Strabismus	(Fimiani et al., 2007; Stephen, Dickson, Kindley, Scott, & Charleton, 2007)	36–47	Clinic-based	27.01% [21.14–33.53]

Nystagmus	(Stephen, Dickson, Kindley, Scott, & Charleton, 2007)	16	Hospital-based	2.84% [1.05–6.09]
Lens opacities/ cataracts	(Fimiani et al., 2007; Stephen, Dickson, Kindley, Scott, & Charleton, 2007)	7.8–11	Hospital-based; Clinic-based	3.32% [1.34–6.71]
Ear and Hearing Problems				
Hearing Loss	(Marder, & Dennis, 2001; Yam, 2008)	31–50	Pediatric departments	10.5% [6.65–15.36]
Glue Ear	N/A			47.6% [40.5–54.36]
Musculoskeletal Problems				
Atlantoaxial instability	(Yam, 2008)	5	Pediatric departments	0.95% [0.11–3.38]
Thyroid Disease	(Yam, 2008)	24	Pediatric departments	13.9% [9.40–19.14]
Hyperthyroidism	N/A	–	–	2.37% [0.77–5.44]
Hypothyroidism	(Gibson et al., 2005; Unachak et al., 2008)	2.8–37.9	Longitudinal Clinic	9.0% [5.51–13.70]
Type 1 Diabetes	(Anwar, Walker, & Frier, 1998; Bergholdt, Eising, Nerup, & Pociot, 2006)	0.7;1.4–10.6	Registers; clinical study estimate	0.95% [0.11–3.38]
Leukemia				1.42% [0.29–4.10]

[a] Weight-to-height ratio greater then 1.2.
[b] z-scores used.

Reference lists of retrieved relevant studies were manually searched but conference proceedings were not. Articles were included if they focused on children aged 18 years or younger with a diagnosis of Down syndrome, and one or more medical comorbidities. Articles were excluded at the title or abstract level if they did not meet the inclusion criteria.

The intention of this review was to provide an overview of the most current and relevant literature on health issues in school-age children but no formal quality appraisal or meta-analysis was undertaken (Mallen, Peat, & Croft, 2006).

3. Results

It is well known that Down syndrome is associated with a variety of birth defects primarily affecting not only the cardiac and gastrointestinal systems but also other systems (Freeman et al., 2009) and that children affected with this disorder may experience a number of medical comorbidities and health-related problems (Leonard, Bower, Petterson, & Leonard, 1999). Medical conditions commonly associated with Down syndrome include cardiac and respiratory disorders, musculoskeletal problems, eye and visual defects, ear and hearing defects, leukemia, thyroid conditions, and frequent episodic illnesses and infections (Leonard et al., 1999). A population-based study of children with Down syndrome born between 1980 and 1991 undertaken in Western Australia in 1997 (Leonard et al., 1999) identified that nearly one-fifth of children experienced four or more medical conditions, as reported by parents, and in only 5% no problems were reported. Moreover over a quarter of children had experienced an ear infection and over one-tenth pneumonia in the previous year. A follow-up study of this cohort but also including children born since 1991 was undertaken 7 years later in 2004 (Thomas, 2009). Data from these two studies (Leonard et al., 1999; Thomas, 2009) and also from a large Hong Kong study (Yam, 2008) ($n = 407$), which had identified children aged below 18 years from about half of the public hospitals and pediatric clinics in Hong Kong, have been used to illustrate population prevalences for the various comorbidities. Where applicable, data from an early UK study based on the Manchester Down's Syndrome Cohort, and on which the Australian study was partially modeled, have also been included (Turner, Sloper, Cunningham, & Knussen, 1990). Odds ratios of specific disorders occurring in young people with Down syndrome when compared with people without Down syndrome, as calculated in a review of comorbidity in the Down syndrome population (van Schrojenstein Lantman-de Valk, Haveman, & Crebolder, 1996), have been provided where applicable. These have been presented alongside some of the more detailed but smaller and clinic-based studies which have tended to focus on individual conditions or systems rather than on the total morbidity load for a child.

3.1. Heart disease

From population-based monitoring systems in Atlanta (Rasmussen et al., 2006), California (Freeman et al., 1998), and Victoria, Australia (Halliday, Collins, Riley, Youssef, & Muggli, 2009) cardiac defects have been reported to be the most commonly occurring birth defect associated with Down syndrome, with prevalence estimates ranging between 40 and 56% (Table 3.3). Estimates of a cardiac condition in 46% were obtained from parent-reported data in the 2004 Western Australian population study of school-aged children with Down syndrome ($n = 208$) (Thomas, 2009) and in 53% from a Hong Kong study reviewing hospital records of children and teenagers with Down syndrome ($n = 407$)(Yam, 2008). This high incidence of congenital heart defects resulted in the American Academy of Pediatrics recommending a cardiology evaluation and echocardiogram for all newborns with Down syndrome (American Academy of Pediatrics, 2001). The most frequently occurring congenital heart defects include atrioventricular septal defect (AVSD), atrial septal defect (ASD), ventricular septal defect (VSD), tetralogy of Fallot (Freeman et al., 2008), and patent ductus arteriosus (PDA) (Nisli et al., 2008), with nearly a quarter of children experiencing multiple defects (Nisli et al., 2008). The National Down Syndrome Project (NDSP), a six-site population-based study representing approximately 11% of all US births, is to date the largest population-based study of Down syndrome (Freeman et al., 2007). Recent research conducted using the NDSP as the source of cases ($n = 1469$) has suggested that there are significant sex and ethnic differences in the prevalence of AVSD in Down syndrome (Freeman et al., 2008). Infant females were twice as likely to be born with AVSD, and black babies and Hispanics experienced twice and one-half the risk of whites, respectively.

Congenital cardiac defects have been a major cause of mortality for children with Down syndrome (Viola & Rosano, 2005; Weijerman et al., 2008) but, for most, successful surgical correction has now been available for some time. However even with these surgical advances, which have resulted in significant improvements in survival and quality of life, congenital heart disease was still a major predictor of mortality in research studies carried out a decade ago in Australia (Leonard et al., 2000) and Sweden (Frid, Drott, Lundell, Rasmussen, & Anneren, 1999). However, more recent research conducted using the same population-based Western Australian source (Thomas, 2009) has found that although parents in 2004 were reporting that slightly more of their children had experienced a heart condition, they were reporting a much lower prevalence of ongoing problems for children born with a cardiac defect than they had done in

1997 (OR 0.32, 95% CI 0.15–0.68). In a population-based study undertaken on a Swedish cohort of children born between 1973 and 1980 and followed for at least 17 years health utilization as measured by hospitalizations was much greater in those with congenital heart disease (Frid, Anneren, Rasmussen, Sundelin, & Drott, 2002). The difference in health utilization was greatest in the first 3 years of life at the time during which cardiac surgery was being performed. However, overall these children were still much more likely than those without congenital heart disease to be admitted for infections. It would be important to repeat such a study on a more recent cohort of children who have had early aggressive surgical treatment for their congenital heart disease. One would predict that such a disparity would now be much less apparent as demonstrated by our Western Australian parent reported data (Thomas, 2009) and by recent data from a population-based study undertaken using record linkage in Victoria, Australia (Halliday et al., 2009). The latter indicated that variation in survival according to the presence of comorbidities was much less evident in a recent 1998–2000 cohort than in an earlier 1988–1990 cohort.

Whilst recognizing the major health benefits that have resulted from early surgical treatment of congenital heart disease it is important to be mindful that adolescents with no known intracardiac disease can still develop mitral valve prolapse and aortic regurgitation (Geggel, O'Brien, & Feingold, 1993). It is also important to reinforce the need for prophylaxis against subacute bacterial endocarditis in those with cardiac or valvular disease (Marder & Dennis, 2001).

3.2. Respiratory problems

Respiratory conditions including pneumonia, bronchitis, and obstructive sleep apnoea are considered a major cause of morbidity among children with Down syndrome. Pneumonia and other respiratory infections were also reported to account for one-third (49/148) of deaths in children under 18 years registered with a state disability service between 1953 and 2000 (Bittles et al., 2006). By asking mothers to report the number of episodes of ill-health in the previous 12 months and by comparison with data from the national Child Development Study, Turner and colleagues were able to support earlier evidence suggesting that the prevalence of respiratory infections was increased in children with Down syndrome (Turner et al., 1990). In a Dutch study investigating the hospitalizations and comorbidity of 196 infants with Down syndrome, respiratory infections were also reported to be the leading cause of hospital admissions beyond the neonatal period and up to 2 years of age, especially for those with congenital heart disease (van Trotsenburg, Heymans, Tijssen, de Vijlder, & Vulsma, 2006). In the early UK study children with current heart problems were also more likely to have suffered from bronchitis or pneumonia during their life (Turner et al., 1990).

A chart review identified 232 admissions of children with Down syndrome to an Australian children's hospital between 1991 and 1998 (Hilton, Fitzgerald, & Cooper, 1999). These admissions related to 86 children and respiratory pathology accounted for over half the admissions. It was determined from the study that the median length of stay and associated costs for these children were two to three times that of a patient without Down syndrome. The presence of congenital heart disease was again associated with longer length of stay and greater severity of illness (Hilton et al., 1999).

Following retrospective evaluation of flexible bronchoscopies of 24 children with Down syndrome with significant respiratory morbidity Bertrand and colleagues (Bertrand, Navarro, Caussade, Holmgren, & Sanchez, 2003) found that, compared to controls, children with Down syndrome had a higher prevalence of airway anomalies. In Down syndrome obstructive sleep apnoea, complete or partial upper-airway obstruction during sleep, may be related to the midface hypoplasia, large adenoids or tonsils, narrow nasopharynx and eustachian tubes, systemic hypotonia (Van Cleve & Cohen, 2006), and inner ear dysplasia (Blaser et al., 2006). Using polysomnography obstructive sleep apnoea was identified in approximately 60% of children with Down syndrome in two clinic-based studies involving 22 (Ng et al., 2006) and 65 (Shott et al., 2006) children. Recurrent upper respiratory infections coupled with adenotonsillar hypertrophy or obesity, conditions also commonly reported in children with Down syndrome, may exacerbate obstructive sleep apnoea further (Schechter, 2002).

Although high prevalences of obstructive sleep apnoea have been reported from two small clinic-based studies (Ng et al., 2006; Shott et al., 2006), much lower prevalences of 7% (Yam, 2008) and 19.8% (Thomas, 2009) have been reported from the population-based studies conducted in Hong Kong and Western Australia. Shott and co-authors (Shott et al., 2006) believe that parents may substantially underestimate the prevalence and severity of obstructive sleep apnoea assuming that irregular breathing during sleep is normal for children with Down syndrome. However, in an Australian study of 33 children with Down syndrome referred to a sleep clinic between 1997 and 2004 because of snoring (Fitzgerald, Paul, & Richmond, 2007) it was reported that all but one were found to have had moderate to severe obstructive sleep apnoea as measured by overnight polysomnography. This extremely high prevalence led Fitzgerald and colleagues to recommend, based on this small non-population-based study, that all children with Down syndrome who snore should be routinely investigated with polysomnography (Fitzgerald et al., 2007). As obstructive sleep apnoea may be associated with complications of general anaesthesia (Mitchell, Call, & Kelly, 2003) and learning (Schechter, 2002) and behavior problems (Melendres, Lutz, Rubin, & Marcus, 2004) in the general population, parents of children with Down syndrome need to be informed about the possibility of sleep apnoea and its associated implications. However, current guidelines would recommend referral to an ENT or sleep specialist rather than the need for every child to have polysomnography (Marder & Dennis, 2001; Van Cleve & Cohen, 2006).

3.3. Gastrointestinal disorders

Children with Down syndrome experience a higher prevalence of gastrointestinal disorders than their peers (Cleves et al., 2007; Schieve, Boulet, Boyle, Rasmussen, & Schendel, 2009). In a large ethnically diverse population-based study conducted from Atlanta, USA using the National Down Syndrome project, the prevalence of congenital gastrointestinal defects in liveborn infants with Down syndrome born between 1989 and 2004 was 6.7% (Freeman et al., 2009)(Table 3.3). The highest rate was for duodenal stenosis/atresia (3.9%) and lower for other defects (anal stenosis/atresia 1.0%, Hirschsprungs 0.8%, esophageal atresia/tracheoesophageal fistula 0.4%, and pyloric stenosis 0.3%). In an earlier study (Keckler, St Peter, Spilde, Ostlie, & Snyder, 2008) but not in this study (Freeman et al., 2009) duodenal atresia and Hirschsprung's disease commonly co-occurred with congenital heart defects. Other common gastrointestinal disorders include gastro-oesophageal reflux (Marder & Dennis, 2001) and celiac disease (Roizen & Patterson, 2003; Van Cleve, Cannon, & Cohen, 2006). Constipation, although not a serious condition, is relatively common occurring in 18.4% of Western Australian school-aged children with Down syndrome (Leonard et al., 1999) (Table 3.3) and often involves prolonged management, placing increased demands on family and carers (Leonard et al., 1999).

The prevalence of celiac disease (including results of screening) in children with Down syndrome has been widely reported in the literature (Bonamico et al., 2001; Book et al., 2001b; Carlsson et al., 1998; Mackey et al., 2001; Uibo et al., 2006; Zachor, Mroczek-Musulman, & Brown, 2000) and appears to be more common than in the general population with prevalences varying from 4.6 to 13% (Table 3.3) compared with approximately 1% in the general population (Maki et al., 2003). On the other hand in the Western Australian population-based study of children with Down syndrome the prevalence was only 1% (Leonard et al., 1999). This variation may be due to the fact that in contrast to the population-based Western Australian survey, most other studies have been much smaller and clinic-based and have involved intensive investigation of their series of patients. Many of the symptoms associated with celiac disease are similar to those common in Down syndrome itself. Some authors (Book et al., 2001a) have recommended that children with Down syndrome should be screened for celiac disease to prevent unnecessary episodes of diarrhoea, constipation or vomiting caused by avoidable ingestion of gluten. At present there are no uniform recommendations for such screening in the Down syndrome population (Cohen, 2006) and screening for celiac disease is not specifically considered in the guidelines for health supervision for children with Down syndrome published by the American Academy of Pediatrics (American Academy of Pediatrics, 2001) or by those recommended in the UK (Marder & Dennis, 2001) or Ireland (Murphy et al., 2005) whilst screening has been recommended in other published clinical guideline resources (Bosch, 2003; Van Cleve et al., 2006). The Down Syndrome Medical Interest Group US recommends an initial screen at age 2 years with IgA tTG and total IgA. In IgA-deficient children IgG AGA should then be measured (Cohen, 2006). It was also mentioned that clinicians should maintain a high index of suspicion when children with Down syndrome present with mild abdominal symptoms, growth failure, anemia, or constipation (Cohen, 2006). On the other hand Swigonski and colleagues comment that although in the general population the ratio between symptomatic and silent forms of celiac disease is 1:8 it is apparently reversed in the Down syndrome population with a ratio of 4:1(Swigonski, Kuhlenschmidt, Bull, Corkins, & Downs, 2006). Using decision analysis they calculated that from the perspective of preventing mortality from non-Hodgkins lymphoma, the most serious complication of celiac disease, it was not cost-effective to screen asymptomatic children with Down syndrome for celiac disease (Swigonski et al., 2006). A further issue however is whether treating celiac disease at an asymptomatic stage does or does not have benefits for other outcomes such as, for instance, growth failure (Kawatu & LeLeiko, 2006). Research of this nature is critically needed but must include evaluation of the burdens both associated with the screening process itself and any further associated invasive procedures as well as with the stringent treatment schedule associated with maintaining a gluten-free diet (Swigonski et al., 2006).

In contrast to the considerable literature relating to celiac disease (Book et al., 2001a; Mackey et al., 2001; Uibo et al., 2006; Zachor et al., 2000), research on the morbidity and long-term effects of congenital gastrointestinal defects is much sparser with few studies following affected children into childhood, further to their having had corrective bowel surgery. The exception is Hirschsprung's disease which was shown to be associated with ongoing incontinence and soiling in a case study of ten patients with Down syndrome surgically treated at an Australian children's hospital between 1974 and 2001 (Catto-Smith, Trajanovska, & Taylor, 2006). In two other studies involving 9 (Hackam et al., 2003; Morabito, Lall, Gull, Mohee, & Bianchi, 2006) and 17 children with Down syndrome, outcomes were similar to those without Down syndrome. In our recent (2004) population-based Western Australian study ($n = 208$) (Thomas, 2009) nearly one-third of parents (31.7%) reported that their chid had had a bowel problem in 2004 and the likelihood was greater than in 1997

(OR 1.69, 95% CI 1.14–2.51). This inflation may relate to better survival of children with gastrointestinal defects. In contrast the prevalence of gastrointestinal problems reported in the clinical record-based Hong Kong study was lower (11%). It is likely that reporting was weighted towards gastrointestinal disorders involving structural defects. Celiac disease was not mentioned as a specific category and it is also probable that constipation was under-reported. However, further population-based research is needed regarding the prevalence and course of congenital and acquired gastrointestinal disorders in school-aged children with Down syndrome.

3.4. Obesity

There is limited research investigating the rate of overweight and obesity in children with Down syndrome, with Australian research focussing only on children with intellectual disability as a whole (De, Small, & Baur, 2008). Other international studies on overweight and obesity in children with Down syndrome have been small ($n=77$) (Ferrara, Capozzi, & Russo, 2008), ($n=34$) (Grammatikopoulou et al., 2008), ($n=20$) (Luke, Sutton, Schoeller, & Roizen, 1996), and ($n=67$) (Magge, O'Neill, Shults, Stallings, & Stettler, 2008). Nevertheless, these studies indicate that children and adolescents with Down syndrome have an increased risk of overweight and obesity and that this risk increases with age (Grammatikopoulou et al., 2008) (Table 3.3).

Two methods have been used to evaluate weight and height in children with Down syndrome. Body mass index (BMI) (Ferrara et al., 2008; Magge et al., 2008; Sharav & Bowman, 1992) and comparison with published growth charts specific (Cronk et al., 1988; Myrelid, Gustafsson, Ollars, & Anneren, 2002; Styles, Cole, Dennis, & Preece, 2002) and non-specific to children with Down syndrome (Grammatikopoulou et al., 2008; Luke et al., 1996) have been used. Additional anthropometric assessments have been conducted to further analyze body composition and reduce the impact of reduced height in children with Down syndrome on BMI and growth chart evaluations. These measurements include waist/hip circumference (Grammatikopoulou et al., 2008; Luke et al., 1996), skinfold thickness (Ferrara et al., 2008; Grammatikopoulou et al., 2008; Luke et al., 1996; Magge et al., 2008), deuterium dilution, bioelectrical impedance (Luke et al., 1996), and dual energy X-ray absorptiometry (Magge et al., 2008).

Factors influencing this increased risk of overweight are biological, environmental, social, and behavioral. In all children parental obesity is a strong risk factor for childhood obesity, particularly obesity of the same-sex parent as the child (Perez-Pastor et al., 2009). Studies comparing BMI between siblings with and without Down syndrome have shown varying results (Magge et al., 2008; Sharav & Bowman, 1992; Whitt-Glover,

O'Neill, & Stettler, 2006) with most showing a higher BMI in siblings with Down syndrome. Ferrara and co-authors (Ferrara et al., 2008) identified a possible genetic link to obesity in children with Down syndrome (allele variability) and Magge and colleagues (Magge et al., 2008) found that leptin levels were higher in children with Down syndrome than in their siblings.

Environmental factors of media exposure and processed food availability as well as the socio-economic status, sedentary behavior, inadequate sleep, dietary habits, and intake of sweetened beverages are all risk factors for childhood overweight and obesity (Crothers, Kehle, Bray, & Theodore, 2009). Specifically for children with Down syndrome, lack of physical activity has been identified as a significant factor (Sharav & Bowman, 1992; Whitt-Glover et al., 2006), whereas dietary evaluation suggests that children with Down syndrome consume less energy than children without Down syndrome (Grammatikopoulou et al., 2008; Luke et al., 1996) although more research is needed in this area due to limited sample size and restrictions in methodology.

The effects of overweight and obesity on health for all children can be significant. If left untreated childhood obesity can have significant mental and physical consequences including cardiovascular, gastrointestinal, endocrine, and musculoskeletal complications (Crothers et al., 2009; Ebbeling, Pawlak, & Ludwig, 2002). Childhood obesity is also a strong risk factor for adult obesity (Field, Cook, & Gillman, 2005), particularly if one or more parents are also obese (Whitaker, Wright, Pepe, Seidl, & Dietz, 1997).

Further research needs to be conducted on the prevalence of overweight and obesity in children with Down syndrome and the determinants behind the statistics. From this, interventions and strategies can be developed to help families prevent and manage overweight and obesity in their children with Down syndrome to reduce the risk of mental and physical complications now and in the future.

3.5. Ophthalmological problems

Ophthalmological problems frequently occur in children with Down syndrome, with one study reporting a prevalence of 100% of ocular abnormalities in a population of Italian children with Down syndrome identified through a family support association ($n = 157$) (Fimiani et al., 2007). Common ophthalmological disorders found in the Italian study included refractive errors (96%), strabismus (36%), nasolacrimal duct obstruction (22%), and lens opacities (11%) (Fimiani et al., 2007) (Table 3.3). In a UK study evaluating guidelines for ophthalmic screening in Down syndrome involving examination of 72 children, 43% had significant refractive errors with 27% having hypermetropia and astigmatism (Stephen, Dickson, Kindley, Scott, & Charleton, 2007). The prevalence of strabismus (47%), nasolacrimal duct obstruction (36%), cataracts (7.8%), and nystagmus (16%)

were also high in this population (Stephen et al., 2007). The high prevalence of refractive errors clearly correlates with the fivefold increased likelihood of children with Down syndrome wearing glasses compared to their typical developing peers as identified in the 1997 Western Australian study (Leonard et al.,1999) (Table 3.3). In this population-based study about three-quarters of parents reported that their children had an eye condition with the prevalence slightly higher in girls than boys. This was similar to the prevalence in the UK study in 1986 where, compared with 1983, it was clear that a larger proportion of vision defects were being identified and managed. In the Hong Kong study the prevalence of visual problems was lower at 48% (Yam, 2008). Strabismus has been reported to occur in one-third to one-half of children with Down syndrome (Fimiani et al., 2007; Haugen & Hovding, 2001; Stephen et al., 2007)(Table 3.3), with one study ($n = 86$) finding a relationship between the prevalence of strabismus and the degree of learning difficulties (Merrick & Koslowe, 2001).

Children with Down syndrome frequently present with poor accommodation shown in one study not to be improved by the wearing of spectacles (Cregg et al., 2001). In contrast a more recent comparative non-randomized intervention study of 34 primary school-aged children found that compared to the prescription of single-vision lenses (to correct refractive error only) bifocal spectacles consistently resulted in more accurate accommodation (Stewart, Margaret Woodhouse, & Trojanowska, 2005). Given that significant underaccommodation results in near vision which is consistently out of focus with the potential for a consequent negative impact on learning (Cregg et al., 2001), children with Down syndrome should be routinely examined for accommodation at near (Stewart et al., 2005).

While emmetropia is positively associated with age in normally developing children (Gordon & Donzis, 1985), children with Down syndrome experience more refractive errors with age (Cregg et al., 2003; Woodhouse, Pakeman, Cregg, & et al., 1997). As visual impairment contributes substantially to secondary disability (Marder & Dennis, 2001) vigilant monitoring of vision is required for all school-aged children with Down syndrome to optimize opportunities for learning and development and to increase quality of life. In the UK, guidelines have been developed by the UK Down Syndrome Medical Interest Group to facilitate such surveillance (Stephen et al., 2007).

3.6. Ear and hearing problems

The prevalence of hearing impairment in children with Down syndrome is high (Maatta, Kaski, Taanila, Keinanen-Kiukaanniemi, & Iivanainen, 2006; Roizen & Patterson, 2003), with as many as 50% (Marder & Dennis, 2001)

(Table 3.3) experiencing a loss from either conductive, sensorineural, or mixed causes (Roizen & Patterson, 2003). While conductive hearing loss occurs frequently in children with Down syndrome due to episodes of otitis media or middle ear dysfunction, sensorineural hearing impairments become increasingly prevalent with age (Driscoll, Kei, Bates, & McPherson, 2003). Further to a small study involving adolescents and young adults with Down syndrome ($n = 26$) and age- and IQ-matched controls Marcell has tentatively suggested that hearing loss may have a more negative impact on cognitive development in young people with Down syndrome than in those with other causes of intellectual disability (Marcell, 1995). It is recommended that children with Down syndrome undergo regular audiological screening for early identification of hearing impairments to remediate and reduce secondary speech problems (Van Cleve & Cohen, 2006).

Anatomical malformations, systemic hypotonia, and an increased susceptibility to infections are all thought to contribute to the high prevalence of otitis media among children with Down syndrome which can lead to glue ear and transient conductive hearing loss (Mitchell et al., 2003). In a recent population-based survey including 146 children with Down syndrome, 604 children with intellectual disability but not Down syndrome, and 96,204 children with neither condition, it was reported that, after adjustment for demographic factors, children with Down syndrome were more than three times more likely to have had an ear infection in the previous year (Schieve et al., 2009). Research using the Western Australian population data source of children with Down syndrome in 2004 ($n = 208$) reported that over half (59.1%) of the children were reported to have had an ear condition, with glue ear occurring the most frequently (in 41.3%) (Thomas, 2009). In the 1997 study, hearing loss had been reported in 10.5% (Leonard et al., 1999) but this had increased to 17.3% in the 2004 study (Thomas, 2009). This is still lower than the prevalence of 31% in Hong Kong (Yam, 2008). In the UK study over half the children had had some hearing loss although this included those in whom the hearing loss was defined as "variable" due to respiratory infections (Turner et al., 1990). The odds ratio for hearing impairment in young people with Down syndrome compared with young people with other types of intellectual disability varied from 2.2 [CI 1.1–4.4] to 18.5 [5.7–64.2] (van Schrojenstein Lantman-de Valk et al., 1996).

Glue ear is commonly treated with insertion of pneumoeustachian tubes (grommets). Two earlier studies undertaken by Selikowitz (Selikowitz, 1993) ($n = 24$) and Lino (Lino, Imamura, Harigai, & Tanaka, 1999) ($n = 28$) reported disappointing results in relation to the efficacy of tympanostomy tube insertion in children with Down syndrome. However, preliminary results at the 1-year follow-up of a 5-year longitudinal study suggested that aggressive evaluation and treatment of chronic otitis media indeed improved the hearing levels in children with Down syndrome

(Shott, Joseph, & Heithaus, 2001). No further follow-up of this study could be identified in the literature. However, a systematic review has since concluded that ventilation tubes are only minimally effective in reversing the hearing loss associated with otitis media with effusion in the general population of children (Lous et al., 2005). As insertion of ventilation tubes in children with Down syndrome was shown to be occurring at a rate 16 times that of the rest of the population in Western Australia (Leonard et al., 1999), further research to guide clinical interventions is clearly needed.

While the role of adenoidectomy in the management of middle ear and sinonasal dysfunction is widely acknowledged in normally developing children over 4 years of age (Casselbrant et al., 2009; Coyte, Croxford, McIsaac, Feldman, & Friedberg, 2001), the efficacy of this intervention has been found to be significantly less than in age- and sex-matched controls in children younger than 16 years with Down syndrome (Price, Orvidas, Weaver, & Farmer, 2004). Since levels of language competence are associated with outcomes such as peer relationship problems in teenagers (Fellinger, Holzinger, Beitel, Launch, & Goldberg, 2009), minimizing the secondary disability associated with hearing problems for children with Down syndrome must be a priority. Clearly more research is also needed in this area.

3.7. Musculoskeletal problems

Children with Down syndrome experience a variety of musculoskeletal disorders (Mik, Gholve, Scher, Widmann, & Green, 2008) due to a predisposition to hypotonia, lax ligaments, and skeletal dysplasias (Marder & Dennis, 2001). Over a third (35.6%) of parents reported that their child had had a musculoskeletal condition in the Western Australian 2004 study (Thomas, 2009) while the prevalence was only 14% in the Hong Kong study (Yam, 2008). However, sourcing from hospital and clinical records (Yam, 2008) may have skewed the identification to the more severe disorders. Commonly occurring musculoskeletal conditions include: patellar instability, metatarsus primus, pes planus (flat foot), scoliosis, and atlantoaxial instability (Mik et al., 2008; Platt, 2001). Minor podiatric anomalies including pes planus, foot pronation, and metatarsus primus, are often overlooked due to a focus on the more severe pathologies associated with Down syndrome (Concolino, Pasquzzi, Capalbo, Sinopoli, & Strisciuglio, 2006). Among children with Down syndrome podiatric anomalies have been associated with subsequent postural alterations (Concolino et al., 2006), which without intervention restricts the gross motor development of these children (Prasher, Robinson, Krishnan, & Chung, 1995). It is recommended that children with Down syndrome receive individual gait analyses to support treatment planning and evaluation (Selby-Silverstein, Hillstrom, & Palisano, 2001). Early identification and treatment of musculoskeletal impairments enables early intervention in biomechanical and postural problems, minimizing resulting disability.

Atlantoaxial instability is thought to occur because of laxity of the transverse ligament which results in instability of the spine at C1–C2 (Ali, Al-Bustan, Al-Busairi, Al-Mulla, & Esbaita, 2006) or in association with hypoplasia or malformations of the odontoid (Platt, 2001). It has been considered to be particularly dangerous due to the potential risk of compression and damage to the spinal cord. This tendency toward instability in the cervical spine is compounded by degenerative changes which increase with age, but occur much earlier in Down syndrome than in the general population (Ali et.al, 2006). In a case review of 12 children with Down syndrome presenting with symptomatic atlantoaxial instability it was concluded that an aggressive surgical approach should be adopted in the management of this condition (Nader-Sepahi, Casey, Hayward, Crockard, & Thompson, 2005).

Although asymptomatic atlantoaxial instability is common in Down syndrome it would not appear to be a significant risk factor for symptomatic atlantoaxial instability which is rare (American Academy of Pediatrics, 2001). Parents of nine children (4.3%) in the Western Australian population-based study reported that their children had been diagnosed with atlantoaxial instability (Thomas, 2009) whilst atlantoaxial subluxation was reported in 5% (Table 3.3) and atlantoaxial dislocation in 1% in the Hong Kong study (Yam, 2008). Historically, the asymptomatic nature of atlantoaxial instability and the potentially catastrophic consequences of spinal cord compression led to recommendations for routine screening and the restriction of certain sporting activities (Marder & Dennis, 2001; Mik et al., 2008). These recommendations have now been revised such that routine screening is mainly indicated for children with Down syndrome who are symptomatic or who participate in contact sports (American Academy of Pediatrics, 2001). However, as concluded by the Committee on Sports Medicine and Fitness, there is a need for higher quality research which examines the combination of symptoms and signs which predicts those who are at the greatest risk of atlantoaxial dislocation (Committee on Sports Medicine and Fitness, 1995).

3.8. Endocrine

Endocrine anomalies, especially thyroid dysfunction (Gibson et al., 2005) and diabetes (Bergholdt, Eising, Nerup, & Pociot, 2006), are reported to be more common among people with Down syndrome than in the general population. Thyroid dysfunction in particular has been widely studied. In 1999 Prasher reviewed the literature and identified over 30 studies measuring the prevalence of thyroid disease in Down syndrome (Prasher, 1999). A couple were confined to neonates and ten were restricted to adults leaving 19 that would have included school-aged children. Case numbers for these studies ranged from 35 to 206 and the majority were cross-sectional or case studies. The end point was an abnormality in T4, T3, or TSH. Estimates varied widely from 0 to 60% and no confidence limits were provided. However, evaluation of the studies suggested a lifetime prevalence of 25–30%. Thyroid disorders have been classified as hypothyroidism, sub-clinical hypothyroidism, and hyperthyroidism (Prasher, 1999). Hypothyroidism can be congenital or acquired and is much more prevalent than hyperthyroidism. Clinical features include tiredness, weight gain, slowing, cold hands, mood change, puffy face, dry brittle hair, dry coarse skin, and constipation some of which are normal features of Down syndrome so that clinical diagnosis can be difficult (Prasher, 1999). However a poor correlation between clinical and biochemical hypothyroidism has been found in adults (Prasher, 1995) and it is likely that these findings can be generalized to children. More recent studies of children and adolescents in the UK (Gibson et al., 2005) and children in Thailand (Unachak et al., 2008) have provided estimates of hypothyroidism varying from approximately 2.8% (Gibson et al., 2005) to 37.9% (Unachak et al., 2008) while in Western Australia (Leonard et al., 1999) 13.9% and in Hong Kong (Yam, 2008) 24% of children were reported to have thyroid problems (Table 3.3). Much of the variation between studies is likely to be due to the operational definition used and whether sub-clinical hypothyroidism is included. In the UK it is estimated that uncompensated hypothyroidism is detected in approximately 10% of school-aged children with Down syndrome (Marder & Dennis, 2001). In a Swedish longitudinal study of children and young adults without congenital hypothyroidism ($n = 85$) who were followed for up to 15 years, 30 developed hypothyroidism and two hyperthyroidism over the study period (Karlsson, Gustafsson, Hedov, Ivarsson, & Anneren, 1998). As the prevalence of hypothyroidism increases with age, and is similar in its presentation to Down syndrome itself, early annual biochemical screening has been previously recommended to identify thyroid disease (American Academy of Pediatrics, 2001). However, some longitudinal studies have demonstrated that sub-clinical hypothyroidism may be transient and likely to resolve spontaneously (Gibson et al., 2005; Prasher & Gomez, 2007) and that screening frequency could thus be reduced. Nevertheless in an elegant population-based record linkage study conducted in Tennessee, USA, rates of medically treated thyroid disease in people with Down syndrome increased 73% after the release of the American Academy of Pediatrics Health Supervision Guidelines (Carroll, Arbogast, Dudley, & Cooper, 2008). This study clearly demonstrates how physician practice can be influenced through the implementation of clinical guidelines.

Diabetes is one condition for which it is recommended that clinicians be vigilant in their patients with Down syndrome (Roizen & Patterson, 2003). However research on exactly how common it may be in school-aged children is lacking. In our Western Australian population-based study the prevalence as reported by parents was 2/211 (0.9%) and in the Hong Kong study (Yam, 2008) it was also 2/407 (<1%). A Scottish study published in 1998 had excellent ascertainment of type 1 diabetes but poor information on the denominator population of Down syndrome thus suggesting a prevalence between 1.4 and 10.6% in individuals with Down syndrome (Anwar, Walker, & Frier, 1998) (Table 3.3). A more recent Danish record linkage study compared the prevalence of Down syndrome in those with type 1 diabetes with the prevalence in the general population and found that there was a 4.2-fold increased prevalence of Down syndrome in the diabetic population (Bergholdt et al., 2006). The increased prevalence for Type 1 diabetes may be genetically linked to the mutation of chromosome 21 which may be associated with the early onset and high frequency of autoimmune diseases (Lammer & Weimann, 2008). As diabetes is relatively common among people with Down syndrome in comparison to the general population, further research should examine the substantial secondary health concerns experienced by children with diabetes, and the increased carer responsibility regarding monitoring of dietary requirements and medication management.

3.9. Leukemia

Although the overall risk of cancer for people with Down syndrome is equal to the general population, the risk of developing leukemia is significantly higher (Patja, Pukkala, Sund, Iivanainen, & Kaski, 2006; Sullivan, Hussain, Glasson, & Bittles, 2007). This increased risk has been demonstrated in data from the Western Australian Cancer Registry where 53% of all cancers recorded in people with Down syndrome resulted from childhood leukemia (Bittles et al., 2006). The increased risk of leukemia for people with Down syndrome has been estimated as 19-fold higher than for the general population in a UK record linkage study (Goldacre, Wotton, Seagroatt, & Yeates, 2004). However, the majority of cases are diagnosed before the age of 5 years (Sullivan et al., 2007) such that using data from the Danish Cytogenetic and Cancer Registers (Hasle, Clemmensen, & Mikkelsen, 2000) and the Western Australian Cancer Registry (Sullivan et al., 2007) the increased risk for preschool children with Down syndrome has been shown to be of the order of 50–60 times greater than for the general population. As acute myeloid leukemia is rare above the age of 5 years (Ross, Spector, Robison, & Olshan, 2005), school-aged children are most likely to experience acute lymphoblastic leukemia, but the majority would be under 10 years at time of onset (Chessells et al., 2001). In the large Nordic study involving 134 patients with Down syndrome diagnosed with acute leukemia the sex ratio for those with acute lymphoblastic anemia was similar to those without Down syndrome with a slight male predominance (Zeller et al., 2005). In a larger Italian study but with a lower proportion (1.9%) of Down syndrome patients compared with 3.9% in the Nordic study, those with Down syndrome were more likely to be females and to be aged 10 years and over (Arico, Ziino, Valsecchi, Cazzaniga, Baronci, Messina, et al., 2008). In a much smaller Finnish study ($n = 28$) there was also a higher prevalence of females (Rajantie & Siimes, 2003). Acute lymphoblastic anemia has been shown to differ in children with Down syndrome from that in children without Down syndrome in terms of the immunophenotype, where there are none with T cell leukemia and in cytogenetics with the absence of the prognostically unfavorable translocations (Whitlock et al., 2005; Zeller et al., 2005). In a large UK trial the survival of children with Down syndrome ($n = 55$) was shown to be inferior to those without Down syndrome ($n = 3596$) due to an increased number of deaths from infection (Chessells et al., 2001), but there was no increase in their risk of relapse. Similarly in the large population-based Nordic study (Zeller et al., 2005) outcomes for children with Down syndrome were also inferior to those without Down syndrome and for the 1993–2001 period they were no better than for the 1984–1992 period, in contrast to the improvement seen for children without Down syndrome. However, in the more recent large Italian study (Arico et al., 2008) treatment results were shown to be improving over time. Children with Down syndrome have also been found to experience higher levels of treatment-related toxicity (Xavier, Ge, & Taub, 2009). This may be associated with their high levels of other comorbidities which may complicate treatment and management regimes.

3.10. Immune dysfunction

Structural abnormalities and an immature immune system may be partly responsible for children with Down syndrome being predisposed to recurrent infections and episodic illnesses. Commonly occurring conditions include upper respiratory infections (Chen, Lander, & Murphy, 2006; Roizen & Patterson, 2003) and otitis media (Roizen & Patterson, 2003; Shott, Joseph, & Heithaus, 2001). The increased susceptibility to infection is likely to be further aggravated by the comorbidity of cardiac and pulmonary diseases and possibly by frequent attendance at health care appointments (Chen et al., 2006).

A recent US population-based study reported that children with Down syndrome had a higher prevalence of ear infections, recent colds/flu, stomach illnesses, and diarrhoea than did children without Down syndrome (Schieve et al., 2009). A major contributor to this increased susceptibility to illnesses may be the array of immune dysfunctions affecting people with Down syndrome (Guazzarotti et al., 2009), including severely diminished expansion of T- and B-lymphocytes (de Hingh et al., 2005). De Hingh and co-authors (de Hingh et al., 2005) found that in children with Down syndrome an absence of T- and B-lymphocyte expansion was present in children under 1. The study found that even though the percentage of T-lymphocytes gradually increased to approach those of children without Down syndrome, B-lymphocytes remained depleted at 88% below the tenth percentile. Although the majority of the episodic illnesses common in children with Down syndrome are not life-threatening, their prevalent and recurrent nature may add significantly to health care utilization, increase the financial and emotional impact on carers, and contribute to an overall decreased quality of life. It may be important to ensure that these children receive influenza vaccinations.

3.11. Oro-facial anomalies and dental disease

The oro-facial development may underlie some of the dental problems seen in the Down syndrome population (Hennequin, Faulks, Veyrune, & Bourdiol, 1999). Hennequin and colleagues (Hennequin et al., 1999) concluded that soft tissue hypotonia was central to skeletal underdevelopment and oro-facial anomalies, which may lead to difficulties in mastication, swallowing, and feeding for persons with Down syndrome. A descriptive cross-sectional study of 102 children with Down syndrome aged up to 15 years from special schools in Chennai, India investigated oral soft and hard tissue findings, including anomalies, in this cohort (Asokan, Muthu, Sivakumar, & Asokan, 2008). Mid-facial deficiency was reported to be the most common (76%) oro-facial anomaly. Relative mandibular prognathism (52%) and high-arched palate associated with posterior crossbite, anterior crossbite, or open bite were other features noted.

In Down syndrome there may be early onset of periodontal disease in primary dentition, with rapid progression and severe generalized gingivitis (Surabian, 2001). A longitudinal study in 34 adolescents with Down syndrome (mean age 16.6 years at baseline and 23.5 years at follow-up) revealed that 35% experienced alveolar bone loss at the onset of the study and this had increased to 74% over 7 years (Agholme, Dahllof, & Modeer, 1999). There was also an increase in the number of patients with pathological periodontal pockets (>4mm) from 41 to 65% over the study period. In addition to motor and behavioral inability to maintain adequate oral hygiene, impaired immunity due to reduction in neutrophil, T-lymphocyte function, and increased production of inflammatory mediators and proteolytic enzymes may contribute to prevalence and severity of periodontal disease in persons with Down syndrome (Morgan, 2007).

The prevalence of taurodontism, partial anodontia, and missing teeth has been reported to be higher in Down syndrome than in the general population (Desai, 1997). Hypoplasia, microdontia, and delayed eruption of deciduous and permanent teeth are common. An age- and gender-matched case–control study involving children with Down syndrome reported a lower prevalence of dental caries in comparison to groups of children with other intellectual disabilities and with no intellectual disability (Stabholz et al., 1991). Anatomic factors such as hypodontia, delayed eruption of teeth, and smaller interproximal areas may contribute to low levels of caries (Desai, 1997). Lower caries prevalence has also been attributed to elevated salivary *S. mutans*-specific IgA (Lee, Kwon, Song, & Choi, 2004) and different profiles of *S. mutans* (Cogulu, Sabah, Uzel, & Ozkinay, 2006) than in the general population. However, irrespective of the caries prevalence, existing literature suggests that dental patients with a disability receive differential treatment to the general population. In sibling-matched studies children with Down syndrome were less likely to receive dental restoration than children without Down syndrome (Allison & Lawrence, 2004; Fung, Lawrence, & Allison, 2008). In general, treatment in the form of extraction has been given preference over restoration. It has also been shown that dental loss is positively correlated with the severity of the intellectual disability in persons with Down syndrome (Maatta et al., 2006). In summary, orofacial deformities associated with Down syndrome itself and inadequate dental hygiene may result in an increased prevalence of dental disease in persons with Down syndrome. These findings reinforce the need for dental screening programs targeting children with Down syndrome in order to minimize preventable dental disease.

4. Discussion

Down syndrome is associated with many co-morbid conditions, health problems, and an increased risk of mortality compared to the general population. Improvements in the medical management of these comorbidities and surgical advances have reduced morbidity and mortality among children with Down syndrome (Bittles et al., 2006). Children with Down syndrome are predisposed to an array of health conditions and impairments, which transcend the sensory, endocrine, cardiovascular, respiratory, immune, gastrointestinal, obesity, oro-facial, musculoskeletal, and hematological systems and vary in their prevalence. Overall, it is evident that high levels of comorbidity significantly impact on the quality of life for children with Down syndrome and their families.

Parents of children with Down syndrome may experience an emotional and financial impact from the medical comorbidities experienced by their child. Parents have reported that their child's increased needs had diminished their finances to the extent that recreational activities and material items were often unaffordable (Mulroy, Robertson, Aiberti, Leonard, & Bower, 2008). Having a child with Down syndrome has also been associated with limited parental time for other children, reduced family socialization (Mulroy et al., 2008), and poor maternal health (Bourke et al., 2008). Parents therefore need a clear understanding of the medical comorbidities associated with Down syndrome to assist in making informed decisions regarding possible terminations of pregnancy (Skotko, Kishnani, & Capone, 2009) or in making future plans for their child and family (Skotko, Capone, & Kishnani, 2009).

Despite the widespread acknowledgement of the comorbidities experienced by children with Down syndrome and their health effect, limited literature is available on medical utilization and health expenditures. The 1997 Western Australian study (Leonard et al., 1999) summarized aspects of service utilization for children with Down syndrome. However, data from the 2004 follow-up survey have also been used to examine socio-demographic and other predictors of service use. In an earlier population-based record linkage study children under 5 years with a medical cause of their intellectual disability (predominantly Down syndrome) were more likely to be admitted to hospital and for longer periods of time than their peers (Williams et al., 2005). In a US study involving a privately insured population mean and median, medical costs for children 0–4 years of age with Down syndrome were 12–13 times higher than for children without Down syndrome. (Boulet, Molinari, Grosse, Honein, & Correa-Villasenor, 2008). Moreover, for infants with Down syndrome and congenital heart disease, mean and median costs were 5–7 times higher than for those with Down syndrome who did not have congenital heart disease. In another US linkage study involving residents of Tennessee born between 1997 and 1999 the hospitalization histories of children with Down syndrome aged 0–3 years were examined (So, Urbano, & Hodapp, 2007). Patterns were similar to the much earlier Swedish study (Frid et al., 2002) with almost half the children having been hospitalized and those with congenital heart disease being over twice as likely to have been admitted. Respiratory illnesses affected almost two-thirds of those with congenital heart disease who had been hospitalized (So et al., 2007) whilst over half of the admissions in the Eastern Australian study had also involved respiratory morbidity (Hilton et al., 1999). However, limited research has examined health service utilization for children over 5 years with Down syndrome or how the need for medical care changes with age. This knowledge would result in a better understanding of the service needs for this population and assist in provision and resource allocation of disability and medical services.

Many of the comorbidities experienced by children with Down syndrome, if left untreated, contribute to substantial secondary disability, resulting in unnecessary hardship and further disadvantage. Sensory defects are a prime example. As vision and hearing contribute to learning, language development, and socialization (Fellinger et al., 2009; Marcell, 1995; Merrick & Koslowe, 2001), the lack of regular screening and subsequent management of impairments not only affects the sensory systems involved but may contribute to a child's chances of academic success and socialization. It is becoming known that children with Down syndrome are disadvantaged in relation to opportunities for socialization and the development of friendships with a third of parents in the Western Australian population-based study reporting that their child had no friends (Oates, 2009). In other studies children with Down syndrome have been reported to have as few as one reciprocal friend (D'Haem, 2008; Guralnick, Neville, Hammond, & Connor, 2007), and to experience limited peer interactions outside school (D'Haem, 2008). Therefore, the importance of minimizing secondary disability is clearly relevant to the development of optimal social relationships for these children. Guidelines for the screening of medical conditions associated with Down syndrome have been published (American Academy of Pediatrics, 2001; Murphy et al., 2005; Van Cleve & Cohen, 2006; Van Cleve et al., 2006). However, in which countries and to what extent these are actually being implemented within schools and the health care system remains unknown. It is likely that in developing countries the medical needs of children with Down syndrome are even less likely to be met (Leonard & Wen, 2002). Further research is needed to provide an understanding of the current screening policies and guidelines being implemented and their effectiveness in both preventing and identifying morbidities experienced by children with Down syndrome worldwide.

Finally, this literature review has important implications for health care professionals and education providers. A clear understanding of the comorbidities experienced by children with Down syndrome provides a base for health care providers to plan and deliver safe and effective intervention programs suitable for each child's physical capacities and limitations. Knowledge of medical conditions is also valuable to health care professionals who are in a position to provide prospective parents with current information to facilitate informed decision-making and future plans. In addition, as teachers play a valuable role in children's development, an understanding of the medical conditions and their functional impact on children with Down syndrome may facilitate the implementation of classroom strategies which minimize disability and foster academic achievement and socialization with peers.

This review has synthesized the most current and relevant literature relating to the medical conditions experienced by school-aged children with Down syndrome; however, its limitations must be acknowledged. As this was not a systematic review the methodological quality of the research was not formally evaluated. Instead, this narrative literature review was undertaken to summarize findings and provide an overview of the common medical conditions experienced by children with Down syndrome. Furthermore, a meta-analysis was not performed due to the dearth of population-based data and heavy reliance on clinic- or hospital-based samples for many of the studies.

5. Conclusion

This review supports the conclusion that many children with Down syndrome are affected by additional birth defects and health-related problems which impact on their quality of life. Medical conditions commonly associated with Down syndrome include heart disease, respiratory problems, gastrointestinal disorders, ophthalmological and ear and hearing problems, musculoskeletal problems, a greater risk of leukemia and thyroid conditions, immune dysfunction, and dental disease. Although there is considerable research documented and describing these conditions predominantly in clinic-based and hospital-based samples, there is limited research examining the impact of levels of comorbidity on everyday functioning and family life. Understanding the impact of high levels of comorbidity would lead to the development of more effective interventions for teachers and health care professionals, and also assist in the provision and resource allocation of disability services.

REFERENCES

Agholme, M., Dahllof, G., & Modeer, T. (1999). Changes in periodontal status in patients with Down syndrome during a 7-year period. *European Journal of Oral Science, 107*, 82–88.

Ali, F. E., Al-Bustan, M. A., Al-Busairi, W. A., Al-Mulla, F. A., & Esbaita, E. Y. (2006). Cervical spine abnormalities associated with Down syndrome. *International Orthopaedics, 30*, 284–289.

Allison, P. J., & Lawrence, H. P. (2004). A paired comparison of dental care in Canadians with Down syndrome and their siblings without Down syndrome. *Community Dentistry & Oral Epidemiology, 32*, 99–106.

American Academy of Pediatrics (2001). Health supervision for children with Down syndrome. *Pediatrics, 107*, 442–449.

Anwar, A. J., Walker, J. D., & Frier, B. M. (1998). Type 1 diabetes mellitus and Down's syndrome: prevalence, management and diabetic complications. *Diabetic Medicine: A Journal Of The British Diabetic Association, 15*, 160–163.

Arico, M., Ziino, O., Valsecchi, M. G., Cazzaniga, G., Baronci, C., Messina, C., et al. (2008). Acute lymphoblastic leukemia and Down syndrome: Presenting features and treatment outcome in the experience of the Italian Association of Pediatric Hematology and Oncology (AIEOP), *Cancer, 113*, 515–521.

Asokan, S., Muthu, M. S., Sivakumar, N., & Asokan, S. (2008). Oral findings of Down syndrome children in Chennai city, India. *Indian Journal of Dental Research, 19*, 230–235.

Australian Bureau Statistics (2006). Australian Social Trends: Trends in women's employment. Retrieved April 15, 2009. from http://www.abs.gov.au/AUSSTATS/abs@.nsf/7d12b0f6763c78caca257061001cc588/858badad39afb98dca2571b000153d73!OpenDocument.

Australian Bureau Statistics (2007). Australian Social Trends: Qualification profile of Australians. Retrieved April 15, 2009. From http://www.abs.gov.au/AUSSTATS/abs@.nsf/Latestproducts/FFEDA0779C20049DCA25732C00207383?opendocument.

Australian Bureau Statistics (2009). Australian Social Trends: Trends in household work. Retrieved April 8, 2009. From http://www.abs.gov.au/AUSSTATS/abs@.nsf/Lookup/4102.0Main+Features40March%202009.

Bell, R., Rankin, J., & Donaldson, L. J. (2003). Down's syndrome: Occurrence and outcome in the north of England, 1985–99. *Paediatric & Perinatal Epidemiology*, *17*, 33–39.

Bergholdt, R., Eising, S., Nerup, J., & Pociot, F. (2006). Increased prevalence of Down's syndrome in individuals with type 1 diabetes in Denmark: A nationwide population-based study. *Diabetologia*, *49*, 1179–1182.

Bertrand, P., Navarro, H., Caussade, S., Holmgren, N., & Sanchez, I. (2003). Airway anomalies in children with Down syndrome: *Endoscopic findings*. *Pediatric Pulmonology*, *36*, 137–141.

Besser, L. M., Shin, M., Kucik, J. E., & Correa, A. (2007). Prevalence of Down syndrome among children and adolescents in metropolitan Atlanta. Birth Defects Research. *Part A, Clinical And Molecular Teratology*, *79*, 765–774.

Binkert, F. (2002). Impact of prenatal diagnosis on the prevalence of live births with Down syndrome in the eastern half of Switzerland 1980–1996. *Swiss medical weekly*, *132*, 478–484.

Bishop, J. (1997). Epidemiologic study of Down syndrome in a racially diverse California population, 1989–1991. *American Journal of Epidemiology*, *145*, 134–147.

Bittles, A. H., Bower, C., Hussain, R., & Glasson, E. J. (2006). The four ages of Down syndrome. *European Journal of Public Health*, *17*, 221–225.

Bittles, A. H., & Glasson, E. J. (2004). Clinical, social and ethical implications of changing life expectancy in Down syndrome. *Developmental Medicine & Child Neurology*, *46*, 282–286.

Blaser, S., Propst, E. J., Martin, D., Feigenbaum, A., James, A. L., Shannon, P., et al. (2006). Inner ear dysplasia is common in children with Down syndrome (trisomy 21). *The Laryngoscope*, *116*, 2113–2119.

Bonamico, M., Mariani, P., Danesi, H. M., Crisogianni, M., Failla, P., Gemme, G., et al. (2001). Prevalence and clinical picture of celiac disease in Italian Down syndrome patients: a multicenter study. *Journal of Pediatric Gastroenterology & Nutrition*, *33*, 139–143.

Book, L., Hart, A., Black, J., Feolo, M., Zone, J., & Neuhausen, S. (2001a). Prevalence and clinical characteristics of celiac disease in Down syndrome in a US study. *American Journal Of Medical Genetics*, *98*, 70–74.

Book, L., Hart, A., Black, J., Feolo, M., Zone, J. J., & Neuhausen, S. L. (2001b). Prevalence and clinical characteristics of celiac disease in Down's syndrome in a US study. *American Journal of Medical Genetics*, *98*, 70–74.

Bosch, J. J. (2003). Health maintenance throughout the life span for individuals with Down syndrome. *Journal of the American Academy of Nurse Practitioners*, *15*, 5–17.

Boulet, S. L., Molinari, N. A., Grosse, S. D., Honein, M. A., & Correa-Villasenor, A. (2008). Health care expenditures for infants and young children with Down syndrome in a privately insured population. *The Journal Of Pediatrics*, *153*, 241–246.

Bourke, J., Ricciardo, B., Bebbington, A., Aiberti, K., Jacoby, P., Dyke, P., et al. (2008). Physical and mental health in mothers of children with Down syndrome. *The Journal Of Pediatrics*, *153*, 320–326.

Bower, C., Callaghan, A., Cosgrove, P., & Quick, J. (2007). Report of the Birth Defects Registry of Western Australia, 1980–2006 (No. 14). Perth, Western Australia: King Edward Memorial Hospital Women and Newborn Health Service.

Bower, C., Leonard, H., & Petterson, B. (2000). Intellectual disability in Western Australia. *Journal of Paediatrics and Child Health*, *36*, 213–215.

Canfield, M., A., Margaret, A. H., Nataliya, Y., Jian, X., Cara, T. M., Julianne, S. C., et al. (2006). National estimates and race/ethnic-specific variation of selected birth defects in the United States, 1999–2001. Birth Defects Research Part A: *Clinical and Molecular Teratology*, *76*, 747–756.

Carlsson, A., Axelsson, I., Borulf, S., Bredberg, A., Forslund, M., Lindberg, B., et al. (1998). Prevalence of IgA-antigliadin antibodies and IgA-antiendomysium antibodies related to celiac disease in children with Down syndrome. *Pediatrics, 101*, 272–275.

Carroll, K., Arbogast, P. G., Dudley, J. A., & Cooper, W. O. (2008) Increase in incidence of medically treated thyroid disease in children with Down's syndrome after rerelease of American Academy of Pediatrics health supervision guidelines. *Pediatrics, 122*, E493–E498.

Casselbrant, M. L., Mandel, E. M., Rockette, H. E., Kurs-Lasky, M., Fall, P. A., & Bluestone, C. D. (2009). Adenoidectomy for otitis media with effusion in 2–3-year-old children. *International Journal of Pediatric Otorhinolaryngology, 73*, 1718–1724.

Catto-Smith, A., Trajanovska, M., & Taylor, R. (2006). Long-term continence in patients with Hirschsprung's disease and Down syndrome. *Journal of Gastroenterology and Hepatology, 21*, 748–753.

Centre for Disease Control (1994). Down syndrome prevalence at birth –United States, 1983–1990. *Morbidity and mortality weekly report, 43*, 617–622.

Chen, M. A., Lander, T. R., & Murphy, C. (2006). Nasal health in Down syndrome: A cross-sectional study. Otolaryngology-head and neck surgery. *Official Journal Of American Academy Of Otolaryngology-Head And Neck Surgery, 134*, 741–745.

Chessells, J. M., Harrison, G., Richards, S. M., Bailey, C. C., Hill, F.G.H., Gibson, B. E., et al. (2001). Down's syndrome and acute lymphoblastic leukaemia: *clinical features and response to treatment. Archives of Disease in Childhood, 85*, 321–325.

Cleves, M. A., Hobbs, C. A., Cleves, P. A., Tilford, J. M., Bird, T. M., & Robbins, J. M. (2007). Congenital defects among liveborn infants with Down syndrome. Birth Defects Research (Part A). *Clinical and Molecular Teratology, 79*, 657–663.

Cogulu, D., Sabah, E., Uzel, A., & Ozkinay, F. (2006). Genotyping of *Streptococcus mutans* by using arbitrarily primed polymerase chain reaction in children with Down syndrome. *Archives of Oral Biology, 51*, 177–182.

Cohen, W. I. (2006). Current dilemmas in Down syndrome clinical care: celiac disease, thyroid disorders, and atlanto-axial instability. *American Journal of Medical Genetics Part C: Seminars in Medical Genetics, 142C*, 141–148.

Collins, V. R., Muggli, E. E., Riley, M., Palma, S., & Halliday, J. L. (2008). Is Down syndrome a disappearing birth defect? *The Journal Of Pediatrics, 152*, 20–24.

Committee on Sports Medicine and Fitness (1995). Atlantoaxial instability in Down syndrome: Subject review. *Pediatrics, 96*, 151–154.

Concolino, D., Pasquzzi, A., Capalbo, G., Sinopoli, S., & Strisciuglio, P. (2006). Early detection of podiatric anomalies in children with Down syndrome. *Acta Paediatrica (Oslo, Norway: 1992), 95*, 17–20.

Coyte, P. C., Croxford, R., McIsaac, W., Feldman, W., & Friedberg, J. (2001). The role of adjuvant adenoidectomy and tonsillectomy in the outcome of the insertion of tympanostomy tubes. *New England Journal of Medicine, 344*, 1188–1195.

Cregg, M., Woodhouse, J. M., Pakeman, V. H., Saunders, K. J., Gunter, H. L., Parker, M., et al. (2001). Accommodation and refractive error in children with Down syndrome: cross-sectional and longitudinal studies. *Investigative Opthalmology & Visual Science, 42*, 55–63.

Cregg, M., Woodhouse, J. M., Stewart, R. E., Pakeman, V. H., Bromham, N. R., Gunter, H. L., et al. (2003). Development of refractive error and strabismus in children with Down syndrome. *Investigative Ophthalmology & Visual Science, 44*, 1023–1030.

Cronk, C., Crocker, A. C., Pueschel, M., Shea, A. M., Zackai, E., Pickens, G., et al. (1988). Growth charts for children with Down Syndrome: 1 month to 18 years of age. *Pediatrics, 81*, 102–110.

Crothers, L. M., Kehle, T. J., Bray, M. A., & Theodore, L. A. (2009). Correlates and suspected causes of obesity in children. *Psychology in the Schools, 46*, 787–796.

D'Haem, J. (2008). Special at school but lonely at home: an alternative friendship group for adolescents with Down syndrome. *Down Syndrome Research and Practice, 12*, 107–111.

de Hingh, Y. C., Vossen, v.d., Gemen, E. F., Mulder, A. B., Hop, W. C., Brus, F., et al. (2005). Intrinsic abnormalities of lymphocyte counts in children with Down syndrome. *Journal of Pediatrics, 147*, 744–747.

De, S., Small, J., & Baur, L. A. (2008). Overweight and obesity among children with developmental disabilities. *Journal of Intellectual and Developmental Disability, 33*, 43–47.

Desai, S. (1997). Down Syndrome: A review of literature. *Oral Surgery, Oral Medicine, Oral Pathology, Oral Radiology and Endodontics, 84*, 279–285.

Driscoll, C., Kei, J., Bates, D., & McPherson, B. (2003). Tympanometry and TEOAE testing of children with Down syndrome in special schools. *The Australian and New Zealand Journal of Audiology, 25*, 85–93.

Ebbeling, C. B., Pawlak, D. B., & Ludwig, D. S. (2002). Childhood obesity: public health crisis, common sense cure. *The Lancet, 360*, 473–482.

Egan, J. F., Benn, P. A., Zelop, C. M., Bolnick, A., Gianferrari, E., & Borgida, A. F. (2004). Down syndrome births in the United States from 1989 to 2001. *Am J Obstet Gynecol, 191*, 1044–1048.

Eurocat (2010). European surveillance of congenital anomolies. Retrieved 26/4/2010, from http://www.eurocat-network.eu/.

Fellinger, J., Holzinger, D., Beitel, C., Launch, M., & Goldberg, D. (2009). The impact of language skills on mental health in teenagers with hearing impairments. *Acta Psychiatrica Scandinavica, 120*, 153–159.

Ferrara, M., Capozzi, L., & Russo, R. (2008). Impact of ER gene polymorphisms on overweight and obesity in Down syndrome. *Central European Journal of Medicine, 3*, 271–278.

Field, A. E., Cook, N. R., & Gillman, M. W. (2005). High normal weight status in childhood as a predictor of being overweight or hypertensive in early childhood. *Obesity Research, 13*, 163–169.

Fimiani, F., Iovine, A., Carelli, R., Pansini, M., Sebastio, G., & Magli, A. (2007). Incidence of ocular pathologies in Italian children with Down syndrome. *European Journal of Ophthalmology, 17*, 817–822.

Fitzgerald, D. A., Paul, A., & Richmond, C. (2007). Severity of obstructive apnoea in children with Down syndrome who snore. *Archives of Disease in Childhood, 92*, 423–425.

Freeman, S. B., Allen, E. G., Oxford-Wright, C. L., Tinker, S. W., Druschel, C., Hobbs, C. A., et al. (2007). The national Down syndrome project: Design and implementation. *Public Health Reports, 122*, 62–72.

Freeman, S. B., Bean, L. H., Allen, E. G., Tinker, S. W., Locke, A. E., Druschel, C., et al. (2008). Ethnicity, sex, and the incidence of congenital heart defects: a report from the National Down Syndrome Project. Genetics In Medicine: *Official Journal Of The American College Of Medical Genetics, 10*, 173–180.

Freeman, S. B., Taft, L. F., Dooley, K. J., Allran, K., Sherman, S. L., Hassold, T. J., et al. (1998). Population-based study of congenital heart defects in Down syndrome. *American Journal of Medical Genetics, 80*, 213–217.

Freeman, S. B., Torfs, C. P., Romitti, P. A., Royle, M. H., Druschel, C., Hobbs, C. A., et al. (2009). Congenital gastrointestinal defects in Down syndrome: A report from the Atlanta and National Down Syndrome Projects. *Clinical Genetics, 75*, 180–184.

Frid, C., Anneren, G., Rasmussen, F., Sundelin, C., & Drott, P. (2002). Utilization of medical care among children with Down's syndrome. *Journal of Intellectual Disability Research, 46*, 310–317.

Frid, C., Drott, P., Lundell, B., Rasmussen, F., & Anneren, G. (1999). Mortality in Down's syndrome in relation to congenital malformations. *Journal of Intellectual Disability Research, 43*, 234–241.

Fryers, T., & Mackay, R. I. (1979). Down syndrome: prevalence at birth, mortality and survival. A 17-year study. *Early Human Development, 3*, 29–41.

Fung, K., Lawrence, H. P., & Allison, P. J. (2008). A paired analysis of correlates of dental restorative care in siblings with and without Down syndrome. *Special Care in Dentistry, 28*, 85–91.

Geggel, R. L., O'Brien, J. E., & Feingold, M. (1993). Development of valve dysfunction in adolescents and young adults with Down syndrome and no known congenital heart disease. *Journal of Pediatrics, 122*, 821–823.

Gibson, P. A., Newton, R. W., Selby, K., Price, D. A., Leyland, K., & Addison, G. M. (2005). Longitudinal study of thyroid function in Down's syndrome in the first two decades. *Archives of Disease in Childhood, 90*, 574–578.

Goldacre, M. J., Wotton, C. J., Seagroatt, V., & Yeates, D. (2004). Cancers and immune related diseases associated with Down's syndrome: A record linkage study. *Archives Of Disease In Childhood, 89*, 1014–1017.

Gordon, R. A., & Donzis, P. B. (1985). Refractive development of the human eye. *Archives of Ophthalmology, 103*, 785–789.

Grammatikopoulou, M. G., Manai, A., Tsigga, M., Tsiligiroglou-Fachantidou, A., Galli-Tsinopoulou, A., & Zakas, A. (2008). Nutrient intake and anthropometry in children and adolescents with Down syndrome – a preliminary study. *Developmental Neurorehabilitation, 11*, 260–267.

Guazzarotti, L., Trabattoni, D., Castelletti, E., Boldrighini, B., Piacentini, L., Duca, P., et al. (2009). T lymphocyte maturation is impaired in healthy young individuals carrying trisomy 21 (Down syndrome). *American Journal On Intellectual And Developmental Disabilities, 114*, 100–109.

Guralnick, M., Neville, B., Hammond, M., & Connor, R. (2007). The friendships of young children with developmental delays: A longitudinal analysis. *Journal of Applied Developmental Psychology, 28*, 64–79.

Hackam, D. J., Reblock, K., Barksdale, E. M., Redlinger, R., Lynch, J., & Gaines, B. A. (2003). The influence of Down's syndrome on the management and outcome of children with Hirschsprung's disease. *Journal Of Pediatric Surgery, 38*, 946–949.

Halliday, J., Collins, V., Riley, M., Youssef, D., & Muggli, E. (2009). Has prenatal screening influenced the prevalence of comorbidities associated with Down syndrome and subsequent survival rates? *Pediatrics, 123*, 256–261.

Hasle, H., Clemmensen, I. H., and Mikkelsen, M. (2000). Risks of leukaemia and solid tumours in individuals with Down's syndrome. *Lancet, 355*, 165–169.

Haugen, O. H., & Hovding, G. (2001). Strabismus and binocular function in children with Down syndrome. A population-based, longitudinal study. *Acta Ophthalmologica Scandinavica, 79*, 133–139.

Hayes, C., Johnson, Z., Thornton, L., Fogarty, J., Lyons, R., O'Connor, M., et al. (1997). Ten-year survival of Down syndrome births. *International Journal of Epidemiology, 26*, 822–829.

Hei-Jen, J., Yih-Shing, K., Jenn-Jeih, H., Ming-Kwang, S., T'Sang-T'ang, H., & Fon-Jou, H. (2005). The evolving national birth prevalence of Down syndrome in Taiwan. A study on the impact of second-trimester maternal serum screening. *Prenatal Diagnosis, 25*, 665–670.

Hennequin, M., Faulks, D., Veyrune, J. L., & Bourdiol, P. (1999). Significance of oral health in persons with Down syndrome: A literature review. *Developmental Medicine & Child Neurology, 41*, 275–283.

Hilton, J. M., Fitzgerald, D. A., & Cooper, D. M. (1999). Respiratory morbidity of hospitalized children with Trisomy 21. *Journal of Paediatrics and Child Health, 35*, 383–386.

Huang, T. (1998). Birth prevalence of Down's syndrome in England and Wales 1990 to 1997. *Journal of Medical Screening, 5*, 213–214.

Karlsson, B., Gustafsson, J., Hedov, G., Ivarsson, S.-A., & Anneren, G. (1998). Thyroid dysfunction in Down syndrome: relation to age and thyroid autoimmunity. *Archives of Disease in Childhood, 79*, 242–245.

Kawatu, D., & LeLeiko, N. S. (2006). Screening for celiac disease in asymptomatic children with Down syndrome: Cost-effectiveness of preventing lymphoma. *Pediatrics, 118*, 816–817.

Keckler, S. J., St Peter, S. D., Spilde, T. L., Ostlie, D. J., & Snyder, C. L. (2008). The influence of trisomy 21 on the incidence and severity of congenital heart defects in patients with duodenal atresia. *Pediatric Surgery International, 24*, 921–923.

Lai, F. M. (2002). Birth prevalence of Down syndrome in Singapore from 1993 to 1998. *Singapore Medical Journal, 43*, 70–76.

Lammer, C., & Weimann, E. (2008). Early onset of type I diabetes mellitus, Hashimoto's thyroiditis and celiac disease in a 7-yr-old boy with Down's syndrome. *Pediatric Diabetes, 9*, 423–425.

Lee, S., Kwon, H., Song, K., & Choi, Y. (2004). Dental caries and salivary immunoglobulin A in Down syndrome children. *Journal of Pediatrics and Child Health, 40*, 530–533.

Leonard, H. (2005). Some socio-demographic trends and technological trends in the developed world and their impact on Down's syndrome. *Italian Journal of Pediatrics, 31*, 213–216.

Leonard, H., & Wen, X. Y. (2002). The epidemiology of mental retardation: Challenges and opportunities in the new millennium. *Mental Retardation and Developmental Disabilities Research Reviews, 8*, 117–134.

Leonard, S., Bower, C., Petterson, B., & Leonard, H. (1999). Medical aspects of school-aged children with Down syndrome. *Developmental Medicine and Child Neurology, 41*, 683–688.

Leonard, S., Bower, C., Petterson, B., & Leonard, H. (2000). Survival of infants born with Down's syndrome: 1980–96. *Paediatric Perinatal Epidemiology, 14*, 163–171.

Lino, Y., Imamura, Y., Harigai, S., & Tanaka, Y. (1999). Efficacy of tympanostomy tube insertion for otitis media with effusion in children with Down syndrome. *International Journal of Pediatric Otorhinolaryngology, 49*, 143–149.

Lous, J., Burton, M., Felding, J., Ovesen, T., Rovers, M., & Williamson, I. (2005). Grommets (ventilation tubes) for hearing loss associated with otitis media with effusion in children. Cochrone Database of Systematic Reviews(1), Article CD001801.

Luke, A., Sutton, M., Schoeller, D. A., & Roizen, N.J.M. (1996). Nutrient intake and obesity in prepubescent children with Down syndrome. *Journal of the American Dietetic Association, 96*, 1262–1267.

Maatta, T., Kaski, M., Taanila, A., Keinanen-Kiukaanniemi, S., & Iivanainen, M. (2006). Sensory impairments and health concerns related to the degree of intellectual disability in people with Down syndrome. *Down Syndrome Research and Practice, 11*, 78–83.

Mackey, J., Treem, W. R., Worley, G., Boney, A., Hart, P., & Kishnani, P. S. (2001). Frequency of celiac disease in individuals with Down syndrome in the United States. *Clinical Pediatrics, 40*, 249–252.

Magge, S. N., O'Neill, K. L., Shults, J., Stallings, V. A., & Stettler, N. (2008). Leptin levels among prepubertal children with Down syndrome compared to their siblings. *Journal of Pediatrics, 152*, 321–326.

Maki, M., Mustalahti, K., Kokkonen, J., Kulmala, P., Haapalahti, M., Karttunen, T., et al. (2003). Prevalence of Celiac disease among children in Finland. *New England Journal of Medicine, 348*, 2517–2524.

Mallen, C., Peat, G., & Croft, P. (2006). Quality assessment of observational studies is not commonplace in systematic reviews. *Journal of Clinical Epidemiology, 59*, 765–769.

Marcell, M. (1995). Relationships between hearing and auditory cognition in Down's syndrome youth. *Down Syndrome Research and Practice, 3*, 75–91.

Marder, E., & Dennis, J. (2001). Medical management of children with Down's syndrome. *Current Paediatrics, 11*, 57–63.

Melendres, M. C., Lutz, J. M., Rubin, E. D., & Marcus, C. L. (2004). Daytime sleepiness and hyperactivity in children with suspected sleep-disordered breathing. *Pediatrics, 114*, 768–775.

Melve, K. K., Lie, R. T., Skjaerven, R., Van Der Hagen, C. B., Gradek, G. A., Jonsrud, C., et al. (2008). Registration of Down syndrome in the Medical Birth Registry of Norway: validity and time trends. *Acta Obstetricia Et Gynecologica Scandinavica, 87*, 824–830.

Merrick, J., & Koslowe, K. (2001). Refractive errors and visual anomalies in Down syndrome. Down's Syndrome, Research And Practice. *The Journal Of The Sarah Duffen Centre / University Of Portsmouth, 6*, 131–133.

Mik, G., Gholve, P., Scher, D., Widmann, R., & Green, D. (2008). Down syndrome: Orthopedic issues. *Current Opinion in Pediatrics, 20*, 30–36.

Mikkelsen, M., Fischer, G., Hansen, J., Pilgaard, B., & Nielsen, J. (1983). The impact of legal termination of pregnancy and of prenatal diagnosis on the birth prevalence of Down syndrome in Denmark. *Annals of Human Genetics, 47*, 123–131.

Mitchell, R. B., Call, E., & Kelly, J. (2003). Ear, nose and throat disorders in children with Down syndrome. *The Laryngoscope, 113*, 259–263.

Morabito, A., Lall, A., Gull, S., Mohee, A., & Bianchi, A. (2006). The impact of Down's syndrome on the immediate and long-term outcomes of children with Hirschsprung's disease. *Pediatric Surgery International, 22*, 179–181.

Morgan, J. (2007). Why is periodontal disease more prevalent and more severe in people with Down syndrome? *Special Care in Dentistry, 27*, 196–201.

Morris, J. K., Mutton, D. E., & Alberman, E. (2002). Revised estimates of the maternal age specific live birth prevalence of Down's syndrome. *Journal of Medical Screening, 9*, 2–6.

Mulroy, S., Robertson, L., Aiberti, K., Leonard, H., & Bower, C. (2008). The impact of having a sibling with an intellectual disability: parental perspectives in two disorders. *Journal Of Intellectual Disability Research, 52*, 216–229.

Murphy, J., Hoey, H.M.C.V., Philip, M., Roche, E. F., Macken, S., Mayne, P., et al. (2005). Guidelines for the medical management of Irish children and adolescents with Down syndrome. *Irish Medical Journal, 98*, 48–52.

Myrelid, A., Gustafsson, J., Ollars, B., & Anneren, G. (2002). Growth charts for Down's Syndrome from birth to 18 years of age. *Archives of Disease in Childhood, 87*, 97–103.

Nader-Sepahi, A., Casey, A.T.H., Hayward, R., Crockard, A., & Thompson, D. (2005). Symptomatic atlantoaxial instability in Down syndrome. *Journal of Neurosurgery: Pediatrics, 103*, 231–237.

Ng, D. K., Hui, H. N., Chan, C. H., Kwok, K. L., Chow, P. Y., Cheung, J. M., et al. (2006). Obstructive sleep apnoea in children with Down syndrome. *Singapore Medical Journal, 47*, 774–779.

Nisli, K., Oner, N., Candan, S., Kayserili, H., Tansel, T., Tireli, E., et al. (2008). Congenital heart disease in children with Down's syndrome: Turkish experience of 13 years. *Acta Cardiologica, 63*, 585–589.

O'Leary, P., Breheny, N., Reid, G., Charles, T., & Emery, J. (2006). Regional variations in prenatal screening across Australia: stepping towards a national policy framework. *The Australian & New Zealand Journal Of Obstetrics & Gynaecology, 46*, 427–432.

Oates, A. (2009). Leisure Participation for School-aged Children with Down Syndrome. Edith Cowan University, Perth.

Olsen, C. L., Cross, P. K., Gensburg, L. J., & Hughes, J. P. (1996). The effects of prenatal diagnosis, population ageing, and changing fertility rates on the live birth prevalence of Down syndrome in New York State, 1983–1992. *Prenatal Diagnosis, 16*, 991–1002.

Patja, K., Pukkala, E., Sund, R., Iivanainen, M., & Kaski, M. (2006). Cancer incidence of persons with Down syndrome in Finland: A population-based study. *International Journal Of Cancer, 118*, 1769–1772.
Perez-Pastor, E. M., Metcalf, B. S., Hosking, J., Jeffery, A. N., Voss, L. D., & Wilkin, T. J. (2009). Assortative weight gain in mother–daughter and father–son pairs: an emerging source of childhood obesity. Longitudinal study of trios (EarlyBird 43). *International Journal of Obesity, 33*, 727–735.
Platt, L. S. (2001). Medical and orthopaedic conditions in special olympics athletes. *Journal Of Athletic Training, 36*, 74–80.
Prasher, V. P. (1995). Reliability of diagnosing clinical hypothyroidism in adults with Down syndrome. *Australia & New Zealand Journal of Developmental Disabilities, 20*, 223–233.
Prasher, V. P. (1999). Down syndrome and thyroid disorders: A review. *Down Syndrome Research and Practice, 6*, 25–42.
Prasher, V. P., Robinson, L., Krishnan, V.H.R., & Chung, M. C. (1995). Podiatric disorders among children with Down syndrome and learning disability. *Developmental Medicine & Child Neurology, 37*, 131–134.
Price, D. L., Orvidas, L. J., Weaver, A. L., & Farmer, S. A. (2004). Efficacy of adenoidectomy in the treatment of nasal and middle ear symptoms in children with Down syndrome. *International Journal of Pediatric Otorhinolaryngology, 68*, 7–13.
Rajantie, J., & Siimes, M. (2003). Long-term prognosis of children with Down's syndrome and leukaemia: A 34-year nation-wide experience. *Journal of Intellectual Disability Research, 47*, 617–621.
Rasmussen, S. A., Wong, L. Y., Correa, A., Gambrell, D., & Friedman, J. M. (2006). Survival in infants with Down syndrome, Metropolitan Atlanta, 1979–1998. *The Journal Of Pediatrics, 148*, 806–812.
Reimand, T., Ounap, K., Zordania, R., Ilus, T., Uibo, O., Sitska, M., et al. (2006). Descriptive epidemiology of Down's syndrome in Estonia. *Paediatric and Perinatal Epidemiology, 20*, 512–519.
Roizen, N., & Patterson, D. (2003). Down's syndrome. *The Lancet, 361*, 1281–1289.
Ross, J. A., Spector, L. G., Robison, L. L., & Olshan, A. F. (2005). Epidemiology of leukemia in children with Down syndrome. *Pediatric Blood & Cancer, 44*, 8–12.
Roussot, M. A., Lawrenson, J. B., Hewitson, J., Smart, R., & de Decker, H. P. (2006). Is cardiac surgery warranted in children with Down syndrome? A case-controlled review. *South African Medical Journal, 96*, 924–930.
Savulescu, J. (2001). Resources, Down's syndrome, and cardiac surgery. *British Medical Journal, 322*, 875–876.
Schechter, M. S. (2002). Technical Report: Diagnosis and Management of Childhood Obstructive Sleep Apnea Syndrome. *Pediatrics, 109*, e69–e69.
Schieve, L. A., Boulet, S. L., Boyle, C., Rasmussen, S. A., & Schendel, D. (2009). Health of children 3 to 17 years of age with Down syndrome in the 1997–2005 National Health Interview Survey. *Pediatrics, 123*, e253–e260.
Selby-Silverstein, L., Hillstrom, H. J., & Palisano, R. J. (2001). The effect of foot orthoses on standing foot posture and gait of young children with Down syndrome. *NeuroRehabilitation, 16*, 183–193.
Selikowitz, M. (1993). Short-term efficacy of tympanostomy tubes for secretory otitis media in children with Down syndrome. *Developmental Medicine and Child Neurology, 35*, 511–515.
Sharav, T., & Bowman, T. (1992). Dietary practices, physical activity and body-mass index in a selected population of Down Syndrome children and their siblings. *Clinical Pediatrics, 31*, 341–344.
Sherman, S., Allen, E., Bean, L., & Freeman, S. (2007). Epidemiology of Down syndrome. *Mental Retardation & Developmental Disabilities Research Reviews, 13*, 221–227.

Shott, S., Amin, R., Chini, B., Heubi, C., Hotze, S., & Akers, R. (2006). Obstructive Sleep Apnea: Should all children with Down syndrome be tested? *Archives of Otolaryngology-Head & Neck Surgery*, *132*, 432–436.

Shott, S. R., Joseph, A., & Heithaus, D. (2001). Hearing loss in children with Down syndrome. *International Journal Of Pediatric Otorhinolaryngology*, *61*, 199–205.

Siffel, C., Correa, A., Cragan, J., & Alverson, C. J. (2004). Prenatal diagnosis, pregnancy terminations and prevalence of Down syndrome in Atlanta. *Birth Defects Research (Part A): Clinical and Molecular Teratology*, *70*, 565–571.

Skotko, B. G., Capone, G. T., & Kishnani, P. S. (2009). Postnatal diagnosis of Down syndrome: synthesis of the evidence on how best to deliver the news. *Pediatrics*, *124*, e751–e758.

Skotko, B. G., Kishnani, P. S., & Capone, G. T. (2009). Prenatal diagnosis of Down syndrome: how best to deliver the news. *American Journal of Medical Genetics A*, *149A*, 2361–2367.

So, S. A., Urbano, R. C., & Hodapp, R. M. (2007). Hospitalizations of infants and young children with Down syndrome: Evidence from inpatient person-records from a statewide administrative database. *Journal of Intellectual Disability Research*, *51*, 1030–1038.

Stabholz, A., Mann, J., Sela, M., Schurr, D., Steinberg, D., & Shapira, J. (1991). Caries experience, periodontal treatment needs, salivary pH, and *Streptococcus mutans* counts in a preadolescent Down syndrome population. *Special Care in Dentistry*, *11*, 203–208.

Stephen, E., Dickson, J., Kindley, A. D., Scott, C. C., & Charleton, P. M. (2007). Surveillance of vision and ocular disorders in children with Down syndrome. *Developmental Medicine and Child Neurology*, *49*, 513–515.

Stewart, R. E., Margaret Woodhouse, J., & Trojanowska, L. D. (2005). In focus: the use of bifocal spectacles with children with Down's syndrome. Ophthalmic & Physiological Optics. *The Journal Of The British College Of Ophthalmic Opticians (Optometrists)*, *25*, 514–522.

Stoll, C., Alembik, Y., Dott, B., & Roth, M. P. (1998). Study of Down syndrome in 238,942 consecutive births. *Annales de Genetique*, *41* 44–51.

Styles, M. E., Cole, T. J., Dennis, J., & Preece, M. A. (2002). New cross-sectional stature, weight, and head circumferences for Down's Syndrome in the UK and Republic of Ireland. *Archives of Disease in Childhood*, *87*, 104–108.

Sullivan, S. G., Hussain, R., Glasson, E., & Bittles, A. H. (2007). The profile and incidence of cancer in Down syndrome. *Journal of Intellectual Disability Research*, *51*, 228–231.

Surabian, S. R. (2001). Developmental disabilities and understanding the needs of patients with mental retardation and Down syndrome. *Journal of the California Dental Association*, *29*, 415–423.

Swigonski, N. L., Kuhlenschmidt, H. L., Bull, M. J., Corkins, M. R., & Downs, S. M. (2006). Screening for celiac disease in asymptomatic children with Down syndrome: Cost-effectiveness of preventing lymphoma. *Pediatrics*, *118*, 594–602.

Thomas, K. (2009). Medical conditions in children with Down syndrome. Edith Cowan University, Perth.

Torfs, C. P., & Christianson, R. E. (1998). Anomalies in Down syndrome individuals in a large population-based registry. *American Journal of Medical Genetics*, 77, 431–438.

Turner, S., Sloper, P., Cunningham, C., & Knussen, C. (1990). Health problems in children with Down's syndrome. Child. *Care, Health & Development*, *16*, 83–97.

Uibo, O., Teesalu, K., Metskula, K., Reimand, T., Saat, R., Sillat, T., et al. (2006). Screening for celiac disease in Down's syndrome patients revealed cases of subtotal villous atrophy without typical for celiac disease HLA-DQ and tissue transglutaminase antibodies. *World Journal Of Gastroenterology*, *12*, 1430–1434.

Unachak, K., Tanpaiboon, P., Pongprot, Y., Sittivangkul, R., Silvilairat, S., Dejkhamron, P., et al. (2008). Thyroid functions in children with Down's syndrome. *Journal of the Medical Association of Thailand, 91*, 56–61.

Van Cleve, S., Cannon, S., & Cohen, W. (2006). Part II: Clinical Practice Guidelines for Adolescents and Young Adults With Down Syndrome: 12 to 21 Years. *Journal of Pediatricric Health Care, 20*, 198–205.

Van Cleve, S., & Cohen, W. (2006). Part 1: Clinical Practice Guidelines for Children with Down Syndrome From Birth to 12 Years. *Journal of Pediatric Health Care, 20*, 47–54.

van Schrojenstein Lantman-de Valk, H. M., Haveman, M. J., & Crebolder, H. F. (1996). Comorbidity in people with Down's syndrome: A criteria-based analysis. *Journal of Intellectual Disability Research, 40*, 385–399.

van Trotsenburg, A. S., Heymans, H. S., Tijssen, J. G., de Vijlder, J. J., & Vulsma, T. (2006). Comorbidity, hospitalization, and medication use and their influence on mental and motor development of young infants with Down syndrome. *Pediatrics, 118*, 1633–1639.

Viola, G., & Rosano, A. (2005). Time trend of survival among infants with Down's syndrome. *Italian Journal of Pediatrics, 31*, 254–260.

Weijerman, M. E., van Furth, A. M., Vonk Noordegraaf, A., van Wouwe, J. P., Broers, C. J., & Gemke, R. J. (2008). Prevalence, neonatal characteristics, and first-year mortality of Down syndrome: a national study. *The Journal Of Pediatrics, 152*, 15–19.

Whitaker, R. C., Wright, J. A., Pepe, M. S., Seidl, K. D., & Dietz, W. H. (1997). Predicting obesity in young adulthood from childhood and parental obesity. *The New England Journal of Medicine, 337*, 869–873.

Whitlock, J. A., Sather, H. N., Gaynon, P., Robison, L. L., Wells, R. J., Trigg, M., et al. (2005). Clinical characteristics and outcome of children with Down syndrome and acute lymphoblastic leukemia: A children's cancer group study. *Blood, 106*, 4043–4049.

Whitt-Glover, M. C., O'Neill, K. L., & Stettler, N. (2006). Physical activity patterns in children with and without Down Syndrome. *Pediatric Rehabilitation, 9*, 158–164.

Williams, K., Leonard, H., d'Espaignet., T., Calvin, L., Slack-Smith, L., & Stanley, F. (2005). Hospitalisations from birth to five years in a population cohort of Western Australian children with intellectual disability. *Archives Of Disease In Childhood, 90*, 1243–1248.

Wilson, M. G., Chan, L. S., & Herbert, W. S. (1992). Birth prevalence of Down syndrome in a predominantly Latino population: A 15-year study. *Teratology, 45*, 285–292.

Woodhouse, J. M., Pakeman, V. H., Cregg, M., et al. (1997). Refractive errors in young children with Down syndrome. *Optometry and Vision Science, 74*, 844–851.

Wortelboer, M.J.M., Wolf, B.T.H.M.d., Verschuuren-Bemelmans, C. C., Reefhuis, J., Mantingh, A., Beekhuis, J. R., et al. (2000). Trends in live birth prevalence of Down syndrome in the Northern Netherlands 1987–96: The impact of screening and prenatal diagnosis. *Prenatal Diagnosis, 20*, 709–713.

Xavier, A. C., Ge, Y., & Taub, J. W. (2009). Down syndrome and malignancies: a unique clinical relationship: a paper from the 2008 William Beaumont Hospital Symposium on molecular pathology. *Journal of Molecular Diagnostics, 11*, 371–380.

Yam, W. (2008). Medical issues among children and teenagers with Down syndrome in Hong Kong. *Down's Syndrome, Research and Practice, 12*, 138–140.

Zachor, D. A., Mroczek-Musulman, E., and Brown, P. (2000). Prevalence of celiac disease in Down syndrome in the United States. *Journal Of Pediatric Gastroenterology and Nutrition, 31*, 275–279.

Zeller, B., Gustafsson, G., Forestier, E., Abrahamsson, J., Clausen, N., Heldrup, J., et al. (2005). Acute leukaemia in children with Down syndrome: a population-based Nordic study. *British Journal of Haematology, 128*, 797–804.

CHAPTER FOUR

Health Conditions Associated with Aging and End of Life of Adults with Down Syndrome

Anna J. Esbensen

Contents

Abstract

Expectations for the life course of individuals with Down syndrome (DS) have changed, with life expectancy estimates increasing from 12 in 1949 to nearly 60 years of age today (Bittles & Glasson, 2004; Penrose, 1949). Along with this longer life expectancy comes a larger population of adults with DS who display premature age-related changes in their health. There is thus a need to provide specialized health care to this aging population of adults with DS who are at

Cincinnati Children's Hospital Medical Center, Division of Developmental and Behavioral Pediatrics, Cincinnati, OH, USA

International Review of Research in Mental Retardation, Volume 39
ISSN 0074-7750, DOI 10.1016/S0074-7750(10)39004-5

high risk for some conditions and at lower risk for others. This review focuses on the rates and contributing factors to medical conditions that are common in adults with DS or that show changes with age. The review of medical conditions includes the increased risk for skin and hair changes, early-onset menopause, visual and hearing impairments, adult-onset seizure disorder, thyroid dysfunction, diabetes, obesity, sleep apnea, and musculoskeletal problems. The different pattern of conditions associated with the mortality of adults with DS is also reviewed.

A highly significant change in the survival of people with Down syndrome (DS) has occurred during the last two generations. In the 1940s, the average life expectancy for individuals with DS was 12 years (Penrose, 1949). With medical breakthroughs and improvements in services, individuals with DS now enjoy life expectancies into their 60s (Bittles & Glasson, 2004). As a result, we are now witness to the first generation of individuals with DS who have benefited from a revolution during their lifetime of better knowledge, health care, advocacy, and services (Yang, Rasmussen, & Friedman, 2002). Along with this longer life expectancy comes a larger population of adults with DS who display premature age-related changes in their health. There is thus a need to provide specialized health care to this aging population of adults with DS who are at high risk for some conditions and at lower risk for others. Adults with DS are at age-related increased risk for dementia, skin and hair changes, early-onset menopause, visual and hearing impairments, adult-onset seizure disorder, thyroid dysfunction, diabetes, obesity, sleep apnea, and musculoskeletal problems. Along with these increased risks for some conditions comes a different pattern of conditions associated with the mortality of adults with DS. This review focuses on the rates and contributing factors to medical conditions that are common in adults with DS or that show changes with age.

1. Skin and Hair Changes

Adults with DS experience a number of dermatological and autoimmune symptoms characteristic of accelerated aging, including premature graying of the hair, hair loss, and wrinkling of the skin (Lott & Lai, 1982). Significant differences in the skin and chronological age of the individual have been found in post-mortem examinations of the skin of adults with DS (Edwards, 1978). Further, sun-exposure may have a greater effect on skin wrinkling for individuals with DS than for the general population, contributing to the appearance of premature skin aging in adults with DS (Brugge, Grove, Clopton, Grove, & Piacquadio, 1993).

Alopecia areata (the loss of hair) is estimated to affect between 6 and 18.4% of adults with DS (du Vivier & Munro, 1975; Prasher, 1994b). In comparison, only 0.1% of individuals with intellectual disability (ID) and 0.1–0.2% of the general population are affected by alopecia areata (du Vivier & Munro, 1975; Safavi, Muller, Suman, Moshell, & Melton, 1995). It is posited that this elevated rate of alopecia areata in adults with DS may be related to immunological deficiency in thymus-dependent function (Carter & Jegasothy, 1976).

Other skin conditions common in adults with DS include atopic dermatitis, fungal infections, seborrhoeic dermatitis, and xerosis, affecting 34–39% of adults (Kerins, Petrovic, Bruder, & Gruman, 2008; Prasher, 1994b; Roizen & Patterson, 2003). These skin conditions are found in higher rates among older than younger adults with DS, and may be due in part to declines in self-care associated with memory loss and dementia that are common in the aging of adults with DS (Kerins et al., 2008).

Several theories have been proposed to account for the premature aging observed in adults with DS. The DNA damage theory of aging focuses on aging as a consequence of unrepaired DNA damage accumulation. The DNA damage theory is supported by lower levels of DNA repair enzymes being found in adults with DS (Madan, Williams, & Lear, 2006). An alternate theory focuses on free-radical metabolism which involves a key enzyme, CuZn superoxide dismutase, which is located on chromosome 21 (Druzhyna, Nair, LeDoux, & Wilson, 1998). Over-expression of this enzyme leads to the altered structure and function of tissue (Sinha, 2005).

2. Menopause

Women with DS are found to experience menopause starting at an earlier age than other women with ID and than women in the general population (Carr & Hollins, 1995; Cosgrave, Tyrrell, McCarron, Gill, & Lawlor, 1999; Schupf et al., 1997). An early report found that 87% of women with DS and 69% of women with ID had stopped menstruating by age 46. All women with DS had stopped menstruating by the age of 51, and all of the women with ID by age 54. An estimate of the median age at menopause for women with DS of 47.1 is 2 years younger than the estimated median age for women with ID of 49.3 (Schupf et al., 1997). These estimates among women with DS and ID are potentially under-estimates as the proportion of women who had never menstruated in the sample was unknown. A recent prospective study using multiple methods of analysis of the age at menopause for women with DS, all of whom had a history of menstruation, reported a median age of 45.8–47.1 (Seltzer, Schupf, & Wu, 2001). No woman with DS older than 52 was menstruating. In comparison, the age at menopause in the general population is 51.3, with perimenopause starting at 47.5 (McKinlay, Brambilla, & Posner, 1992), indicating that women with DS have a median age of menopause that is 4–6 years earlier than women in the general population.

The earlier onset of menopause in women with DS has implications for their health as menopause is a risk factor for heart disease, depression, osteoporosis, breast-cancer, and dementia in the general population (Harlow & Ephross, 1995), and is associated with cognitive declines and dementia in women with DS (Patel, Seltzer, Wu, & Schupf, 2001; Schupf et al., 2003). Some studies have found thyroid deficiency contributing to earlier onset of menopause (Carr & Hollins, 1995), whereas others have not replicated the findings in part due to appropriate thyroid treatment being available to the women sampled (Schupf et al., 1997; Seltzer et al., 2001). As such, the contribution of thyroid conditions to earlier menopause is still uncertain.

3. Vision Impairments

Visual impairments (44–71%) and eye abnormalities are common among aging adults with DS (Gardiner, 1967; Jacobson, 1988; McCarron, Gill, McCallion, & Begley, 2005). The prevalence of visual impairments does not appear to be related to level of intellectual functioning among individuals with DS, and is greater than the prevalence (8–50%) observed in older adults with ID without DS (Gardiner, 1967; Haveman, Maaskant, & Sturmans, 1989; Janicki & Jacobson, 1986; Moss, 1991). Comparable to visual acuity in the general population, visual impairment deteriorates among adults with DS, with the prevalence of severe visual impairment increasing from 18% among 30–39 year olds to 28% among 40–49 year olds and to 45% among 50–59 year olds (Van Buggenhout et al., 1999). Of greater concern than the prevalence of visual impairment are reports of only 53% of cases of impairment being diagnosed, and only 50% of individuals with DS receiving correction for their visual impairment (Jacobson, 1988).

Cataracts (11–33%), strabismus (23–37%), refraction problems (30–34%), and keratoconus (15%) are common ophthalmological problems (Aitchison, Easty, & Jancar, 1990; Prasher, 1994b; Van Allen, Fung, & Jurenka, 1999; Van Buggenhout et al., 1999). A small study of 19 adults with DS over the age of 40 reported even higher rates of ophthalmological problems, with 55% suffering from strabismus and 75% from refraction problems (Hesmes, Sand, & Fostad, 1991). The prevalence of cataracts is greater in adults than in children with DS and is comparable to or higher than the prevalence of 17% found in adults in the general population

(Congdon et al., 2004). Higher rates of cataracts among adults with DS have been reported (30–68%), with few warranting surgery (Hesmes et al., 1991; Pueschel, 1990; Van Allen et al., 1999). Even when surgery is performed, visual problems and impairments may persist related to aphakia (absence of the lens of the eye) and to poor use of bifocals (Van Allen et al., 1999). Senile cataracts appear to develop earlier in adults with DS than in the general population and increase in prevalence with age (Pueschel, 1990; Robb & Marchevsky, 1978; Van Allen et al., 1999). These senile cataracts, characterized by a gradual thickening of the lens, tends to occur at a younger age in DS compared to other individuals with ID, possibly due to the accelerated aging process present in individuals with DS and the increased amounts of free-radical reactions (Ellis, 2002).

Keratoconus, a deterioration of the structure of the cornea with gradual bulging from the normal round shape to a cone shape, also increases in prevalence with age, from 11% in middle-age to 20% in the elderly (Van Allen et al., 1999). One small study reported that 37% of adults over the age of 40 had keratoconus (Hesmes et al., 1991).

4. Hearing Impairments

Age-related hearing loss is more common among adults with DS compared to the general population, and appears to have an earlier age of onset. High-frequency sensorineural hearing impairments (such as presbycusis) in adults with DS onsets about 20–30 years earlier than in their peers with ID, and about 30–40 years earlier than in the general population (Buchanan, 1990). Rates of hearing loss among adults with DS range from 12 to 72% (Howells, 1989; Prasher, 1994b; Van Buggenhout et al., 1999), and may depend on the nature of the hearing assessment. Using detailed audiometric methods, Van Buggenhout et al. (1999) found 53% of adults with DS to have moderate hearing loss, 17% to have a severe hearing loss, and 2% to have a profound hearing loss. These rates of hearing loss were reported to increase with age and the hearing loss to become more severe (Buchanan, 1990; Van Buggenhout et al., 1999). While the rate of hearing loss is not related to level of ID, it has been found to be higher among adults with co-morbid dementia (McCarron et al., 2005).

Howells (1989) reported that 55% of adults over age 21 may have sensorineural hearing loss. For adults over 35 years of age, 68% of ears tested were reported to have cochlear hearing loss, with conductive hearing loss found in 5% of ears and mixed hearing loss found in 13% of ears (Evenhuis, Van Zanten, Procaar, & Roerdinkholder, 1992). Van Buggenhout et al. (1999) similarly found a low rate of conductive hearing loss (10%) in their sample of adults with DS, and a comparable number with sensorineural and mixed hearing loss (45 and 44%, respectively). However, Evenhuis et al. (1992) argues that we do not know how much the rate and degree of hearing impairment in adults with DS is related to previous middle ear pathology, such as otitis media. With the life expectancy of adults with DS growing longer, it is important to understand how medical conditions common early in the life course may influence the health of the individual later in life.

While hearing impairments are common among adults with DS, few are identified or treated. Of individuals identified with hearing impairments during research testing who did not use hearing devices, 80% of their care providers and general practitioners were unaware of the hearing loss (Van Buggenhout et al., 1999). Additionally, only 41% of individuals with hearing impairments identified during research testing were using hearing devices (Van Buggenhout et al., 1999). Half of this sample had severe to profound ID which may have contributed to a difficulty in using hearing devices.

5. Seizure Disorder

The rate of seizures increases with age for individuals with DS, especially for individuals suffering from comorbid dementia. Early reports of the rate of seizures were significantly lower than more recent prevalence estimates. One early estimate of the rate of seizures was 12.2% for adults with DS over the age of 55 and 15.8% for adults over the age of 60 (Veall, 1974). However, early estimates were consistent with more recent estimates that abnormal readings reflective of seizure activity are high, with 71.4% of adults over 55 showing this abnormal activity (Tangye, 1979). Although these early reports underestimated current prevalence estimates, perhaps consistent with the shorter life expectancy of the time, these studies consistently reported a rise in the rate of seizures with age from adolescents to young adults to later adulthood. This increase in the rate of seizures across the lifespan is supported by other later research. Cohort differences show that 8% of adolescents or young adults with DS suffer from seizures as compared to 24–28% of seniors aged 50 and older (Johannsen, Christensen, Goldstein, Nielsen, & Mai, 1996; McDermott et al., 2005). McVicker, Shanks, and McClelland (1994) also supported a lower rate of seizures among younger individuals (7%) as compared to adults older than 50 (46%). A lifespan study of individuals with DS found that approximately 8% of individuals with DS suffer from seizures, and of these 40% experienced seizures after the age of 20 (Pueschel, Louis, & McKnight, 1991). The higher rate of seizures observed in individuals with DS may be related to the gene for myoclonus epilepsy being mapped to chromosome 21;

however, this form of seizure is more commonly found in children and adolescents (Hattori et al., 2006). Older patients with DS typically have tonic–clonic (formerly known as grand mal), complex partial or simple partial seizures (Pueschel et al., 1991). Alternatively, structural abnormalities and biochemical aberrations of the CNS in adults with DS may in part be responsible for increased seizure frequency (Pueschel et al., 1991).

The increase in seizures related to age parallels the increase in the general population, although the rate of seizures is lower in the general population than among individual with DS (McDermott et al., 2005). However, it should be noted that the rate of seizure activity among individuals with DS is lower than the reported rate among individuals with ID in general (McDermott et al., 2005). More recent estimates of the rate of seizures among adults with DS range from 9.4 to 26.5%, with a mean onset of seizures over the age of 30, around age 37 (Johannsen et al., 1996; McDermott et al., 2005; McVicker et al., 1994; Puri, Ho, & Singh, 2001).

In addition to increasing with age, the rate of epilepsy and seizures is also related to the onset of dementia among adults with DS (Prasher & Corbett, 1993; Puri et al., 2001). In one study, 80% of the adults with seizures also presented with symptoms consistent with a clinical diagnosis of dementia (McVicker et al., 1994). In another study, 53% of individuals with dementia were reported to have seizures and the onset of seizures appeared to presage the onset of cognitive deterioration and symptoms of dementia (Lott & Lai, 1982). Indeed, the onset of seizures has been reported to occur at a younger age for individuals with DS who do not suffer from dementia (age 29) as compared to those who do (age 45). Dementia may be an important risk factor for late-onset seizures in adults with DS, but not for the high rate of seizures among all individuals with DS (Menéndez, 2005).

6. Thyroid Dysfunction

Comparable to how the rate of seizures increases with age in adults with DS, the rate of individuals with DS at risk for thyroid disease also increases with age (Korsager, Chatham, & Ostergaard-Kristensen, 1978), although some samples have indicated no increase with age (Murdoch, Ratcliffe, McLarty, Rodger, & Ratcliffe, 1977; Šare, Ruvalcaba, & Kelley, 1978). Approximately 35–40% of adults with DS are reported to have abnormal thyroid function, although only 7–8% had active hypothyroidism (Dinani & Carpenter, 1990; Prasher, 1994a, b). Also comparable to seizure findings, the rate of thyroid disease in adults with DS is greater than that found in the general population (Coleman, 1994).

The high rate of abnormal thyroid function highlights the need for consistent and routine monitoring of thyroid functioning for adults with DS. Routine monitoring is particularly important as some individuals tested with abnormal thyroid functioning were identified with thyroid disease and were receiving too much or too little medication to manage their disease (Prasher, 1994a).

7. Other Medical Conditions

7.1. Diabetes

There are a few reports of an increased risk of Type 1 diabetes among individuals with DS and of increased risk of mortality due to Type 1 diabetes as compared to the general population (Anwar, Walker, & Frier, 1998; Hill et al., 2003). The age of onset of Type 1 diabetes appears to be increasing in individuals with DS. Earlier studies of Type 1 diabetes from the 1960s focused on children (Burch & Milunsky, 1969; Farquhar, 1962; Milunsky & Neurath, 1968) and reported that the age of onset peaked at 8 years of age for individuals with DS. However, the life expectancy of individuals with DS in the 1960s was 18 years (Collmann & Stoller, 1963). With increasing life expectancies for individuals with DS, more recent age of onset estimates of 22 years are comparable to the onset of type 1 diabetes in the general population (Anwar et al., 1998) and consistent with more individuals being diagnosed with adult-onset diabetes than juvenile diabetes. However, contrary reports suggest that adults with DS are at lower risk for mortality due to Type 1 diabetes than the general population and than adults with ID due to other causes (Haveman et al., 1989; Yang et al., 2002). Few reports are available regarding Type 2 diabetes in adults with DS, but the rate reported in a preliminary report appears to be lower than that in the general population (Silverman, 2010). There is a need for more detailed population studies on the rate of Type 1 and Type 2 diabetes in individuals with DS to confirm these findings.

7.2. Obesity

A significant proportion of adults with DS are reported to be overweight or obese according to the body mass index (BMI). Between 45 and 79% of males and between 56 and 96% of females with DS are reported to be overweight (Bell & Bhate, 1992; Melville, Cooper, McGrother, Thorp, & Collacott, 2005; Prasher, 1995; Rubin, Rimmer, Chicoine, Braddock, & McGuire, 1998), while the prevalence in the general population that is overweight was reported to be approximately a third during the time period of these studies (Rubin et al., 1998). Contributing factors to the high rate of overweight and obese individuals with DS may include a combination of eating behavior, intake, metabolic rate, hypothyroidism, and reduced exercise (Prasher, 1995).

BMIs are found to increase with age in the general population. Conversely, BMIs of cohorts of adults with DS are observed to be smaller with increasing age (Prasher, 1995; Rubin et al., 1998). Contributing factors to the lower BMIs found in older adults with DS are speculative, but may include residential setting and healthier weights contributing to longevity (Rubin et al., 1998).

7.3. Sleep apnea

Obstructive sleep apnea (OSA) is present in approximately 30–55% of children with DS (de Miguel-Díez, Villa-Asensi, & Álvarez-Sala, 2003; Stebbens, Dennis, Samuels, Croft, & Southall, 1991). The known risk factors for OSA in children include facial (midfacial hypoplasia, mandibular hypoplasia) and other physical features (glossoptosis, an abnormally small upper airway, superficially positioned tonsils, relative tonsillar and adenoidal encroachment, hypotonia of upper airway) (Marcus, Keens, Bautista, von Pechmann, & Ward, 1991; Roizen & Patterson, 2003). Other risk factors have yet to be identified. Adults with DS are at increased risk for OSA as these risk factors observed in children continue into adulthood, and other risk factors become more prevalent. Obesity (reviewed previously) is a risk factor for OSA that puts adults with DS at increased risk for developing this disorder. The rate of hypothyroidism (reviewed previously) increases with age in adults with DS, and is associated with OSA. The few studies that have examined the rate of OSA among adults with DS report that up to 94% of adults suffer from the disorder (Trois et al., 2009). Despite the increase in the number of risk factors predisposing adults with DS to OSA, increasing age is found to be the strongest risk factor, particularly when other risk factors are not present (Resta et al., 2003).

7.4. Musculoskeletal

Musculoskeletal problems often result from premature degenerative bone and joint disease (Dacre & Huskisson, 1988; Olive, Whitecloud, & Bennet, 1988). Osteoporosis is common among adults with DS and adults are at greater risk as they age (Center, Beange, & McElduff, 1998). There are several factors that may contribute to this increased risk for osteoporosis in adults with DS, including early menopause, deceased physical activity, low muscle tone, and decreased strength. Degenerative osteoarthritis is also common among adults with DS, with osteoarthritis of the spine affecting 22% of middle-age adults and 40% of elderly adults (Van Allen et al., 1999).

Typical symptoms include numbness, weakness, and pain. It is often difficult to detect these symptoms in individuals with ID, and thus the rate of degenerative osteoarthritis may be underreported. Orthopedic problems, such as flat feet (a congenital condition), are the most common musculoskeletal abnormality observed in adults with DS, affecting approximately 70% of individuals (Prasher, 1994b).

7.5. Mitral valve prolapse

Mitral valve prolapse is common among adults with DS, occurring in between 46 and 57% of individuals (Barnhart & Connolly, 2007; Roizen & Patterson, 2003). Even though children with DS have a high risk of congenital heart disease, this previous cardiac pathology is not linked to the high rate of mitral valve prolapse later in life. Early signs of mitral valve prolapse are comparable to those observed in the general population and include fatigue, weight gain, and irritability (Barnhart & Connolly, 2007).

8. Mortality

Health problems present in adults, reviewed earlier in this chapter such as sensory handicaps, thyroid disorders, and degenerative spine disease, may contribute to the earlier mortality observed in adults with DS (Kapell et al., 1998; Lantman-de Valk, Haveman, & Crebolder, 1996). However, their direct effect on mortality is not yet well documented. The life expectancy of adults with DS has a similar pattern until the age of 40 as compared to their age peers with other types of ID, and elevated mortality rates thereafter (Haveman et al., 1989; Maaskant, Gevers, & Wierda, 2002; Strauss & Eyman, 1996).

The life expectancy of adults with DS is increasing and now averages around the mid- to late-50s. Still, this life expectancy is substantially below that of the general population and that of their peers with ID (Glasson et al., 2002; Janicki, Dalton, Henderson, & Davidson, 1999). Also, while women with DS are observed to have shorter life expectancies than men with DS, the opposite pattern is seen in the general population and among individuals with other types of ID (Carter & Jancar, 1983; Glasson et al., 2002; Glasson et al., 2003; Tyrer, Smith, & McGrother, 2007). A gender difference in mortality among individuals with DS is still speculative as other studies have not replicated this finding (Day, Strauss, Shavelle, & Reynolds, 2005; Janicki et al., 1999). If valid, earlier menopause may be a contributing factor to earlier mortality in women with DS as compared to men with DS (Schupf et al., 1997).

The evidence is mixed regarding other risk factors found to predict mortality of adults with DS. Some studies have found that functional abilities predict mortality in adults with DS (Chaney & Eyman, 2000; Esbensen, Seltzer, & Greenberg, 2007; Eyman, Call, & White, 1991; Strauss & Zigman, 1996), comparable to findings in their peers with ID (Bittles et al., 2002; Strauss & Eyman, 1996). Prior levels of functional abilities and declines in functional abilities were found to predict mortality in a sample of adults with and without DS (Esbensen et al., 2007). However, the relationship between functional abilities and mortality among adults with DS is not always supported (Glasson et al., 2002; Strauss & Eyman, 1996; Strauss & Zigman, 1996). Age has consistently been found to be a predictor of mortality for adults with DS (Esbensen et al., 2007; Eyman, Call, & White, 1989; Hayden, 1998), and new research suggests that worsening of behavior problems is another predictor of mortality (Esbensen et al., 2007).

Common causes of death in this population include leukemia, respiratory illness, congenital circulatory defects, diseases of the digestive system, dementia, and Alzheimer's disease, and are reported to vary with age (Day et al., 2005; Hermon, Alberman, Beral, & Swerdlow, 2001; Hill et al., 2003; Thase, 1982). Although a common cause of death among children with DS is leukemia (behind respiratory illness and congenital heart defects), this risk is found to decrease with age (Hasle, Clemmensen, & Mikkelsen, 2000; Yang et al., 2002). In contrast, the risk of mortality due to cancer in adults with DS is equal to or lower than that in the general population or among their peers with ID (Day et al., 2005; Hasle et al., 2000; Patja, Eero, & Iivanainen, 2001a; Sullivan, Hussain, Glasson, & Bittles, 2007; Yang et al., 2002). In particular, the risk of mortality due to solid tumors among adults with DS is considerably lower than among their peers and the general population (Hasle et al., 2000; Hill et al., 2003; Sullivan, et al., 2007). In contrast, the risk for dementia was found to increase with age (Yang et al., 2002). Respiratory problems, congenital anomalies (other than congenital heart anomalies), and ischemic heart disease were also found to vary with age in their relation to mortality in individuals with DS. Among older adults with DS, respiratory problems and congenital anomalies are reported to be more common and ischemic heart disease less common than expected (Yang et al., 2002). That cardiovascular and circulatory defects are common causes of death among individuals with DS is not unexpected given the biological phenotype of this syndrome (Roizen, 1996). In comparison, the common causes of mortality found among individuals with ID include cardiovascular diseases, respiratory diseases, and cancers (Patja, Mölsä, & Iivanainen, 2001b), and these have been found to be comparable to causes of mortality among a sample of only adults with DS (Esbensen et al., 2007).

9. Medical Conditions with Low Risk

While adults with DS are at risk for several medical conditions just described, they are also at low risk for other medical conditions. In a review of cancers among individuals with DS, malignant solid tumors were reported to be underrepresented (Satgé et al., 1998). In particular, common epithelial tumors were underrepresented in adults, as are breast, uterine, digestive, genital, skin, bronchial, ear/nose/throat, or urinary tract cancers (Hasle et al., 2000; Hill et al., 2003; Jancar & Jancar, 1976; Oster, Mikkelsen, & Nielsen, 1975; Scholl, Stein, & Hansen, 1982). However, a greater risk for testicular cancer has been reported among males with DS as compared to typically developing males (Dieckmann, Rube, & Henke, 1997; Hasle et al., 2000).

Possible explanations for the decreased risk of some cancers among adults with DS are that accurate population morbidity studies are rare. It has also been proposed that individuals with DS may be less exposed to environmental contributors to cancer risk (Satgé et al., 1998). Decreased alcohol and tobacco use, early menopause and other lifestyle and environmental factors may contribute to lower cancer risk. However, obesity and the lack of physical activity common in adults with DS would contribute to an increased risk of cancers. The shorter life expectancy of individuals with DS has also been suggested to contribute to lower risk for cancer (Satgé et al., 1998). However, as the life expectancy of individuals with DS has increased dramatically over the last few decades, shorter life expectancy becomes a less probable explanation for the apparent lower risk of solid tumors. Several tumor-suppressor genes have been identified on chromosome 21, potentially contributing to the decreased risks for many solid tumors (Lee, Park, Park, & Park, 2003). Copper-zinc superoxide dismutase, also located on chromosome 21, and its contribution to the metabolism of oxygen free radicals are further hypothesized to reduce the risk of carcinogens (De La Torre et al., 1996).

While the rate of mitral valve prolapse is high, there is a lower risk for cardiovascular and cerebrovascular disease observed in adults with DS as compared to the general population (Marino & Pueschel, 1996) and lower rates of emphysema, fractures, hypercholesterolemia, and heart disease as compared to adults with ID due to other causes (Haveman et al., 1989; Kerins et al., 2008). Further, individuals with DS are found to have lower resting heart rates and lower blood pressure than the general population (Prasher, 1994b; Richards & Enver, 1979). The rise in blood pressure seen with age in the general population is not as great among individuals with DS, and hypertension is an uncommon problem reported in adults with DS (Kerins et al., 2008; Prasher, 1994b).

While upper respiratory infections are common among adults with DS, significant respiratory problems are not common (Minihan & Dean, 1990; Prasher, 1994b; Wilson & Haire, 1990). Further, as mobility declines with age, recurrent pneumonia with incomplete recovery has been found to occur more often (Van Allen et al., 1999). This is particularly noteworthy as respiratory illness is a common cause of mortality in adults with DS. It may be that chronic respiratory problems contribute to mortality more so than acute respiratory problems.

10. Health Care

There are excellent guidelines for the health care of individuals with DS across the lifespan, including guidelines specific to adults (Cohen, 2002). They provide recommendations to health care professionals of what conditions to screen for and how frequently. However, little is known about the pattern of screening, health care use and access, or barriers to health care experienced by adults with DS specifically, although efforts are currently being made to explore these questions.

The literature on health care service use by adults with ID indicates that this population experiences significant health disparities in access to health care in comparison to the general population (Horwitz, Kerker, Owens, & Zigler, 2000). As an example, few adults with ID receive care from specialists despite a high percentage of individuals, such as individuals with DS, having medical needs that require specialty care. An agenda has been set by the federal government for promoting the health of individuals with ID, improving their quality of and access to health care, and training health care providers to the specific needs of individuals with ID (U.S. Public Health Service, 2001).

11. Conclusions

As individuals with DS continue to experience longer lives, the need to understand their aging and associated health conditions becomes more critical. The chronic disorders that onset in adults with DS, and the age-related change in other disorders, have important implications for health care management of this aging population. Health care providers need to be informed of the health conditions more common among adults with DS as they age, to be alert for declines earlier than expected in the general population, and the implication that early-life medical conditions may have in the later life of the individual. For example, chronic and inadequately treated middle ear infections in childhood may have an impact on later hearing loss in adults with DS.

The different pattern of health conditions in aging adults with DS also has implications for family members and support providers. Over 60% of adults with ID co-reside with their families (Fujiura, 1998). As such, families and support providers of adults with DS need to be informed of what symptoms to be alert for in order to better communicate changes in health to medical providers, such as lethargy, irritability, and fatigue. The health care provider is then responsible for determining whether these common symptoms are due to hypothyroidism, mitral valve prolapse, symptoms of menopause, pain, poor sleep, or to depression resulting from disorientation due to sensory impairments. Deteriorations in health can also be associated with an increase in behaviors, particularly if the individual with DS has communication difficulties in expressing problems or medical complaints. And finally, adults with DS should be provided with appropriate information to better understand, and counseling to cope with, changes in their own level of ability or health.

Acknowledgments

This manuscript was prepared with support from the National Institute on Child Health and Human Development (R03 HD59848).

REFERENCES

Aitchison, C., Easty, D. L., & Jancar, J. (1990). Eye abnormalities in the mentally handicapped. *Journal of Mental Deficiency Research*, *34*, 41–48.

Anwar, A. J., Walker, J. D., & Frier, B. M. (1998). Type 1 diabetes mellitus and Down's syndrome: Prevalence, management and diabetic complications. *Diabetic Medicine*, *15*, 160–163.

Barnhart, R. C., & Connolly, B. (2007). Aging and Down syndrome: Implications for physical therapy. *Physical Therapy*, *87*, 1399–1406.

Bell, A. J., & Bhate, M. S. (1992). Prevalence of overweight and obesity in Down syndrome and other mentally handicapped adults living in the community. *Journal of Intellectual Disability Research*, *36*, 359–364.

Bittles, A. H., & Glasson, E. J. (2004). Clinical, social, and ethical implications of changing life expectancy in Down syndrome. *Developmental Medicine and Child Neurology*, *46*, 282–286.

Bittles, A. H., Petterson, B. A., Sullivan, S. G., Hussain, R., Glasson, E. J., & Montgomery, P. D. (2002). The influence of intellectual disability on life expectancy. *Journal of Gerontology: Medical Sciences*, *57A*, M470–M472.

Brugge, K. L., Grove, G. L., Clopton, P., Grove, M. J., & Piacquadio, D. J. (1993). Evidence for accelerated skin wrinkling among developmentally delayed individuals with Down's syndrome. *Mechanics of Ageing and Development*, *70*, 213–225.

Buchanan, L. H. (1990). Early onset of presbyacusis in Down syndrome. *Scandinavian Audiology, 19*, 103–110.

Burch, P. R. J., & Milunsky, A. (1969). Early-onset diabetes mellitus in the general and Down's syndrome populations: Genetics, aetiology, and pathogenesis. *The Lancet, 293*, 554–558.

Carr, J., & Hollins, S. (1995). Menopause in women with learning disabilities. *Journal of Intellectual Disability Research, 39*, 137–139.

Carter, D. M., & Jegasothy, B. V. (1976). Alopecia areata and Down syndrome. *Archives of Dermatology, 112*, 1397–1399.

Carter, G., & Jancar, J. (1983). Mortality in the mentally handicapped: A 50 year survey at the Stoke Park group of hospitals (1930–1980). *Journal of Mental Deficiency Research, 27*, 143–156.

Center, J., Beange, H., & McElduff, A. (1998). People with mental retardation have an increased prevalence of osteoporosis: a population study. *American Journal on Mental Retardation, 103*, 19–28.

Chaney, R. H., & Eyman, R. K. (2000). Patterns in mortality over 60 years among persons with mental retardation in a residential facility. *Mental Retardation, 38*, 289–293.

Cohen, W. I. (2002). Health care guidelines for individuals with Down syndrome—1999 revision. In W. I. Cohen, L. Nadel, & M. E. Madnick (Eds.), *A Vision for the 21st Century: Down Syndrome* (pp. 237–245). New York, NY: Wiley-Liss.

Coleman, M. (1994). Thyroid dysfunction in Down's syndrome: A review. *Down Syndrome Research and Practice, 2*, 112–115.

Collmann, R. D., & Stoller, A. (1963). Data on mongolism in Victoria, Australia: Prevalence and life expectation. *Journal of Mental Deficiency Research, 17*, 117–122.

Congdon, N., Vingerling, J. R., Klein, B. E., West, S., Friedman, D. S., Kempen, J., O'Colmain, B., Wu, S. Y., & Taylor, H. R. (2004). Prevalence of cataract and pseudophakia/aphakia among adults in the United States. *Archives of Ophthalmology, 122*, 487–494.

Cosgrave, M. P., Tyrrell, J., McCarron, M., Gill, M., & Lawlor, B. A. (1999). Age at onset of dementia and age of menopause in women with Down's syndrome. *Journal of Intellectual Disability Research, 43*, 461–465.

Dacre, J. E., & Huskisson, E. D. (1988). Arthritis in Down syndrome. *Annals of Rheumatic Disease, 47*, 254–255.

Day, S. M., Strauss, D. J., Shavelle, R. M., & Reynolds, R. J. (2005). Mortality and causes of death in persons with Down syndrome in California. *Developmental Medicine and Child Neurology, 47*, 171–176.

De La Torre, R., Casado, A., Lopez-Fernández, E., Carrascosa, D., Ramirez, V., & Saez, J. (1996). Overexpression of copper-zinc superoxide dismutase in trisomy 21. *Experientia, 52*, 871–873.

Dieckmann, K. P., Rube, C., & Henke, R. P. (1997). Association of Down's syndrome and testicular cancer. *Journal of Urology 157*, 1701–1704.

Dinani, S., & Carpenter, S. (1990). Down's syndrome and thyroid disorder. *Journal of Mental Deficiency Research, 34*, 187–193.

Druzhyna, N., Nair, R. G., LeDoux, S. P., & Wilson, G. L. (1998). Defective repair of oxidative damage in mitochondrial DNA in Down's syndrome. *Mutation Research, 409*, 81–89.

Edwards, J. S. H. (1978). Skin age in Down's syndrome: A note on the findings of Murdoch and Evans. *Journal of Mental Deficiency Research, 22*, 223.

Ellis, F. J. (2002). Management of pediatric cataract and lens opacities. *Current Opinion in Pediatrics, 13*, 33–37.

Esbensen, A. J., Seltzer, M. M., & Greenberg, J. S. (2007). Factors predicting mortality in midlife adults with and without Down syndrome living with family. *Journal of Intellectual Disability Research, 51*, 1039–1050.

Evenhuis, H. M., Van Zanten, G. A., Brocaar, M. P., & Roerdinkholder, W. H. M. (1992). Hearing loss in middle-age persons with Down syndrome. *American Journal on Mental Retardation, 97*, 47–56.

Eyman, R. K., Call, T. L., & White, J. F. (1989). Mortality of elderly mentally retarded persons in California. *Journal of Applied Gerontology, 8*, 203–215.
Eyman, R. K., Call, T. L., & White, J. F. (1991). Life expectancy of persons with Down syndrome. *American Journal on Mental Retardation, 95*, 603–612.
Farquhar, J. W. (1962). Diabetic children in Scotland and the need for care. *Scottish Medical Journal, 7*, 119–124.
Fujiura, G. T. (1998). Demography of family households. *American Journal on Mental Retardation, 103*, 225–235.
Gardiner, P. A. (1967). Visual defects in cases of Down's syndrome and in other mentally handicapped children. *British Journal of Ophthalmology, 51*, 469–474.
Glasson, E. J., Sullivan, S. G., Hussain, R., Petterson, B. A., Montgomery, P. D., & Bittles, A. H. (2002). The changing survival profile of people with Down's syndrome: Implications for genetic counselling. *Clinical Genetics, 62*, 390–393.
Glasson, E. J., Sullivan, S. G., Hussain, R., Petterson, B. A., Montgomery, P. D., & Bittles, A. H. (2003). Comparative survival advantage of males with Down syndrome. *American Journal of Human Biology, 15*, 192–195.
Harlow, S. D., & Ephross, S. A. (1995). Epidemiology of menstruation and its relevance to women's health. *Epidemiologic Reviews, 17*, 265–286.
Hasle, H., Clemmensen, I. H., & Mikkelsen, M. (2000). Risks of leukaemia and solid tumors in individuals with Down's syndrome. *Lancet, 355*, 165–169.
Hattori, M., Fujiyama, A., Taylor, T. D., Watanabe, H., Yada, T., Park, H.-S., Toyoda, A., Ishii, K., Totoki, T., Choi, D.-K., Soeda, E., Ohki, M., et al., (2006). The DNA sequence of human chromosome 21. *Nature, 405*, 311–319.
Haveman, M., Maaskant, M. A., & Sturmans, F. (1989). Older Dutch residents of institutions, with and without Down syndrome: Comparisons of mortality and morbidity trends and motor/social functioning. *Australia and New Zealand Journal of Development Disabilities, 15*, 241–255.
Hayden, M. F. (1998). Mortality among people with mental retardation living in the United States: Research review and policy application. *Mental Retardation, 36*, 345–359.
Hermon, C., Alberman, E., Beral, V., & Swerdlow, A. J. (2001). Mortality and cancer incidence in persons with Down's syndrome, their parents and siblings. *Annals of Human Genetics, 65*, 167–176.
Hesmes, A., Sand, T., & Fostad, K. (1991). Ocular findings in Down's syndrome. *Journal of Mental Deficiency Research, 35*, 194–203.
Hill, D. A., Gridley, G., Cnattingius, S., Mellemkjaer, L., Linet, M., Adami, H-.O., Olsen, J. H., Nyren, O., & Fraumeni, J. F. (2003). Mortality and cancer incidence among individuals with Down syndrome. *Archives of Internal Medicine, 163*, 705–711.
Horwitz, S. M., Kerker, B. D., Owens, P. L., & Zigler, E. (2000). *The health status and needs of individuals with mental retardation*. Washington, DC: Special Olympics.
Howells, G. (1989). Down's syndrome and the general practitioner. *Journal of the Royal College of General Practitioners, 39*, 470–475.
Jacobson, L. (1988). Ophthalmology in mentally retarded adults. A clinical survey. *Acta Ophthalmologica, 66*, 457–462.
Jancar, M. P., & Jancar, J. (1976). Cancer and mental retardation. *Bristol Medico-Chirurgical Journal, 92*, 3–7.
Janicki, M. P., Dalton, A. J., Henderson, C. M., & Davidson, P. W. (1999). Mortality and morbidity among older adults with intellectual disability: Health services considerations. *Disability and Rehabilitation, 21*, 284–294.
Janicki, M. P., & Jacobson, J. W. (1986). General trends in sensory, physical, and behavioral abilities among older mentally retarded persons. *American Journal of Mental Deficiency, 90*, 490–500.

Johannsen, P., Christensen, J. E. J., Goldstein, H., Nielsen, V. K., & Mai, J. (1996). Epilepsy in Down syndrome: Prevalence in three age groups. *Seizure, 5*, 121–125.

Kapell, D., Nightingale, B., Rodriguez, A., Lee, J. H., Zigman, W. B., & Schupf, N. (1998). Prevalences of chronic medical conditions in adults with mental retardation: Comparison with the general population. *Mental Retardation, 36*, 269–279.

Kerins, G., Petrovic, K., Bruder, M. B., & Gruman, C. (2008). Medical conditions and medication use in adults with Down syndrome: A descriptive analysis. *Down Syndrome Research and Practice, 12*, 141–147.

Korsager, S., Chatham, E. M., & Ostergaard-Kristensen, H. P. (1978). Thyroid function tests in adults with Down's syndrome. *Acta Endocrinology, 88*, 48–54.

Lantman-de Valk, H. M. J., Haveman, M. J., & Crebolder, H. F. J. M. (1996). Comorbidity in people with Down's syndrome: A criteria-based analysis. *Journal of Intellectual Disability Research, 40*, 385–399.

Lee, E. B., Park, T. I., Park, S. H., & Park, J. Y. (2003). Loss of heterozygosity on the long arm of chromosome 21 in non-small cell lung cancer. *Annals of Thoracic Surgery, 75*, 1597–1600.

Lott, I. T., & Lai, F. (1982). Dementia in Down's syndrome: Observations from a neurology clinic. *Applied Research in Mental Retardation, 3*, 233–239.

Maaskant, M. A., Gevers, J. P. M., & Wierda, H. (2002). Mortality and life expectancy in Dutch residential centres for individuals with intellectual disability, 1991–1995. *Journal of Applied Research in Intellectual Disabilities, 15*, 200–212.

Madan, V., Williams, J., & Lear, J. T. (2006). Dermatological manifestations of Down's syndrome. *Clinical and Experimental Dermatology, 31*, 623–629.

Marcus, C. L., Keens, T. G., Bautista, D. B., von Pechmann, W. S., & Ward, S. L. D. (1991). Obstructive sleep apnea in children with Down syndrome. *Pediatrics, 88*, 132–139.

Marino, B., & Pueschel, S. M. (1996). *Heart disease in persons with Down syndrome*. Baltimore: Paul H. Brooks.

McCarron, M., Gill, M., McCallion, P., & Begley, C. (2005). Health co-morbidities in ageing persons with Down syndrome and Alzheimer's dementia. *Journal of Intellectual Disability Research, 49*, 560–566.

McDermott, S., Moran, R., Platt, T., Wood, H., Isaac, T., & Dasari, S. (2005). Prevalence of epilepsy in adults with mental retardation and related disabilities in primary care. *American Journal on Mental Retardation, 110*, 48–56.

McKinlay, S. M., Brambilla, D. J., & Posner, J. G. (1992). The normal menopause transition. *Maturitas, 14*, 103–115.

McVicker, R. W., Shanks, O. E. P., & McClelland, R. J. (1994). Prevalence and associated features of epilepsy in adults with Down's syndrome. *British Journal of Psychiatry, 164*, 528–532.

Melville, C. A., Cooper, S.-A., McGrother, C. W., Thorp, C. F., & Collacott, R. (2005). Obesity in adults with Down syndrome: A case–control study. *Journal of Intellectual Disability Research, 49*, 125–133.

Menéndez, M. (2005). Down syndrome, Alzheimer's disease and seizures. *Brain & Development, 27*, 246–252.

de Miguel-Díez, J., Villa-Asensi, J. R., & Álvarez-Sala, J. (2003). Prevalence of sleep-disordered breathing in children with Down syndrome: Polygraphic findings in 108 children. *Sleep, 26*, 1006–1009.

Milunsky, A., & Neurath, P. W. (1968). Diabetes mellitus in Down's syndrome. *Archives of Environmental Health, 17*, 373–376.

Minihan, P. M., & Dean, D. H. (1990). Meeting the needs for health services of persons with mental retardation living in the community. *American Journal of Public Health, 80*, 1043–1048.

Moss, S. C. (1991). Age and functional abilities of people with a mental handicap: evidence from the Wessex Mental Handicap Register. *Journal of Mental Deficiency Research, 35*, 430–445.

Murdoch, J. C., Ratcliffe, W. A., McLarty, D. G., Rodger, J. C., & Ratcliffe, J. G. (1977). Thyroid function in adults with Down's syndrome. *Journal of Clinical Endocrinology and Metabolism, 44*, 453–458.

Olive, P. M., Whitecloud, T. S., & Bennet, J. T. (1988). Lower cervical spondylosis and myelopathy in adults with Down syndrome. *Spine, 13*, 781–784.

Oster, J., Mikkelsen, M., & Nielsen, A. (1975). Mortality and life-table in Down's syndrome. *Acta Paediatrica Scandinavica, 64*, 322–326.

Patel, B. N., Seltzer, G. B., Wu, H.-S., & Schupf, N. (2001). Effect of menopause on cognitive performance in women with Down syndrome. *Cognitive Neuroscience and Neuropsychology, 12*, 2659–2662.

Patja, K., Eero, P., & Iivanainen, M. (2001a). Cancer incidence among people with intellectual disability. *Journal of Intellectual Disability Research, 45*, 300–307.

Patja, K., Mölsä, P., & Iivanainen, M. (2001b). Cause-specific mortality of people with intellectual disability in a population-based, 35 year follow-up study. *Journal of Intellectual Disability Research, 45*, 30–40.

Penrose, L. S. (1949). The incidence of Mongolism in the general population. *Journal of Mental Science, 95*, 685–688.

Prasher, V. P. (1994a). Prevalence of thyroid dysfunction and autoimmunity in adults with Down syndrome. *Down Syndrome Research and Practice, 2*, 67–70.

Prasher, V. P. (1994b). Screening of medical problems in adults with Down syndrome. *Down Syndrome Research and Practice, 2*, 59–66.

Prasher, V. P. (1995). Overweight and obesity amongst Down's syndrome adults. *Journal of Intellectual Disability Research, 39*, 437–441

Prasher, V. P., & Corbett, J. A. (1993). Onset of seizures as a poor indicator of longevity in people with Down syndrome and dementia. *International Journal of Geriatric Psychiatry, 8*, 923–927.

Pueschel, S. M. (1990). Clinical aspects of Down syndrome from infancy to adulthood. *American Journal of Medical Genetics Supplement, 7*, 52–56.

Pueschel, S. M., Louis, S., & McKnight, P. (1991). Seizure disorders in Down syndrome. *Archives of Neurology, 48*, 318–320.

Puri B. K., Ho, K. W., & Singh, I. (2001). Age of seizure onset in adults with Down's syndrome. *International Journal of Clinical Practice, 55*, 442–444.

Resta, O., Barbaro, M. P. F., Giliberti, T., Caratozzolo, G., Cagnazzo, M. G., Scarpelli, F., & Nocerino, M. C. (2003). Sleep related breathing disorders in adults with Down syndrome. *Down Syndrome Research and Practice, 8*, 115–119.

Richards, B. W., & Enver, F. (1979). Blood pressure in Down's syndrome. *Journal of Mental Deficiency Research, 23*, 123–135.

Robb, R. M., & Marchevsky, A.(1978). Pathology of the lens in Down's syndrome. *Archives of Ophthalmology, 96*, 1039–1042.

Roizen, N. J. (1996). Down syndrome and associated medical disorders. *Mental Retardation and Developmental Disabilities Research Reviews, 2*, 85–89.

Roizen, N. J., & Patterson, D. (2003). Down's syndrome. *Lancet, 361*, 1281–1289.

Rubin, S. S., Rimmer, J. H., Chicoine, B., Braddock, D., & McGuire, D. E. (1998). Overweight prevalence in persons with Down syndrome. *Mental Retardation, 36*, 175–181.

Safavi, K. H., Muller, S. A., Suman, V. J., Moshell, A. N., & Melton, L. J. (1995). Incidence of alopecia areata in Olmsted County, Minnesota, 1975 through 1989. *Mayo Clinic Proceedings, 70*, 628–633.

Šare, Z., Ruvalcaba, R. H. A., & Kelley, V. C. (1978). Prevalence of thyroid disorder in Down syndrome. *Clinical Genetics, 14*, 154–158.

Satgé, D., Sommelet, D., Geneix, A., Nishi, M., Malet, P., & Vekemans, M. (1998). A tumor profile in Down syndrome. *American Journal of Medical Genetics, 78*, 207–216.

Scholl, T., Stein, Z., & Hansen, H. (1982). Leukemia and other cancers, anomalies and infections as causes of death in Down's syndrome in the United States during 1976. *Developmental Medicine & Child Neurology*, *24*, 817–829.

Schupf, N., Pang, D., Patel, B. N., Silverman, W., Schubert, R., Lai, F., Kline, J. K., Stern, Y., Ferin, M., Tycko, B., & Mayeux, R. (2003). Onset of dementia is associated with age at menopause in women with Down's syndrome. *Annals of Neurology*, *54*, 433–438.

Schupf, N., Zigman, W., Kapell, D., Lee, J. H., Kline, J., & Levin, B. (1997). Early menopause in women with Down's syndrome. *Journal of Intellectual Disability Research*, *41*, 264–267.

Seltzer, G. B., Schupf, N., & Wu, H.-S. (2001). A prospective study of menopause in women with Down's syndrome. *Journal of Intellectual Disability Research*, *45*, 1–7.

Silverman, W. (2010, January). *Dementia among adults with Down syndrome: Individual differences in risk and progression.* Webinar presented through the American Association on Intellectual and Developmental Disabilities Aging and End of Life Webinar Series.

Sinha, S. (2005). Anti-oxidant gene expression imbalance, aging and Down syndrome. *Life Sciences*, *76*, 1407–1426.

Stebbens, V. A., Dennis, J., Samuels, M. P., Croft, C. B., & Southall, D. P. (1991). Sleep related upper airway obstruction in a cohort with Down's syndrome. *Archives of Disease in Childhood*, *66*, 1333–1338.

Strauss, D., & Eyman, R. K. (1996). Mortality of people with mental retardation in California with and without Down syndrome, 1986–1991. *American Journal on Mental Retardation*, *100*, 643–653.

Strauss, D., & Zigman, W. B. (1996). Behavioral capabilities and mortality risk in adults with and without Down syndrome. *American Journal on Mental Retardation*, *101*, 269–281.

Sullivan, S. G., Hussain, R., Glasson, E. J., & Bittles, A. H. (2007). The profile and incidence of cancer in Down syndrome. *Journal of Intellectual Disability Research*, *51*, 228–231.

Tangye, S. R. (1979). The EEG and incidence of epilepsy in Down's syndrome. *Journal of Mental Deficiency Research*, *23*, 17–24.

Thase, M. E. (1982). Longevity and mortality in Down's syndrome. *Journal of Mental Deficiency Research*, *26*, 177–192.

Trois, M. S., Capone, G. T., Lutz, J. A., Melendres, M. C., Schwartz, A. R., Collop, N. A., & Marcus, C. L. (2009). Obstructive sleep apnea in adults with Down syndrome. *Journal of Clinical Sleep Medicine*, *15*, 317–323.

Tyrer, F., Smith, L. K., & McGrother, C. W. (2007). Mortality in adults with moderate to profound intellectual disability: A population-based study. *Journal of Intellectual Disability Research*, *51*, 520–527.

U.S. Public Health Service (2001). *Closing the Gap: A National Blueprint for Improving the Health of Individuals with Mental Retardation. Report of the Surgeon General's Conference on Health Disparities and Mental Retardation.* Washington: DC.

Van Allen, M. I., Fung, J., & Jurenka, S. B. (1999). Health care concerns and guidelines for adults with Down syndrome. *American Journal of Medical Genetics*, *89*, 100–110.

Van Buggenhout, G.J. C.M., Trommelen, J. C. M., Schoenmaker, A., de Bal, C., Verbeek, J. J. M. C., Smeets, D. F. C. M., Ropers, H. H., Devriendt, K., Hamel, B. C. J., & Fryns, J. P. (1999). Down syndrome in a population of elderly mentally retarded patients: Genetic-diagnostic survey and implications for medical care. *American Journal of Medical Genetics*, *85*, 376–384.

Veall, R. M. (1974). The prevalence of epilepsy among Mongols related to age. *Journal of Mental Deficiency Research*, *18*, 99–106.

du Vivier, A., & Munro, D. D. (1975). Alopecia areata, autoimmunity, and Down's syndrome. *British Medical Journal*, *1*, 191–192.

Wilson, D. N., & Haire, A. (1990). Health care screening for people with mental handicap living in the community. *British Medical Journal, 301*, 1379–1381.

Yang, Q., Rasmussen, S. A., & Friedman, J. M. (2002). Mortality associated with Down's syndrome in the USA from 1983 to 1997: A population-based study. *Lancet, 359*, 1019–1025.

Systems and Diseases in DS

CHAPTER FIVE

Cancer among Persons with Down Syndrome

Johann K. Hitzler

Contents

Division of Hematology/Oncology, Clinician-Scientist, Developmental and Stem Cell Biology, The Hospital for Sick Children, 555 University Avenue, Toronto, Ontario M5G 1X8, Canada

International Review of Research in Mental Retardation, Volume 39
ISSN 0074-7750, DOI 10.1016/S0074-7750(10)39005-7

Abstract

The overall incidence of cancer in children and adults with Down syndrome (DS) appears the same as in the general population. The distribution of tumor types, however, is markedly different. The risk for leukemia in children with DS is 10–20-fold higher than in children without DS. In contrast, solid tumors both of childhood and adult age are markedly less frequent in people with DS. Leukemia is the predominant type of cancer in DS. In children with DS under the age of 5 years, acute myeloid leukemia (AML) is approximately 150-fold and acute lymphoblastic leukemia (ALL) approximately 40-fold more common than in the general pediatric population. The leukemic cells of AML in DS commonly have a platelet precursor phenotype and harbor somatic mutations of the hematopoietic transcription factor *GATA1*. AML cells of children with DS show increased sensitivity to some chemotherapeutic agents such as cytarabine. Event-free survival (EFS) rates after treatment for AML in DS range between 70 and 90% and are significantly higher than for non-DS children with AML. Newborns with DS in 10% of cases develop a transient leukemia which typically resolves after the first months of life without treatment. Approximately 20% of infants with transient leukemia, however, go on to develop AML later in life.

ALL in children with DS is considered the same disease as in the general pediatric population. After treatment outcomes in the past lagged behind that for children without DS, currently the success rate of treatment for ALL in DS is now considered comparable to that for non-DS ALL. The risk for severe adverse events during treatment, specifically life-threatening infections, is increased in children with DS and ALL. Increased expression of the gene *CRLF2* (cytokine receptor-like factor 2) and activating mutations of JAK2 have been recently identified as more frequently associated with ALL in DS. The incidence of most solid tumors of childhood and adult age has been found to be significantly lower in individuals with DS. Although the mechanisms underlying both the increased frequency of leukemia and the decreased incidence of solid tumors in DS remain to be determined, intriguing hypotheses have been proposed.

1. Introduction

Down syndrome (DS) affects approximately 1 in 1000 live born children (Roizen & Patterson, 2003). Early on the probability of children with DS to develop leukemia was suspected to be higher than in the general pediatric population (Krivit & Good, 1957). Numerous case reports and some large series entertained the possibility that the incidence of solid tumors was increased for certain types and overall decreased in DS (Satge et al., 1998a; Windham, Bjerkedal, & Langmark, 1985). Circumventing the concern of potential reporting bias, a landmark study from Denmark pursued the approach to determine the incidence of cancer in people with DS by linking population-wide registries of all residents, cancer diagnoses (supplemented by a review of death certificates), and cytogenetic data between 1968 and 1995 (Hasle, 2001; Hasle, Clemmensen, & Mikkelsen, 2000). The observed number of cancer cases among the 2814 individuals with DS (male/female ratio 1:2) who were identified was compared with the number expected for the entire Danish population specific for age, sex, and time period. Based on the results, age-and sex-specific standardized incidence ratios (SIR; of observed to expected cases) could be calculated for cancer in individuals with DS.

Although the overall risk of cancer in people with DS surprisingly was the same as in the general population (SIR 1.2, 95% confidence interval (CI) 0.92–1.55; 60 cases of cancer observed vs. 49.8 expected), the distribution of tumor types was very unusual. Leukemia accounted for 60% of all cancer cases (and for 97% in children younger up to 15 years of age), whereas solid tumors were significantly less frequent than in the general population. The leukemia risk was particularly high among young children (under 5 years of age) with DS (see Section 2.2.1). Similar findings have since then been reported by other record linking studies (Goldacre, Wotton, Seagroatt, & Yeates, 2004; Hill et al., 2003; Patja, Eero, & Iivanainen, 2001; Sullivan, Hussain, Glasson, & Bittles, 2007).

2. Leukemia in DS

2.1. Overview

Leukemia is the predominant type of cancer in DS and accounts for 95% of cancer cases in children with DS (younger than 15 years of age) (Hasle et al. , 2000). The association of leukemia and DS was early recognized (Krivit & Good, 1957). The relative risk to develop leukemia was calculated to be 10–20-fold increased (18-fold in a large epidemiological study (Hasle et al., 2000) for children and adults with DS compared to the population average. About 1 in 150 individuals with DS develop leukemia (Russell et al., 2009). Children with DS account for approximately 2% of all children diagnosed with acute lymphoblastic leukemia (ALL) (Malinge, Izraeli, & Crispino, 2009) and 10% of those diagnosed with acute myeloid leukemia (AML) (Rabin & Whitlock, 2009).

The averaging of the risk for leukemia over all age groups and leukemia subtypes, however, does not reveal the unique features of leukemia in individuals with DS. The incidence of leukemia in DS shows a marked dependence on age. The risk for any leukemia in DS is highest among children during the first 4 years of life (SIR 56). It decreases to approximately 10-fold population average until early adulthood. Strikingly, no case of leukemia was observed in individuals with DS aged 30 years [in a cohort of 2814 individuals with DS (Hasle et al., 2000)]. Accordingly, the cumulative risk for leukemia in DS by age 30 years (2.7%) is almost entirely accounted for by the cumulative risk for leukemia by age 5 years (2.1%) (Hasle et al., 2000).

The relative risk for AML is significantly higher in young children with DS than that for ALL. The relative risk for AML and ALL is 153-fold and 41-fold increased, respectively, in children with DS under the age of 5 years compared to the age-matched population averages. In the age group between 5 and 29 years, both forms of leukemia are observed 10-fold more often than expected in the general population.

ALL is the more common form of childhood leukemia in the general population with ALL cases outnumbering those of AML 6.7 to 1 (under 15 years of age). In children with DS this ratio drops to 1.7 in keeping with the increased relative risk of AML in young children with DS. Due to the markedly higher incidence of ALL in the general population, however, the absolute number of ALL cases remains higher than that of AML even in children under 5 years of age with leukemia and DS (15 cases of ALL and 10 AML observed vs. 0.34 and 0.06 expected, respectively (Hasle et al., 2000).

AML and ALL in young children therefore is the most significantly overrepresented cancer in people with DS.

2.2. AML in children with DS

A markedly increased incidence of AML ("myeloid" is here used to denote all forms of nonlymphoid leukemia, including those of megakaryoblastic and erythroid lineage) among children with DS has been consistently demonstrated by population-based studies (Hasle, 2001; Hasle et al., 2000; Lie et al., 1996). In large contemporary treatment trials of pediatric AML conducted by cooperative groups, 11–18% of enrolled patients have DS (Creutzig, Reinhardt et al., 2005; Lange et al., 1998; Lie et al., 1996).

In addition to a higher frequency, AML in children DS (DS-AML) has a distinct clinical presentation, treatment response, and underlying disease mechanism(s).

2.2.1. Age

AML in children with DS occurs at a significantly younger age [median 1.8 years compared to 7–8 years in those without DS (Craze, Harrison, Wheatley, Hann, & Chessells, 1999; Creutzig, Reinhardt et al., 2005; Kojima et al., 2000; Lange et al., 1998)] and the vast majority (94%) of children with DS are under 4 years of age when they develop AML (Creutzig et al., 1996; Gamis et al., 2003; Kojima et al., 2000).

2.2.2. Blast lineage phenotype

The leukemic blasts in AML display one of several hematopoietic lineage phenotypes. The platelet precursor or megakaryoblastic phenotype of AML [also referred to as acute megakaryoblastic leukemia, AMKL, or AML FAB-M7 (Bennett et al., 1985)] is rare in the general population but with a 500-fold increased incidence in DS-AML (Creutzig et al., 1996) constitutes the predominant blast immunophenotype [>60% of cases (Lange et al., 1998)]. Contemporary diagnostic procedures for AMKL include a bone marrow aspirate and the flowcytometric detection by specific antibodies of megakaryoblastic lineage markers such as CD41 and CD61 on the surface of the leukemic blasts. It is possible that the prevalence of AMKL in DS previously was underestimated due to a low percentage of leukemic cells in the bone marrow (see Section 2.2.4.), the lack of readily available flow cytometric detection of megakaryoblastic surface marker on leukemic cells, the presence of multiple lineage markers (Slordahl et al., 1993), and inappropriately high diagnostic cut-off values.

2.2.3. Blast cytogenetics

Acquired chromosomal abnormalities of AML blasts form the basis for current risk stratification in (non-DS) AML (Gibson et al., 2005). The chromosomal rearrangements typical of non-DS AML, such as t(8;21), t(15;17), inv(16), however, are very uncommon in DS-AML (Creutzig et al., 1996; Forestier et al., 2008; Kojima et al., 2000; Lange et al., 1998). Instead additional copies of chromosome 8, 21, dup(1q), and del(7q) were reported (Creutzig et al., 1996; Forestier et al., 2008; Kojima et al., 2000; Lange et al., 1998) without an prognostic implication. The t(1;22)(p13; q13) occurs in approximately one third of cases of human AMKL, the AML subtype in which the blasts display a platelet precursor phenotype. This translocation, which generates the *RBM15-MKL1* (Ma et al., 2007; Ma et al., 2001) also termed *OTT-MAL* (Mercher et al., 2001; Mercher et al., 2009) fusion gene, is specific for AMKL, particularly in infants (Bernstein et al., 2000), but is not found in AMKL or AML of children with DS (Lorsbach, 2004).

2.2.4. Preceding myelodysplastic syndrome

Whereas the majority of pediatric AML occurs *de novo*, without a preceding hematological disorder, AML in DS in an estimated 20–60% proportion of cases follows a myelodysplastic syndrome (MDS) (Creutzig et al., 1996; Lange et al., 1998), which is defined by anemia and thrombocytopenia and may precede overt AML by up to 19 months (Creutzig et al., 1996; Lange et al., 1998). The latter is now diagnosed when the blast percentage in the bone marrow exceeds 20%. Since there are no biological, prognostic, and therapeutic differences between MDS and AML in DS, the unifying term "myeloid leukemia of DS" (Hasle et al., 2003) has been proposed to denote that both are manifestations of the same disease entity in DS.

2.3. A specific disease mechanism in leukemic blasts of DS-AML: somatic *GATA1* mutations

The *GATA1* gene maps to the X chromosome and encodes a hematopoietic transcription factor that is normally expressed in erythroid, megakaryocytic, eosinophilic, multipotential hematopoietic progenitor cells, and mast cells (Evans & Felsenfeld, 1989; Martin, Zon, Mutter, & Orkin, 1990; Romeo et al., 1990; Tsai et al., 1989; Zon et al., 1993). Lack of *GATA1* function in cells of megakaryocytic lineage results in impaired differentiation and the paradoxical accumulation of immature megakaryocytic cells (Shivdasani, Fujiwara, McDevitt, & Orkin, 1997) with increased proliferative potential *in vitro* (Vyas, Ault, Jackson, Orkin, & Shivdasani, 1999). This phenotype [reviewed in (Gurbuxani, Vyas, & Crispino, 2004)] has striking similarities DS-AML and a pathogenetically related precursor lesion termed TL (Hitzler & Zipursky, 2005; Zipursky, 2003) (see Section 2.5.). Somatic *GATA1* mutations have been shown to be specific for DS-AML(Wechsler et al., 2002). Short deletions, insertions, and point mutations, which cluster in exon 2 (Cabelof et al., 2009; Crispino, 2004; Hitzler, Cheung, Li, Scherer, & Zipursky, 2003; Muntean & Crispino, 2005; Rainis et al., 2003; Xu et al., 2003), are sufficiently diverse to serve as clonal markers of DS-AML (Pine et al., 2005). Despite this clone-specific diversity, *GATA1* mutations in DS-AML uniformly result in the expression of a truncated (40 kD) mutant GATA1 protein, termed GATA1s, which lacks an N-terminal transcriptional activation domain of wild-type GATA1 (47 kD)(Wechsler et al., 2002). *GATA1* mutations have been detected in the vast majority of DS-AML cases examined (Baum, Weissman, Tsukamoto, Buckle, & Peault, 1992; Groet et al., 2003; Hitzler et al., 2003; Mundschau et al., 2003; Rainis et al., 2003; Xu et al., 2003) suggesting they are a key event that cooperates with cellular trisomy 21 and yet unknown additional events in the development of DS-AML. Germ line mutations of *GATA1* resulting in the expression of the truncated mutant protein, GATA1s, in the absence of DS is associated with anemia and neutropenia but not leukemia (Hollanda et al., 2006) further supporting the concept of an essential functional cooperation between trisomy 21 and acquired mutations of *GATA*1.

2.4. Increased sensitivity of DS-AML blast to specific chemotherapeutic agents

After the success rate of AML therapy in children with DS was found to be significantly higher than in the general pediatric population (see Section 2.4.1.), investigations of underlying mechanisms showed that the leukemic blasts of DS-AML (AMKL) were 2–23-fold more sensitive to chemotherapeutic such as cytarabine, anthracyclines, and etoposide *in vitro* (Taub et al.,

1999; Zwaan et al., 2002). Subsequent studies supported a model in which activation of cytarabine to the active intracellular metabolite ara-CTP was enhanced (Ge et al., 2006; Taub & Ge, 2005) while transcripts for cytidine deaminase, the enzyme responsible for its degradation, were significantly lower in AML blasts from children with DS compared to non-DS AML (Ge et al., 2004). Interestingly the phenotype of increased sensitivity to cytarabine in DS-AML cells could be related to the presence of GATA1 mutations as shown by the restoration of normal, lower drug sensitivity levels following the forced expression of wild-type GATA1 protein (Ge et al., 2005). Alternative hypotheses for the observed increased sensitivity of DS-AML blasts to selected chemotherapeutic agents such as a higher generation of cytotoxic reactive oxygen species or a predisposition of DS-AML cells to undergo apoptosis (see Section 4.) await experimental confirmation.

2.4.1. Treatment outcomes

The development of AML therapy in children with DS has not only achieved a gratifying level of treatment efficacy but also illustrates the value of clinical research and unbiased treatment approaches. Before 1990 the prognosis of any acute leukemia in children with DS was considered very poor [with a 5 years EFS 28% (Levitt, Stiller, & Chessells, 1990)]. Possible causes include a reluctance to use intensive chemotherapy in children with DS based on a concern about toxicity. However, following the enrollment of children with DS and AML in clinical trials, the results revealed that children with DS-AML could achieve superior EFS when treated with appropriately tailored chemotherapy compared to children without DS (Ravindranath, 2005; Ravindranath et al., 1992). This initially unexpectedly favorable outcome of treatment for DS-AML has been corroborated by multiple study groups (Athale et al., 2001; Creutzig, Reinhardt et al., 2005; Gamis et al., 2003; Kojima et al., 2000; Lie et al., 1996) (Table 5.1) and current EFS rates range between 70 and 90% compared to 50 and 60% for AML in the general pediatric population (Creutzig, Zimmermann et al., 2005; Gibson et al., 2005).

Survival of children with DS-AML, which predominantly has a megakaryoblastic cellular phenotype (see above), was markedly higher than that of AML with a megakaryoblastic phenotype (AMKL) in the general population (Athale et al., 2001). Based on available information on clinical phenotype, genetic mechanism, and drug response, however, what appears to be a common phenotype (i.e., AMKL) in this case denotes two fundamentally different diseases (DS-AML vs. a specific form of non-DS AML).

2.4.2. Prognostic factors in DS-AML

Among children with DS-AML the described favorable outcomes are predominantly achieved in the age group under 4 years. Older children

Table 5.1 Summary of treatment trials for AML in children with DS EFS in cooperative group studies in DS AML

Study protocol (yrs)	*n* (DS)	EFS (DS)	EFS (non-DS)	Comments	Study
AML-BFM 98 (1998–2003)	66	89% ± 4% (3 yr)	53% ± 2% (p=.0001)		Creutzig et al. [9]
CCG 2891 (1989–1999)	161	77% (6 yr)	33% (p<.0001)		Gamis et al. [7]
Japan (1987–1997)	33	80% ± 7%	DS protocol	All <4 yrs old	Kojima et al. [34]
Japan (2000–2004)	72	83.3% ± 9.1% (4 yr)	DS protocol	70/72 <4 yrs old	Kudo et al. [35]
MRC AML 10 (1987–1995)	23	70% ± 9.6% (5 yr)	59% ± 4.6% (p=.6)	OS, not EFS	Craze et al. [89]
NOPHO 88 (1988–1992)	15	47% (not given)			Abildgaard et al. [32]
NOPHO 93 (1993–2002)	37	81% ± 6% (5 yr)			Lie et al. [90]
POG 8498 (1984–1989)	12	100% (4 yr)	33% (p=.0001)		Ravindranath et al. [27]
POG 8821 (1988–1993)	27	77% ± 2.1% (3 yr)	34% ± 2.5%		Ravindranath et al. [91]
POG 9421 (1995–1999)	57	76.9% (5 yr)	51.9% (p<.001)		O'Brien et al. [74]
Toronto (1990–2003)	18	67% ± 11% (5 yr)	DS protocol		Al-Ahmari et al. [36]

AML acute megakaryoblastic leukemia; BFM, Berlin-Frankfurt-Münster; CCG, Children's Cancer Group; DS, Down syndrome; EFS, event-free survival; MRC, Medical Research Council; NOPHO, Nordic Society of Paediatric Haematology and Oncology; OS, overall survival; POG, Pediatric Oncology Group.

Source: From Rabin and Whitlock (2009).

with DS and AML have significantly lower EFS rates [28% vs. >70% for the younger age group (Gamis et al., 2003)]. A possible explanation was recently provided by the observation that AML blasts in children 4 years or older with DS often lack GATA1 mutations (Hasle et al., 2008). The disease mechanism, treatment response, and prognosis of AML in older children with DS, therefore, appear to more closely resemble the less favorable AML phenotype in the non-DS population. Whether GATA1 mutational status in DS-AML can be used for prognostic stratification remains to be demonstrated prospectively.

2.4.3. Treatment intensity

Maximization of treatment intensity has resulted in a marked improvement of survival for children with non-DS AML (Creutzig, Zimmermann et al., 2005; Gibson et al., 2005) but had adverse effects when extrapolated to children with DS (Gamis, 2005). Use of intensively timed administration of chemotherapy regimens prior to bone marrow recovery from previous therapy resulted in a 32% rate of mortality compared to 11% in those without DS (Lange et al., 1998). Based on the lower risk of relapse in DS-AML, and the increased risk of treatment-related death during highly intensive chemotherapy regimens, distinct chemotherapy protocols for the treatment of AML in children with DS have been developed.

The common principles are the use of an intermediate intensity of treatment (Abildgaard et al., 2006; Gamis, 2005; Kojima et al., 2000; Kudo et al., 2007; Rao et al., 2006; Webb, 2005) and decreased chemotherapy directed at CNS involvement with leukemia, which in DS-AML is very infrequent. Provocatively, the use of ultra low-dose cytarabine [10 mg/m^2 q12h s.c. every other week for 2 years (Al-Ahmari, Shah, Sung, Zipursky, & Hitzler, 2006)], which was used in a small nonrandomized series reported retrospectively and builds upon the hypersensitivity of DS-AML blasts to this agent, suggests that further dose reduction in the treatment of DS-AML may be feasible and should be further studied.

Current trials by the Children's Oncology Group in North America and the BFM group in Europe incorporate dose reductions of anthracyclines and do not use cranial irradiation or stem cell transplantation (Zwaan, Reinhardt, Hitzler, & Vyas, 2008) in first remission of AML. In contrast to the treatment of MDS in children without DS by stem cell transplantation, MDS in children with DS is considered the same disease entity as DS-AML and has a high probability of responding to chemotherapy alone. Stem cell transplantation for the treatment of leukemia in children with DS has been shown to be feasible but is associated with a lower survival than in the general population due to excessive complications of the transplant procedure particularly involving the lungs (Rubin, Mick, & Johnson, 1996) and leukemic relapse (Meissner et al., 2007) and is not part of primary leukemia therapy in DS.

2.5. Transient leukemia of DS

Unique to children with DS, approximately 10% of newborns with DS have blasts of megakaryoblastic lineage circulating in their peripheral blood (Zipursky, 2003). This condition has been termed transient leukemia (TL), transient myeloproliferative disorder (MD), or transient abnormal myelopoiesis (TAM). The author favors the term TL since it captures the fact that the underlying blast population as in leukemia is clonal may infiltrate organs such as heart, lung, and liver and in a proportion of cases is fatal (Al-Kasim, Doyle, Massey, Weinstein, & Zipursky, 2002; Klusmann et al., 2008).

2.5.1. Presentation and treatment

The clinical presentation of TL (Klusmann et al., 2008; Massey et al., 2006) may be limited to the presence of these abnormal blood cells in an otherwise healthy infant. Hepatosplenomegaly and skin rashes may be present. In severe cases, ascites, pericardial, and pleural effusions, conjugated hyperbilirubinemia with progressive liver failure and a life-threatening cardio-pulmonary syndrome (Al-Kasim et al., 2002) develop.

The diagnosis of TL is based on the clinical setting of a newborn with DS and the immunophenotyping of the blasts population in a peripheral blood sample. Expression of megakaryocytic antigens (CD41, CD42b, CD61) in combination with myeloid antigens (CD33, CD13), stem cell-associated antigens (CD34, CD117) and, in the majority of cases, T-cell antigens (CD7, CD4) is typical (Klusmann et al., 2008; Massey et al., 2006; Zipursky, 2003; Zipursky, Brown, Christensen, Sutherland, & Doyle, 1997). The diagnosis does not require bone marrow aspiration and a minimal blast percentage but is dependent on the context of constitutional trisomy 21 (or trisomy 21 mosaicism) and occurrence in the first 3 months of life. TL in a newborn with trisomy 21 mosaicism may not be associated with physical features of DS and thus pose particular diagnostic challenges until the karyotype of the infant's leukemic and nonleukemic cells (e.g., buccal smear, lymphocytes, skin fibroblasts) are available. TL in an infant with DS or trisomy 21 mosaicism has to be distinguished from that of congenital or infant leukemia by the absence of trisomy 21.

The most striking feature of TL in DS, which distinguishes it from any other form of childhood leukemia, is its spontaneous reversibility. In the majority of cases blasts disappear from the periphery and blood counts normalize on average within 2 and 3 months, respectively (Massey et al., 2006). Despite this favorable prognosis for the majority, in a large series of 146 infants with TL, early death occurred in 15% of cases resulting in a 5 years overall and EFS of 85 and 63%, respectively (Klusmann et al., 2008). High white cell count, ascites, preterm delivery and bleeding tendency at diagnosis and development of liver fibrosis, cholestasis, and renal failure during TL were associated with a high probability of a fatal course (Klusmann et al., 2008).

Survival in this high-risk group of TL could be increased from 28 to 52% (Klusmann et al., 2008) by treatment with low-dose cytarabine (0.3–1.5 mg/kg for 3–12 days) (Al-Kasim et al., 2002; Klusmann et al., 2008; Tchernia et al., 1996).

2.5.2. The role of TL in the development of AML

Although TL resolves spontaneously during early infancy in majority of cases, approximately one in five children, who had TL as an infant, go onto develop DS-AML later on in life (Klusmann et al., 2008; Massey et al., 2006; Zipursky, 2003), typically by 4 years of age (see above). This observation raised the possibility that TL in DS represents a precursor stage to AML. Such a disease model was supported when somatic GATA1 mutations, which initially were detected in the megakaryocytic blasts of DS-AML (Wechsler et al., 2002), were also shown to be present in the blast of TL (Groet et al., 2003; Hitzler et al., 2003; Mundschau et al., 2003; Rainis et al., 2003; Xu et al., 2003). According to a widely held concept, the transformation of normal hematopoietic cells into AML results from a multistep process involving at least two sets of cooperating genetic events, which impair cell differentiation and increase cell proliferation and survival (Speck & Gilliland, 2002). Typically, we have no access to the stages of leukemic transformation in AML because the process is too rapid and intermediate stages cannot be discerned. The unique condition of TL as a precursor of AML in DS, therefore, provides a singular opportunity to study the molecular mechanisms and the cellular target of AML.

2.5.2.1. Initiation of TL

At least three factors appear to cooperate in the development of TL: cellular trisomy 21, acquired mutations of GATA1, and the tissue environment of prenatal blood cell formation (Fig. 5.1).

The detection of TL immediately after birth and the detection of TL blasts (based on *GATA1* mutations) in fetal liver tissue as early as 23 weeks of gestation (Taub et al., 2004) demonstrate that the preleukemic condition TL originates *in utero* during fetal blood cell development. Similar to the prenatal timing of genetic events that may initiate lymphoblastic leukemia (Greaves, Maia, Wiemels, & Ford, 2003; Greaves & Wiemel, 2003), *GATA1* mutations identified in the blasts of childhood DS-AML were already detectable in neonatal blood spot sample collected from the same individuals within days after birth (Ahmed et al., 2004). Of note, although the majority of TL blast populations are clonal based on the presence of a single clone-specific GATA1 mutation, cases of oligoclonal GATA1-positive blood cell population in newborns with DS have been described (Ahmed et al., 2004) suggesting the possible subsequent selection of a predominant TL clone. The expression of the mutant GATA1 protein

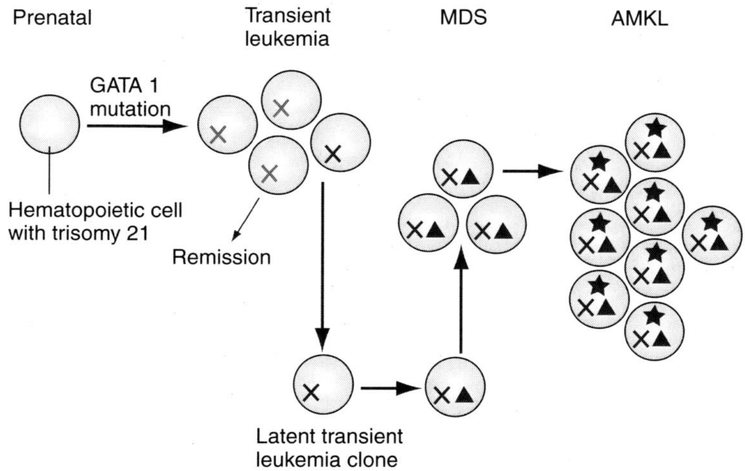

Figure 5.1 Model of the multistep mechanism underlying the development of AML in children with DS [from (Hitzler & Zipursky, 2005)]. AMKL, acute megakaryoblastic leukemia, MDS, myelodysplastic syndrome.

GATA1s, similar to a lack of wild-type protein (Shivdasani et al., 1997; Vyas et al., 1999), is thought to underlie the accumulation of abnormally differentiated cells of megakaryocytic lineage or TL blasts in the fetal liver, blood, bone marrow, and occasionally other organs such as heart and lung. It is plausible that there is functional cooperation between mutant GATA1 and gene product(s) encoded on chromosome 21 but this even in its preliminary outline remains to be defined. Some clues as to the target cells for GATA1 mutations were provided by observations of an increased number of megakaryocyte–erythroid progenitors cells among DS fetal liver cells (Tunstall-Pedoe et al., 2008) and a high proliferative potential conferred to hematopoietic fetal liver cells by the expression of mutant GATA1 protein in a murine model (Li et al., 2005). Of great interest and potential relevance for mechanism-based anti-leukemic intervention are the mechanisms underlying the resolution of TL. The latter observations raise the intriguing possibility that the normal developmental regulation of blood cell formation particularly the cessation of fetal liver hematopoiesis after birth may play a role in the resolution of TL after the newborn period.

2.5.1.2. *Progression of TL to AML*

The detection of the identical clone-specific GATA1 mutations in TL and subsequent AML in the same individual (Hitzler et al., 2003; Rainis et al., 2003) is consistent with the development of AML from a subclone of TL. Which additional events cooperate with GATA1 mutations in the 20% subset of TL who goes on to develop AML later in life is of significant interest. Cytogenetic abnormalities of TL blasts in addition constitutional trisomy 21 are present in approximately 20% of cases but were not found to be prognostic for survival or subsequent AML (Klusmann et al., 2008) but were more prevalent in blasts of DS-AML than TL (Massey et al., 2006). Genomic approaches comparing genome-wide expression in TL and DA-AML blasts have not yet yielded conclusive results likely due to small sample sizes and unpurified blast populations (Lightfoot, Hitzler, Zipursky, Albert, & Macgregor, 2004; McElwaine et al., 2004). Mutations in the genes encoding JAK2, JAK3, c-MPL, c-KIT, FLT3, N-RAS, and K-RAS have been examined in small cohorts of TL and DS-AML (Kiyoi, Yamaji, Kojima, & Naoe, 2007; Klusmann et al., 2007; Malinge et al., 2008; Norton et al., 2007; Walters et al., 2006). In essence, activating JAK3 mutations were detected in only a small portion of DS-AML (2 of 23) as well as non-DS-AML of megakaryocytic lineage (1 of 16) and 1 of 15 TL cases and none of the other candidate genes examined. Mutation of *N-RAS* was recently detected in 1 of 9 DS-AML and none of 11 TL samples (Chen et al., 2010).

The available information can be integrated into the following model. The clonal TL cell population that is present at birth becomes spontaneously extinct in approximately 80% of newborns with TL who do not go on to develop AML later in life. In contrast, in approximately 20% of children with TL, a subclone of TL cells persists during the first 3 years of life below the threshold of routine diagnostic detection and after acquiring additional mutations gives rise to DS-AML (Fig. 5.2).

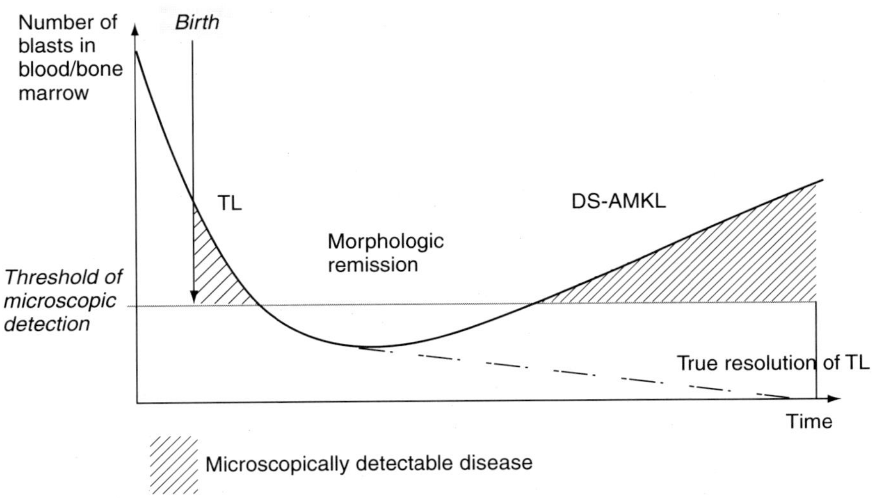

Figure 5.2 Hypothetical time course of the development of AML in children with Down syndrome arising from latently persisting cells of transient leukemia (TL). *Source*: From Hitzler and Zipursky (2005).

The observation of an intermediate phase of myelodysplasia (MDS) prior to the onset of overt DS-AML (see 2.2.4.) is likely to add an additional layer of complexity to our understanding of events underlying the path from TL to DS-AML.

In addition to inspiring intriguing mechanistic model of AML, the existence of the TL phenotype and the sequence of events as determined so far leads to some clinically highly relevant questions:

Can the subgroup of TL newborns at highest risk for transformation into DS-AML be identified by tracking the size of the remaining TL cell clone [based on GATA1 mutations (Pine et al., 2005)] over time?

If TL is the precursor to AML in children with DS, can AML be prevented by directing available TL treatment, such as low-dose cytarabine (see Section 2.5.1.), to a broader group of newborns with TL rather than the subset with immediate complications? Studies aiming to answer these questions are currently underway (Reinhardt et al., 2009).

2.6. Acute lymphoblastic leukemia in DS

DS is diagnosed in 1 of 1000 live births (Roizen & Patterson, 2003). A concomitant diagnosis of DS is present in approximately 1–3% of all children with ALL (Chessells et al., 2001; Dordelmann et al., 1998; Malinge et al., 2009; Pui et al., 1993; Whitlock et al., 2005; Zeller et al., 2005). In contrast to acute AML which is clinically and biologically different from AML in non-DS individuals, ALL in DS is commonly considered the same disease as non-DS ALL, although clinical presentation and blast characteristic show distinct features in children with DS (reviewed in (Whitlock, 2006)).

2.6.1. Presentation

Large case series have been reported that show a consistent absence of infants (under 1 year of age) with DS who are diagnosed with ALL (Chessells et al., 2001; Dordelmann et al., 1998; Hasle et al., 2000; Kalwinsky et al., 1990; Levitt et al., 1990; Pui et al., 1993; Ragab et al., 1991; Rajantie & Siimes, 2003; Robison et al., 1984; Whitlock et al., 2005; Zeller et al., 2005). Otherwise, the age distribution of ALL in DS is generally described as similar to the general population with a slightly older peak age (5 years) in DS (Bassal et al., 2005; Dordelmann et al., 1998; Malinge et al., 2009; Pui et al., 1993; Whitlock et al., 2005).

As in ALL in the general pediatric population, the leukemic blasts predominantly express a B precursor phenotype. In contrast, ALL with a T-cell lineage (T-ALL) or mature B-cell phenotype (Burkitt leukemia) is virtually absent in children with DS (Chessells et al., 2001; Dordelmann et al., 1998; Levitt et al., 1990; Pui et al., 1993; Rabin & Whitlock, 2009; Rajantie & Siimes, 2003; Whitlock, 2006; Whitlock et al., 2005; Zeller et al., 2005). Similarly, a lower frequency of leukemic involvement of the CNS is reported for DS-ALL by the majority (Chessells et al., 2001; Dordelmann et al., 1998; Levitt et al., 1990; Pui et al., 1993; Rajantie & Siimes, 2003; Zeller et al., 2005).

2.6.2. Cytogenetics and genomics

Both prognostically favorable and unfavorable chromosomal aberrations are less frequently present in leukemic blast of DS-ALL than those of ALL in the general pediatric population. The two most common favorable cytogenetic features of pediatric ALL, high hyperdiploidy (>50 chromosomes), and the t(12;21), which results in the expression of a *ETV6-RUNX1* fusion gene, formerly termed *TEL-AML1*, are each found in approximately 25% of cases in the general population (Forestier et al., 2008; Pui, Relling, & Downing, 2004). In contrast, they were significantly underrepresented in DS-ALL [10% each of 215 cases of DS-ALL (Forestier et al., 2008)] in keeping with previous reports (Arico et al., 2008; Bassal et al., 2005; Lanza et al., 1997), although the chromosomal distribution in hyperdiploid blasts of DS-ALL was not different from non-DS-ALL (Forestier et al., 2008). Likewise, chromosomal translocations associated with unfavorable outcome in pediatric ALL such as those resulting in the expression of the BCR-ABL1 fusion gene and rearrangements of the MLL gene are significantly less frequent in DS-ALL (Bassal et al., 2005; Chessells et al., 2001; Dordelmann et al., 1998; Forestier et al., 2008; Whitlock et al., 2005). Cytogenetic abnormalities that are overrepresented in blasts of DS-ALL include +X, t(8;14)(q11;q32) and del(9p) (Forestier et al., 2008; Kaleem et al., 2000; Pui et al., 1993).

Analysis of gene expression in blasts of DS-ALL using an unsupervised algorithm revealed a very heterogeneous pattern that lacked the clustering of cases comparable to that of distinct cytogenetic subgroups in non-DS ALL (Hertzberg et al., 2010) and led the authors to conclude that DS-ALL, unlike DS-AML, is not a disease entity defined by a unique molecular mechanism. This approach, however, did identify genes in DNA damage response pathway to be overrepresented in the gene expression profile of DS-ALL blasts.

A landmark study reporting the genome-wide analysis of leukemic blasts using high-resolution, single-nucleotide polymorphism arrays, and genomic DNA sequencing has shown that genes regulating normal B-cell development are affected by deletions in approximately 40% of cases of pediatric (non-DS) ALL (Mullighan et al., 2007). A comparable frequency (53%) was found in DS-ALL including deletions of IKZF1 (Hertzberg et al., 2010) (see Section 2.7.2.).

2.7. Specific disease mechanism in DS-ALL

2.7.1. JAK mutations

Abnormal activation of kinase-mediated cell signaling in DS-ALL was investigated as a disease mechanism after a mutation in the gene encoding the kinase, and signaling molecule JAK2 was detected in the leukemic blasts of a boy with DS and B precursor ALL (Malinge et al., 2007).

Subsequent mutational analyses of ALL blasts from 183 children with DS and B precursor ALL confirmed the presence of JAK2 mutations in 18–28% of cases of DS-ALL (Bercovich et al., 2008; Gaikwad et al., 2009; Kearney et al., 2009) compared to only one of 156 in the non-DS All control group (incidentally this patient's ALL blasts had an isochromosome 21q and germ line material was unavailable, suggesting the possibility of undiagnosed DS mosaicism). The mutations of the JAK2 were predominantly point mutations changing arginine residue 683, located in the JH2 pseudokinase domain of the JAK2 protein, whose normal function is thought to negatively regulate the activity of the kinase domain and may mediate protein–protein interactions, into glycine (R683G) or less frequently serine, lysine and threonine (Bercovich et al., 2008; Gaikwad et al., 2009; Kearney et al., 2009). The mutations were somatic, as indicated by their absence from remission samples, and typically heterozygous. The mutant JAK2 protein is a constitutively active JAK2 kinase activating intracellular JAK/STAT signaling. Functional studies demonstrate that mutant JAK2 protein confers the capacity of cytokine-independent proliferation onto a murine B lineage cell line (Bercovich et al., 2008; Kearney et al., 2009; Mullighan et al., 2009b) and of serial myeloid colony formation to primary murine hematopoietic progenitors (c-Kit+lin-) *in vitro* (Bercovich et al., 2008). The mutations result in constitutive activation of the JAK/STAT signaling pathway as shown by (constitutive) tyrosine phosphorylation of Jak2 and Stat5.

Although the functional effect of mutant JAK2 protein *in vitro* required the association with a cytokine receptor, for example, that for erythropoietin and thrombopoietin (Bercovich et al., 2008), a cooperating cytokine receptor chain in B precursor ALL suspected to bind and activate mutated JAK2 (Bercovich et al., 2008; Malinge et al., 2007) was not evident (see Section 2.7.2.).

Of note the JAK2 mutations found in blasts of DS-ALL, chiefly JAK2 R683G are distinct from the JAK2 V617F mutations previously identified in over 90% of polycythemia vera and approximately half of other MD in non-DS individuals (James et al., 2005).

Although reports vary regarding the association of JAK2 mutations in DS-ALL with younger age (Bercovich et al., 2008) or male gender (Gaikwad et al., 2009), they consistently found that JAK2 mutation status was not correlated with the probability of EFS and thus lacked prognostic value in DS-ALL. These observations raised the question whether lymphoid-type JAK2 mutations (as represented by R683G) are a genetic event that is specific for lymphoblastic leukemia in children with DS, similar to the DS-specific role of GATA1 mutations in myeloid leukemia (Wechsler et al., 2002). A large genome-wide analysis of DNA copy number alterations, transcriptional profiling, and gene resequencing (Mullighan et al., 2009b) in 187 children (including 9 with DS) with high-risk B precursor ALL (as defined by age and white blood cell count at diagnosis recently provided an unexpected answer). Although 2 of the 9 children with ALL and DS had JAK mutations (all in the *JAK2* gene), 10.7% of the remaining (non-DS) children with high-risk B precursor ALL had mutations of JAK2 (in the majority affecting arginine 683 of pseudokinase domain as in DS-ALL), and less frequently JAK1 (pseudokinase domain) and JAK3. The subgroup with ALL blasts harboring JAK mutations significantly more often showed other prognostically adverse features such as a deletion or mutation of the IKAROS gene (IKZF1) (Mullighan et al., 2009a), a regulator of B-cell development (present in 70% of JAK mutated vs. only 25.6% of non-JAK mutated ALL), a deletion of the tumor suppressor gene and cell cycle regulator CDKN2A/B and an overall gene expression profile of the leukemic blasts resembling that of the very high-risk subtype of ALL defined by the BCR-ABL1 fusion gene. As a result the probability of leukemic relapse in this group was high (77% if both IKZF and JAK were altered; 54 and 33% if IKZF1 and JAK alone were altered, respectively; and 23% in the absence of both mutations). Due to the close association with IKZF1 alterations, JAK mutation status had no independent prognostic value (Mullighan et al., 2009b).

In summary, somatic JAK mutations are not specific for DS-ALL. They occur not only in approximately 20% of DS-ALL but also in approximately 10% of high-risk ALL in non-DS children [equivalent to approximately 3% of unselected childhood ALL (Mullighan et al., 2009b)]. Association with IKZF1 and CDKN2A/B alterations indicate that genetic lesion targeting multiple cellular pathways including lymphoid differentiation, cell cycle control, and activation of tyrosine kinases such as JAK cooperate to induce aggressive leukemia. Knowledge of this disease mechanisms in ALL has led to efforts aiming at pharmacological inhibition of JAK/STAT activation as induced by JAK pseudokinase domain mutations, e.g., by novel JAK inhibitor compounds for the treatment of ALL.

2.7.2. Increased expression of CRLF2 in DS-ALL

Two chromosomal abnormalities involving the pseudoautosomal region 1 (PAR1) on the X and Y chromosome (Xp22.3 and Yp11.3) have recently been found to be particularly frequent in ALL blasts of children with DS (Russell et al., 2009). One is a translocation of the entire coding region of the CRLF2 gene, which maps to PAR1, into the IGH@ locus (on 14q32) (Russell et al., 2009). The second is an interstitial deletion within PAR1 (Russell et al., 2009) which generates a fusion gene (Mullighan et al., 2009) by juxtaposing the CRLF2 coding sequence with the first, noncoding exon of another gene mapping to PAR1 termed P2RY8 (Fujiwara et al., 2007). Both the translocation and deletion result in increased expression of CRFL2 mRNA and protein in ALL blasts. These chromosomal rearrangements occur only in 5–7% of unselected cases of childhood ALL (Mullighan et al., 2009; Russell et al., 2009) but in 50–60% of DS-ALL (Hertzberg et al., 2010; Mullighan et al., 2009), where the PAR1 deletion mechanism predominates (Russell et al., 2009). In contrast, activating mutations within the CRLF2 gene are rare (3/87 DS-ALL samples (Hertzberg et al., 2010)).

CRLF2 interacts with the interleukin-7 receptor alpha chain to form the heterodimeric receptor for thymic stromal lymphopoietin (TSLP), whose function includes mediation of B-cell precursor proliferation and survival *in vitro* (Ziegler & Liu, 2006) and a role in T-cell, dendritic cell development, inflammation, and allergic disease but which may not be required for normal B-cell development (Carpino et al., 2004).

Expression of human CRLF2 in murine fetal liver cells increased the proliferation of primary lymphoid progenitors, expanded cells with immature immunophenotype, and resulted in phosphorylation of STAT5 (Russell et al., 2009).

Interestingly, CRLF2 alterations in DS ALL are strongly associated with JAK mutations. Overall, the blasts of approximately 25% of children with ALL and DS harbor activating JAK mutations (see above), targeting mostly the pseudokinase domain of JAK2 (R683G) (Hertzberg et al., 2010; Mullighan et al., 2009), JAK2 kinase domains, and JAK1 pseudokinase domain (Mullighan et al., 2009). This proportion increases to 45–60% in the DS-ALL subset with increased CRLF2 expression (Mullighan et al., 2009; Russell et al., 2009) compared to <1% in DS-ALL lacking CRLF2 alterations (Mullighan et al., 2009). Together with the recent observation of increased *CRLF2* expression in all of 22 cases of non-DS B precursor ALL with somatic *JAK2* mutations(Yoda et al., 2010), these findings strongly suggest a functional cooperation between CRLF2 and JAK signaling in ALL that applies to individuals with and without DS.

Of note, in DS-ALL no prognostic association was found between CRLF2 and/or JAK mutations status and outcome (Mullighan et al., 2009). In contrast CRLF2 rearrangements are overrepresented among B precursor ALL with high-risk features in the general population and in this context correlated with other adverse prognostic features such as *IKZF1* deletions and a significantly increased risk of relapse (Harvey et al., 2010). Interestingly, increased *CRLF2* expression due to the deletion mechanism within PAR1 (see above) was recently found to correlate with a very high risk of relapse (67%) (Cario et al., 2010) in children with B precursor ALL classified to have "standard risk" disease based on the currently available prognostic variables.

Not surprisingly, the observation that JAK2/STAT5 signaling is constitutively activated *in vitro* by expression of CRLF2 and JAK2 mutations (Hertzberg et al., 2010; Mullighan et al., 2009; Russell et al., 2009) has placed this signaling pathway on the list of targets for mechanism-based innovative leukemia therapy in children with and without DS.

2.8. Treatment and outcomes for DS-ALL

In contrast to ML, the sensitivity of ALL blasts to chemotherapeutic agents *in vitro* does not significantly differ between children with and without DS (Zwaan et al., 2002). Historically, however, the probability of EFS for children with ALL and Ds was reported as lower than that for children without DS in most series (Chessells et al., 2001; Dordelmann et al., 1998; Kalwinsky et al., 1990; Levitt et al., 1990; Pui et al., 1993; Ragab et al., 1991; Robison et al., 1984) (for a recent review see Rabin and Whitlock (2009); Whitlock (2006)]. In some studies this difference of outcomes between DS-ALL and non-DS-ALL did not reach statistical significance (Dordelmann et al., 1998) or was absent in subgroups receiving more intensive treatment protocols (Ragab et al., 1991; Whitlock et al., 2005). In children with DS-ALL treatment included reductions of treatment intensity in almost half of the patients (Dordelmann et al., 1998). Importantly, EFS rates were found to be comparable for ALL in children with and without DS, if the analysis takes into account the lower prevalence of prognostically favorable cytogenetic risk groups, such as high hyperdiploidy (>50 chromosomes) and expression of the ETV6-RUNX1 (or TEL-AML1) (see above) in DS-ALL (Bassal et al., 2005; Whitlock, 2006).

With current therapy, the probability of EFS of ALL in DS, which has ranged between 63 and 84% (Table 5.2), is expected to be similar to that of ALL in the general pediatric population.

2.9. Higher risk for adverse events during treatment of ALL in children with DS

Children with DS, however, have a significantly higher risk for significant adverse effects during chemotherapy for ALL. Administration of methotrexate results in a higher frequency of severe mucositis and myelosuppression in children with DS (Bassal et al., 2005; Garre et al., 1987), likely due to host factors such as delayed methotrexate clearance (Dordelmann et al., 1998; Garre et al., 1987) and the increased expression of cellular transport proteins for methotrexate such as the reduced folate carrier encoded on chromosome 21 (Taub & Ge, 2005; Whitlock, 2006). Transient hyperglycemia after treatment with asparagines and glucocorticoids is more

Table 5.2 Summary of treatment trials for ALL in children with DS EFS in cooperative group studies in DS ALL

Study protocol(yrs)	*n* (DS)	EFS (DS)	EFS (non-DS)	Comments	Study
BFM (1981–1995)	61	58% ± 8% (6 yr)	70 ± 1% (p = .14)	3.3% induction deaths; 6.6% "treatment deaths"	Dordelmann et al. [56]
CCG (1989–1995)	179	68.1% ± 3.9% (10 yr)	77.2 ± 0.5% (p < .001)	3% induction deaths	Whitelock et al. [60]
CCG 1961 (1996–2002)	51	69.1% ± 8.4% (5 yr)	70.4% ± 1.5%	High-risk patients only; 8.7% induction deaths	Hastings et al. [66]
CCG 1952 (1996–2000)	59	79.6%	84.3% (p = .04)	Standard-risk patients only; more hospitalizations	Bassal et al. [59]
MRC UKALL X, XI (1985–1997)	55	53%	63% (p = .1)	11% remission deaths	Chessells et al. [57]
NOPHO (1984–2001)	64	51% ± 7% (10 yr)	70% ± 1%	3.1% remission deaths	Zeller et al. [58]
POG and St Jude (1979–1992)	37	65% ± 14.5% (4 yr)	74% ± 1.6% (p = .21)		Pui et al. [55]

ALL, acute lymphoblastic leukemia; BFM, Berlin-Frankfurt-Münster; CCG, Children's Cancer Group; DS, Down syndrome; EFS, event-free survival; MRC, Medical Research Council; NOPHO, Nordic Society of Paediatric Haematology and Oncology; POG, Pediatric Oncology Group.

Source: From Rabin and Whitlock (2009).

common in children with DS (Bassal et al., 2005; Dordelmann et al., 1998; Kalwinsky et al., 1990). Overall, the increased frequency of adverse effects of treatment results in a higher number of hospital days in children with DS treated for ALL (Bassal et al., 2005; Shah et al., 2009).

Of greatest concern is the significantly increased risk for fatal infection during ALL therapy in children with DS. Treatment-related deaths of children with ALL and DS have been reported during (Levitt et al., 1990; Robison et al., 1984; Wheeler, Chessells, Bailey, & Richards, 1996) and after the induction phase of treatment (Wheeler et al., 1996). A similar experience was recently reported for contemporary North American treatment trials of DS-ALL (Rabin & Whitlock, 2009). Given that DS has been associated with a degree of immunodeficiency due to dysgammaglobulinemia, impaired T-cell mediated immunity, low NK activity, and decreased chemotaxis of neutrophils and monocytes in DS [reviewed in Ugazio, Maccario, Notarangelo, and Burgio (1990)], it is a priority to optimize the supportive care of children with DS undergoing treatment for ALL.

Little is known about specific late effects of ALL therapy in children with DS. The risk of abnormal cardiac function after treatment for leukemia was reported to be three-fold increased in children with DS (Krischer et al., 1997) resulting symptomatic cardiomyopathy in 17% of children with DS following treatment for AML (O'Brien et al., 2008), whereas others reported the same low frequency (4%) as in the children without DS (Creutzig, Diekamp, Zimmermann, & Reinhardt, 2007).

Some children with DS have undergone cranial irradiation as part of their treatment. Whether this intervention results in specific neurocognitive late effects in children with DS has not been determined.

The challenge of successful ALL therapy in children with DS, therefore, is to strike the right balance between intensification of treatment and avoidance of undue treatment toxicity. This requires careful data collection not only regarding survival but also the frequency of severe adverse effects, resulting treatment modifications and their impact on treatment success in children with DS.

3. Solid Tumors in DS

The risk for leukemia is significantly increased in people with DS, particular during early childhood (see above). Yet the same overall cancer incidence in DS compared to the population average has been observed in population-based studies (Boker et al., 2001; Goldacre et al., 2004; Hasle, 2001; Hasle et al., 2000; Hill et al., 2003; Patja et al., 2001; Sullivan et al., 2007). The finding is explained by an equally significant decrease of the incidence of solid tumors in individuals with DS.

Available information on solid tumors in individuals with DS is derived from case reports, large series, and population-based studies.

The landmark study by Hasle et al. (Hasle, 2001; Hasle et.al., 2000) provides SIR for solid tumors in individuals with DS. By linking a population, cancer, and cytogenetics registries the number and type of cancers observed in 2814 individuals (1536 male 1278 female; 1.2) with DS in Denmark between 1968 and 1995 are compared with the number expected for each cancer type based on sex- and age-specific cancer rates in the general population at the same time.

Only 24 solid tumors (vs. 47.8 expected) were observed resulting in a significantly decreased SIR for solid tumors of SIR 0.50 (95% CI 0.32–0.75) (Table 5.3). Solid tumors were less frequent in individuals with

Table 5.3 Observed and expected site-specific number of cancer cases in 2814 individuals with DS in Denmark (the solid tumor diagnoses in DS include lung (squamous cell) cancer, ovarian dysgerminoma, seminomas, and embryonal carcinoma of the testis, uterine adenocarcinoma, retroperitoneal germ cell tumor, unilateral retinoblastoma, and one glioblastoma)

Site (ICD-7)	Observed	Expected	SIR (95% CI)
All sites (140–205)	60	49.83	1.20 (0.92–1.55)
Buccal cavity (140–148)	0	1.04	0.00 (0.0–2.88)
Digestive system (150–159)	4	6.52	0.61 (0.17–1.57)
Stomach (151)	1	0.91	1.10 (0.01–6.14)
Colon (153)	2	2.24	0.89 (0.10–3.23)
Peritoneum (158–159)	1	0.01	67.77 (0.89–377)
Respiratory system (160–164)	1	4.96	0.20 (0–1.12)
Lung (162)	1	4.22	0.24 (0–1.32)
Breast (170)	0	7.32	0.00 (0.0–0.41)
Female genital organs (171–176)	4	5.68	0.70 (0.19–1.80)
Uterus (172)	1	1.20	0.83 (0.01–4.63)
Ovary (175)	3	1.52	1.97 (0.40–5.77)
Male gental organs (177–179)	4	2.82	1.42 (0.38–3.63)
Testis (178)	4	2.15	1.86 (0.50–4.77)
Urinary tract (180–181)	4	2.97	1.35 (0.36–3.45)
Kidney (180)	1	1.19	0.84 (0.01–4.66)
Bladder (181)	3	1.78	1.69 (0.34–4.93)
Skin (190–191)	2	8.14	0.25 (0.03–0.89)
Non-melanoma	2	5.76	0.35 (0.04–1.25)

(Continued)

Table 5.3 *(Continued)*

Site (ICD-7)	Observed	Expected	SIR (95% CI)
Other specified sites (192–197)	2	4.75	0.42 (0.05–1.52)
Eye (192)	1	0.27	3.68 (0.05–20.5)
Brain (193)	1	3.32	0.30 (0–1.68)
Secondary and unspecified sites (198–199)	3	0.92	3.27 (0.66–9.56)
Non-Hodgkin lymphoma (200, 202)	0	1.41	0.00 (0.0–2.13)
Hodgkin's disease (201)	0	0.92	0.00 (0.0–3.25)
All solid tumors (140–202)	24	47.77	0.50 (0.32–0.75)
Leukemia (204)	36	2.04	17.63 (12.4–24.4)
ALL	20	0.82	24.36 (14.9–37.6)
AML	12	0.59	20.28 (10.5–35.4)
Acute unspecified leukemia	3	0.11	26.86 (5.4–78.5)
Leukemia not otherwise specified	1	0.52	1.93 (0.03–10.8)

Source: From Hasle et al. (2000).

DS in all age groups. The SIR for solid tumor was 0.44 (CI 0.09–1.28) in the age group under 30 years and 0.51 (CI 0.32–0.78) in individuals aged 30 years and older. Only three solid tumors were observed in individuals with DS younger than 30 years, retinoblastoma, dysgerminoma, and embryonal testicular carcinoma.

The majority of all malignancies in DS (including leukemia) were found in males (37 in males and 23 in females, ratio 1.6). Solid tumors were particularly rare among girls and women with DS (seven solid tumor observed vs. 27.13 expected; SIR 0.26; CI 0.10–0.53) compared to males (SIR 0.82, CI 0.48–1.32). Strikingly, no case of breast cancer was observed in women with DS when 7.3 cases had been expected (Hasle, 2001; Hasle et al., 2000).

A study from Western Australia using the same approach confirmed the significantly decreased SIR for all solid tumors (0.44; 95% CI 0.19–0.86) in people with DS but did not find a significantly lower incidence of solid tumors SIR in females (SIR 0.70(0.26–1.53) (Sullivan et al., 2007). The malignancies observed in DS included three gastrointestinal tumors (adenosquamous carcinoma of the gallbladder, cancer of ileum, cancer of floor of mouth) a brain tumor, melanoma, testicular teratoma, cancer of conjunctiva, and Waldenstrom macroglobulinemia, but the small number of solid tumors precluded interpretation of SIRs for individual cancers. Similarly, reports of an excess of gastric (Boker et al., 2001), gall balder, and liver cancer in DS (Boker et al., 2001; Hill et al., 2003) are based on small numbers.

Beyond population-based studies, case reports and large series have commented on the possibly increased incidence of certain solid tumors in DS.

3.1. Lymphoma

A large retrospective cases series of solid tumors in DS included 20 cases of lymphoma (Satge et al., 1998b), including seven cases of Hodgkin lymphoma (see also Sandoval, Hudson, Ozkaynak, Tugal, and Jayabose (2000). Most occurred in males (8 of 9 patients with available information) and occurred between 3 weeks and 54 years of age, including two cases of neonatal T-cell lymphoma. Outcomes are difficult to assess since not all patients were treated. Although an overrepresentation of lymphoma in DS was suggested, the population-based cancer incidence data described above did not identify a single case of Hodgkin or non-Hodgkin lymphoma in their large cohort of people with DS (Hasle et.al., 2000). These authors concluded that a major increase in risk of lymphoma was unlikely.

3.2. Germ cell tumors

Frequent previous case reports are reviewed by Satge (Satge et al., 1998b). Of 24 testicular tumors, 20 are characterized as germ cell tumors, predominantly seminoma and far less frequently as endodermal sinus tumor and embryonal carcinoma. Intratubular germ cell neoplasia in the testes of an 18-week fetus with trisomy 21 has been described. The report of extragonadal teratomas in children with a retroperitoneal (5 of 9) and intracranial (7 of 27) location suggested DS may predispose to germ cell tumors. In contrast the SIR for testicular cancer in the Danish registry study was not statistically significantly increased in DS (1.86; CI 0.5–4.77) leading to the conclusion that the relative risk of germ cell tumors in males and females with DS has not been definitely answered.

3.3. Retinoblastoma

Brichard reported a series of 16 cases of retinoblastoma in DS (Brichard, Vermylen, De Potter, & Casteels, 2003). One third of patients (5 of 16) had the hereditary form of retinoblastoma compared to 40–50% in general population. Whether the excess of nonhereditary retinoblastoma represents a predisposition in DS for retinoblastoma, however, is difficult to conclude due to the small number of cases. Of note, hyperplastic and dysplastic retinal lesions in DS have been described (Ginsberg, Bofinger, & Roush, 1977). Two large epidemiological studies in Norway and Denmark (Hasle et al., 2000; Windham et al., 1985) mention a possible association between DS and retinoblastoma. Since 1 eye tumor was observed and 0.27 expected, the resulting SIR is 9 with a broad CI (0.1–51) (Hasle et al., 2000).

3.4. Brain tumors

The distribution of brain tumors in children with DS appears unique. They are mainly glial cell tumors and germ cell tumors, without medulloblastoma or any kind of neural cell neoplasm (Satge & Rickert, 2009). Among 16 children with brain tumors and DS [reviewed in Satge et al. (1998b)], neither medulloblastoma nor meningioma were found. In contrast, germ cell tumors make up one third of the total, significantly exceeding expected relative frequencies in this age group (1.3%). Males are significantly overrepresented (11 vs. 5 in female patients). The incidence of brain tumors in DS according to data from the population-based study from Denmark appears low but any potential decrease was not statistically significant (SIR 0.3; CI 0–1.7) (Hasle et al., 2000).

3.5. Skin tumors

Syringomas are small benign adenomatous tumors of sweat ducts, usually restricted to eyelids, and may occur early and be extensive. The incidence in DS is estimated to be 20-fold increased in DS (Satge et al., 1998b).

3.6. Common solid tumors of children and adults are underrepresented in DS

Breast cancer is the most common malignant disease in women. No case, however, was detected in 1278 women with DS when 7.3 were expected (Hasle et al., 2000). Neuroblastoma and Wilms tumors appear underrepresented among solid tumors of children with DS. Among 5854 patients in the National Wilms Tumor Study, no patient with DS was identified (Olson, Hamilton, & Breslow, 1995). Similarly, none of 6724 infants and children diagnosed in 11 European countries with neuroblastoma has DS (Satge et al., 1998b).

4. Mechanistic Hypotheses

4.1. Increased risk for leukemia in DS

The increased incidence of leukemia in the context of cellular trisomy 21 is consistent with a concept in which one or more genes encoded on chromosome 21 (Hattori et al., 2000) are over expressed through a gene-dosage effect and thus bring about the leukemic transformation of hematopoietic cells. The list of candidate genes on chromosome 21 includes hematopoietic transcription factors (*RUNX1/AML1, ETS2*), regulators of apoptosis (SON), and metastasis (TIAM1) as well as signaling molecules such as interferon receptors and provides attractive targets for further functional studies. Since only a small proportion of individuals with DS develop leukemia, it is plausible that other nongenetic factors are involved. Altered folate metabolism in DS (Gurbuxani et al., 2004) associated with increased cystathionine β-synthase expression (encoded on chromosome 21) or intrauterine folate deficiency, due to reduced activity of MTHFR in mothers of children with DS, have been considered (Rabin & Whitlock, 2009) but does not explain the decreased frequency of non-hematological cancers.

4.2. Decreased incidence of solid tumors in DS

Lower exposure to environmental carcinogens such tobacco, alcohol, and occupational carcinogens in DS has been proposed as a mechanism (Hasle, 2001) but would have to be restricted to carcinogens for nonleukemic tumors. Hormonal factors due to earlier menopause in women with DS are expected to decrease the risk for breast cancer. Since pregnancy and its protective effect against breast cancer are rare in women with DS, it seems unlikely that hormonal factors alone account for the decreased incidence of breast cancer in this group.

Analogous to the postulate of leukemia-inducing gene on chromosome 21, one or more yet to be defined tumor suppressor genes on chromosome 21 could explain for the observed lack of solid tumors in children and adults with DS. Such a mechanism is supported by the observation that tumor frequency in a murine model of intestinal neoplasia is lowered by the expression of genes syntenic to those on human chromosome 21 (Sussan, Yang, Li, Ostrowski, & Reeves, 2008).

Increased activity of copper zinc superoxide dismutase, the product of a gene on chromosome 21, has been demonstrated in red blood cells of individuals with DS (De La Torre et al., 1996). Conceivably increased enzymatic activity may reduce the susceptibility of DS cells to the carcinogenic effects of reactive oxygen species. In contrast, increased generation of reactive oxygen species was found in DS neurons and resulted in increased apoptosis in this tissue (Busciglio & Yankner, 1995), which could represent an alternative mechanism of tissue protection against malignant transformation. Increased differentiation of neural cells due to overproduction of S-100b, encoded on chromosome 21, was postulated as another explanation for the decreased incidence of neuroblastoma in DS (Satge et al., 1998a).

Since serum levels of endostatin are higher in people with DS (Zorick et al., 2001), endostatin is a cleavage product of collagen XVIII, encoded by *COL18A1* on chromosome 21, and acts as a potent inhibitor of angiogenesis in solid tumors, constitutionally impaired angiogenesis may play a role in the decreased incidence of solid tumors in DS. Additional support for this mechanism was recently provided by the observation that *Dscr1* (DS candidate region 1), a gene encoded on chromosome 21 and overexpressed in human DS tissues, suppresses tumor growth in mice through decreased tumor angiogenesis (as a consequence of suppression of calcineurin signaling) (Baek et al., 2009; Ryeom, Baek, & Zaslavsky, 2009; Ryeom & Folkman, 2009).

5. Outlook

The treatment of cancers in children and adults with DS continues to teach lessons on how cancers develop and how this development can be interfered with. The experience of increased side effects during some cancer treatments in children with DS makes it clear that cancer therapy must not only concern itself with optimally targeting the cancer cell population but also with supporting the host, the child, or adult with DS. Even a brief history of cancer therapy in children with DS teaches that anecdote is rarely the basis for progress and that unbiased research can result in unexpected success. The current challenge is to identify the most effective cancer treatments with the least amount of side effects for children and adults with DS while translating new knowledge into better, mechanism-based cancer drugs.

REFERENCES

Abildgaard, L., Ellebaek, E., Gustafsson, G., Abrahamsson, J., Hovi, L., Jonmundsson, G., et al. (2006). Optimal treatment intensity in children with Down syndrome and myeloid leukaemia: Data from 56 children treated on NOPHO-AML protocols and a review of the literature. *Annals of Hematology*, *85*(5), 275–280.

Ahmed, M., Sternberg, A., Hall, G., Thomas, A., Smith, O., O'Marcaigh, A., et al. (2004). Natural history of GATA1 mutations in Down Syndrome. *Blood*, *103*(7), 2480–2489.

Al-Ahmari, A., Shah, N., Sung, L., Zipursky, A., & Hitzler, J. (2006). Long-term results of an ultra low-dose cytarabine-based regimen for the treatment of acute megakaryoblastic leukaemia in children with Down syndrome. *British Journal of Haematology*, *133*(6), 646–648.

Al-Kasim, F., Doyle, J. J., Massey, G. V., Weinstein, H. J., & Zipursky, A. (2002). Incidence and treatment of potentially lethal diseases in transient leukemia of Down syndrome: Pediatric Oncology Group Study. *Journal of Pediatric Hematology/oncology*, *24*(1), 9–13.

Arico, M., Ziino, O., Valsecchi, M. G., Cazzaniga, G., Baronci, C., Messina, C., et al. (2008). Acute lymphoblastic leukemia and Down syndrome: Presenting features and treatment outcome in the experience of the Italian Association of Pediatric Hematology and Oncology (AIEOP). *Cancer*, *113*(3), 515–521.

Athale, U. H., Razzouk, B. I., Raimondi, S. C., Tong, X., Behm, F. G., Head, D. R., et al. (2001). Biology and outcome of childhood acute megakaryoblastic leukemia: A single institution's experience. *Blood*, *97*(12), 3727–3732.

Baek, K. H., Zaslavsky, A., Lynch, R. C., Britt, C., Okada, Y., Siarey, R. J., et al. (2009). Down's syndrome suppression of tumour growth and the role of the calcineurin inhibitor DSCR1. *Nature, 459*(7250), 1126–1130.

Bassal, M., La, M. K., Whitlock, J. A., Sather, H. N., Heerema, N. A., Gaynon, P. S., et al. (2005). Lymphoblast biology and outcome among children with Down syndrome and ALL treated on CCG-1952. *Pediatric Blood & Cancer, 44*(1), 21–28.

Baum, C., Weissman, I., Tsukamoto, A., Buckle, A., & Peault, B. (1992). Isolation of a candidate human hematopoietic stem-cell population. *PNAS, 89*(7), 2804–2808.

Bennett, J. M., Catovsky, D., Daniel, M. T., Flandrin, G., Galton, D. A., Gralnick, H. R., et al. (1985). Criteria for the diagnosis of acute leukemia of megakaryocyte lineage (M7). A report of the French-American-British Cooperative Group. *Annals of Internal Medicine, 103*(3), 460–462.

Bercovich, D., Ganmore, I., Scott, L. M., Wainreb, G., Birger, Y., Elimelech, A., et al. (2008). Mutations of JAK2 in acute lymphoblastic leukaemias associated with Down's syndrome. *Lancet, 372*(9648), 1484–1492.

Bernstein, J., Dastugue, N., Haas, O., Harbott, J., Heerema, N., Huret, J., et al. (2000). Nineteen cases of the t(1;22)(p13;q13) acute megakaryoblastic leukemia of infants/children and a review of 39 cases: Report from a t(1;22) study group. *Leukemia, 14*(1), 216–217.

Boker, L. K., Blumstein, T., Sadetzki, S., Luxenburg, O., Litvak, I., Akstein, E., et al. (2001). Incidence of leukemia and other cancers in Down syndrome subjects in Israel. *International Journal of Cancer, 93*(5), 741–744

Brichard, B., Vermylen, C., De Potter, P., & Casteels, I. (2003). Down syndrome: Possible predisposition to retinoblastoma. *Medical and Pediatric Oncology, 41*(1), 73–74.

Busciglio, J., & Yankner, B. A. (1995). Apoptosis and increased generation of reactive oxygen species in Down's syndrome neurons in vitro. *Nature, 378*(6559), 776–779.

Cabelof, D. C., Patel, H. V., Chen, Q., van Remmen, H., Matherly, L. H., Ge, Y., et al. (2009). Mutational spectrum at GATA1 provides insights into mutagenesis and leukemogenesis in Down syndrome. *Blood, 114*(13), 2753–2763.

Cario, G., Zimmermann, M., Romey, R., Gesk, S., Vater, I., Harbott, J., et al. (2010). Presence of the P2RY8-CRLF2 rearrangement is associated with a poor prognosis in non-high-risk precursor B-cell acute lymphoblastic leukemia in children treated according to the ALL-BFM 2000 protocol. *Blood, 115*(26), 5393–5397.

Carpino, N., Thierfelder, W. E., Chang, M. S., Saris, C., Turner, S. J., Ziegler, S. F., et al. (2004). Absence of an essential role for thymic stromal lymphopoietin receptor in murine B-cell development. *Molecular and Cellular Biology, 24*(6), 2584–2592.

Chen, J., Li, Y., Doedens, M., Wang, P., Shago, M., Dick, J., et al. (2010). Functional differences between myeloid leukemia-initiating and transient leukemia cells in Down's syndrome. *Leukemia, 24*, 1012–1017.

Chessells, J. M., Harrison, G., Richards, S. M., Bailey, C. C., Hill, F. G., Gibson, B. E., et al. (2001). Down's syndrome and acute lymphoblastic leukaemia: Clinical features and response to treatment. *Archives of Disease in Childhood, 85*(4), 321–325.

Craze, J. L., Harrison, G., Wheatley, K., Hann, I. M., & Chessells, J. M. (1999). Improved outcome of acute myeloid leukaemia in Down's syndrome. *Archives of Disease in Childhood, 81*(1), 32–37.

Creutzig, U., Diekamp, S., Zimmermann, M., & Reinhardt, D. (2007). Longitudinal evaluation of early and late anthracycline cardiotoxicity in children with AML. *Pediatric Blood & Cancer, 48*(7), 651–662.

Creutzig, U., Reinhardt, D., Diekamp, S., Dworzak, M., Stary, J., & Zimmermann, M. (2005). AML patients with Down syndrome have a high cure rate with AML-BFM therapy with reduced dose intensity. *Leukemia, 19*(8), 1355–1360.

Creutzig, U., Ritter, J., Vormoor, J., Ludwig, W., Niemeyer, C., Reinisch, I., et al. (1996). Myelodysplasia and acute myelogenous leukemia in Down's syndrome. A report of 40 children of the AML-BFM study group. *Leukemia, 10*, 1677–1686.

Creutzig, U., Zimmermann, M., Ritter, J., Reinhardt, D., Hermann, J., Henze, G., et al. (2005). Treatment strategies and long-term results in paediatric patients treated in four consecutive AML-BFM trials. *Leukemia, 19*(12), 2030–2042.

Crispino, J. D. (2004). GATA1 mutations in Down syndrome: Implications for biology and diagnosis of children with transient myeloproliferative disorder and acute megakaryoblastic leukemia. *Pediatric Blood & Cancer,* doi 10.1002/pbc.20066.

De La Torre, R., Casado, A., Lopez-Fernandez, E., Carrascosa, D., Ramirez, V., & Saez, J. (1996). Overexpression of copper-zinc superoxide dismutase in trisomy 21. *Experientia, 52*(9), 871–873.

Dordelmann, M., Schrappe, M., Reiter, A., Zimmermann, M., Graf, N., Schott, G., et al. (1998). Down's syndrome in childhood acute lymphoblastic leukemia: Clinical characteristics and treatment outcome in four consecutive BFM trials. Berlin-Frankfurt-Munster Group. *Leukemia, 12*(5), 645–651.

Evans, T., & Felsenfeld, G. (1989). The erythroid-specific transcription factor Eryf1: A new finger protein. *Cell, 58*(5), 877–885.

Forestier, E., Izraeli, S., Beverloo, B., Haas, O., Pession, A., Michalova, K., et al. (2008). Cytogenetic features of acute lymphoblastic and myeloid leukemias in pediatric patients with Down syndrome: An iBFM-SG study. *Blood, 111*(3), 1575–1583.

Fujiwara, S., Yamashita, Y., Choi, Y. L., Watanabe, H., Kurashina, K., Soda, M., et al. (2007). Transforming activity of purinergic receptor P2Y, G protein coupled, 8 revealed by retroviral expression screening. *Leukemia and Lymphoma, 48*(5), 978–986.

Gaikwad, A., Rye, C. L., Devidas, M., Heerema, N. A., Carroll, A. J., Izraeli, S., et al. (2009). Prevalence and clinical correlates of JAK2 mutations in Down syndrome acute lymphoblastic leukaemia. *British Journal of Haematology, 144*(6), 930–932.

Gamis, A. S. (2005). Acute myeloid leukemia and Down syndrome evolution of modern therapy—state of the art review. *Pediatric Blood & Cancer, 44*(1), 13–20.

Gamis, A. S., Woods, W. G., Alonzo, T. A., Buxton, A., Lange, B., Barnard, D. R., et al. (2003). Increased age at diagnosis has a significantly negative effect on outcome in children with Down syndrome and acute myeloid leukemia: A report from the children's Cancer Group Study 2891. *Journal of Clinical Oncology, 21*(18), 3415–3422.

Garre, M. L., Relling, M. V., Kalwinsky, D., Dodge, R., Crom, W. R., Abromowitch, M., et al. (1987). Pharmacokinetics and toxicity of methotrexate in children with Down syndrome and acute lymphocytic leukemia. *Journal of Pediatrics, 111*(4), 606–612.

Ge, Y., Dombkowski, A. A., LaFiura, K. M., Tatman, D., Yedidi, R. S., Stout, M. L., et al. (2006). Differential gene expression, GATA1 target genes, and the chemotherapy sensitivity of Down syndrome megakaryocytic leukemia. *Blood, 107*(4), 1570–1581.

Ge, Y., Jensen, T. L., Stout, M. L., Flatley, R. M., Grohar, P. J., Ravindranath, Y., et al. (2004). The role of cytidine deaminase and GATA1 mutations in the increased cytosine arabinoside sensitivity of Down syndrome myeloblasts and leukemia cell lines. *Cancer Research, 64*(2), 728–735.

Ge, Y., Stout, M. L., Tatman, D. A., Jensen, T. L., Buck, S., Thomas, R. L., et al. (2005). GATA1, cytidine deaminase, and the high cure rate of Down syndrome children with acute megakaryocytic leukemia. *Journal of the National Cancer Institute, 97*(3), 226–231.

Gibson, B. E., Wheatley, K., Hann, I. M., Stevens, R. F., Webb, D., Hills, R. K., et al. (2005). Treatment strategy and long-term results in paediatric patients treated in consecutive UK AML trials. *Leukemia, 19*(12), 2130–2138.

Ginsberg, J., Bofinger, M. K., & Roush, J. R. (1977). Pathologic features of the eye in Down's syndrome with relationship to other chromosomal anomalies. *American Journal of Ophthalmology, 83*(6), 874–880.

Goldacre, M. J., Wotton, C. J., Seagroatt, V., & Yeates, D. (2004). Cancers and immune related diseases associated with Down's syndrome: A record linkage study. *Archives of Disease in Childhood, 89*(11), 1014–1017.

Greaves, M. F., Maia, A. T., Wiemels, J. L., & Ford, A. M. (2003). Leukemia in twins: Lessons in natural history. *Blood, 102*(7), 2321–2333.

Greaves, M. F., & Wiemel, J. (2003). Origins of chromosome translocations in childhood leukaemia. *Nature Reviews Cancer, 3*(9), 639–649.

Groet, J., McElwaine, S., Spinelli, M., Rinaldi, A., Burtscher, I., Mulligan, C., et al. (2003). Acquired mutations in GATA1 in neonates with Down's syndrome with transient myeloid disorder. *Lancet, 361*(9369), 1617–1620.

Gurbuxani, S., Vyas, P., & Crispino, J. D. (2004). Recent insights into the mechanisms of myeloid leukemogenesis in Down syndrome. *Blood, 103*, 399–406.

Harvey, R. C., Mullighan, C. G., Chen, I. M., Wharton, W., Mikhail, F. M., Carroll, A. J., et al. (2010). Rearrangement of CRLF2 is associated with mutation of JAK kinases, alteration of IKZF1, Hispanic/Latino ethnicity, and a poor outcome in pediatric B-progenitor acute lymphoblastic leukemia. *Blood, 115*, 5312–5321.

Hasle, H. (2001). Pattern of malignant disorders in individuals with Down's syndrome. *Lancet Oncology, 2*(7), 429–436.

Hasle, H., Abrahamsson, J., Arola, M., Karow, A., O'Marcaigh, A., Reinhardt, D., et al. (2008). Myeloid leukemia in children 4 years or older with Down syndrome often lacks GATA1 mutation and cytogenetics and risk of relapse are more akin to sporadic AML. *Leukemia, 22*(7), 1428–1430.

Hasle, H., Clemmensen, I. H., & Mikkelsen, M. (2000). Risks of leukaemia and solid tumours in individuals with Down's syndrome. *Lancet, 355*(9199), 165–169.

Hasle, H., Niemeyer, C. M., Chessells, J. M., Baumann, I., Bennett, J. M., Kerndrup, G., et al. (2003). A pediatric approach to the WHO classification of myelodysplastic and myeloproliferative diseases. *Leukemia, 17*(2), 277–282.

Hattori, M., Fujiyama, A., Taylor, T. D., Watanabe, H., Yada, T., Park, H. S., et al. (2000). The DNA sequence of human chromosome 21. *Nature, 405*(6784), 311–319.

Hertzberg, L., Vendramini, E., Ganmore, I., Cazzaniga, G., Schmitz, M., Chalker, J., et al. (2010). Down syndrome acute lymphoblastic leukemia, a highly heterogeneous disease in which aberrant expression of CRLF2 is associated with mutated JAK2: A report from the International BFM Study Group. *Blood, 115*(5), 1006–1017.

Hill, D. A., Gridley, G., Cnattingius, S., Mellemkjaer, L., Linet, M., Adami, H. O., et al. (2003). Mortality and cancer incidence among individuals with Down syndrome. *Archives of Internal Medicine, 163*(6), 705–711.

Hitzler, J., & Zipursky, A. (2005). GATA 1 mutations as clonal markers of minimal residual disease in acute megakaryoblastic leukemia of Down syndrome—a new tool with significant potential applications. *Leukemia Research, 29*(11), 1239–1240.

Hitzler, J. K., Cheung, J., Li, Y., Scherer, S. W., & Zipursky, A. (2003). GATA1 mutations in transient leukemia and acute megakaryoblastic leukemia of Down syndrome. *Blood, 101*(11), 4301–4304.

Hitzler, J. K., & Zipursky, A. (2005). Origins of leukaemia in children with Down syndrome. *Nature Reviews Cancer, 5*(1), 11–20.

Hollanda, L. M., Lima, C. S., Cunha, A. F., Albuquerque, D. M., Vassallo, J., Ozelo, M. C., et al. (2006). An inherited mutation leading to production of only the short isoform of GATA-1 is associated with impaired erythropoiesis. *Nature Genetics, 38*(7), 807–812.

James, C., Ugo, V., Le Couedic, J. P., Staerk, J., Delhommeau, F., Lacout, C., et al. (2005). A unique clonal JAK2 mutation leading to constitutive signalling causes polycythaemia vera. *Nature, 434*(7037), 1144–1148.

Kaleem, Z., Shuster, J. J., Carroll, A. J., Borowitz, M. J., Pullen, D. J., Camitta, B. M., et al. (2000). Acute lymphoblastic leukemia with an unusual t(8;14)(q11.2;q32): A Pediatric Oncology Group Study. *Leukemia, 14*(2), 238–240.

Kalwinsky, D. K., Raimondi, S. C., Bunin, N. J., Fairclough, D., Pui, C. H., Relling, M. V., et al. (1990). Clinical and biological characteristics of acute lymphocytic leukemia in children with Down syndrome. *American Journal of Medical Genetics. Supplement*, 7, 267–271.

Kearney, L., Gonzalez De Castro, D., Yeung, J., Procter, J., Horsley, S. W., Eguchi-Ishimae, M., et al. (2009). Specific JAK2 mutation (JAK2R683) and multiple gene deletions in Down syndrome acute lymphoblastic leukemia. *Blood*, *113*(3), 646–648.

Kiyoi, H., Yamaji, S., Kojima, S., & Naoe, T. (2007). JAK3 mutations occur in acute megakaryoblastic leukemia both in Down syndrome children and non-Down syndrome adults. *Leukemia*, *21*(3), 574–576.

Klusmann, J. H., Creutzig, U., Zimmermann, M., Dworzak, M., Jorch, N., Langebrake, C., et al. (2008). Treatment and prognostic impact of transient leukemia in neonates with Down syndrome. *Blood*, *111*(6), 2991–2998.

Klusmann, J. H., Reinhardt, D., Hasle, H., Kaspers, G. J., Creutzig, U., Hahlen, K., et al. (2007). Janus kinase mutations in the development of acute megakaryoblastic leukemia in children with and without Down's syndrome. *Leukemia*, *21*(7), 1584–1587.

Kojima, S., Sako, M., Kato, K., Hosoi, G., Sato, T., Ohara, A., et al. (2000). An effective chemotherapeutic regimen for acute myeloid leukemia and myelodysplastic syndrome in children with Down's syndrome. *Leukemia*, *14*(5), 786–791.

Krischer, J. P., Epstein, S., Cuthbertson, D. D., Goorin, A. M., Epstein, M. L., & Lipshultz, S. E. (1997). Clinical cardiotoxicity following anthracycline treatment for childhood cancer: The Pediatric Oncology Group experience. *Journal of Clinical Oncology*, *15*(4), 1544–1552.

Krivit, W., & Good, R. A. (1957). Simultaneous occurrence of mongolism and leukemia; report of a nationwide survey. *AMA Journal of Diseases of Children*, *94*(3), 289–293.

Kudo, K., Kojima, S., Tabuchi, K., Yabe, H., Tawa, A., Imaizumi, M., et al. (2007). Prospective study of a pirarubicin, intermediate-dose cytarabine, and etoposide regimen in children with Down syndrome and acute myeloid leukemia: The Japanese childhood AML cooperative Study Group. *Journal of Clinical Oncology*, *25*(34), 5442–5447.

Lange, B. J., Kobrinsky, N., Barnard, D. R., Arthur, D. C., Buckley, J. D., Howells, W. B., et al. (1998). Distinctive demography, biology, and outcome of acute myeloid leukemia and myelodysplastic syndrome in children with Down syndrome: Children's Cancer Group Studies 2861 and 2891. *Blood*, *91*(2), 608–615.

Lanza, C., Volpe, G., Basso, G., Gottardi, E., Perfetto, F., Cilli, V., et al. (1997). The common TEL/AML1 rearrangement does not represent a frequent event in acute lymphoblastic leukaemia occuring in children with Down syndrome. *Leukemia*, *11*(6), 820–821.

Levitt, G. A., Stiller, C. A., & Chessells, J. M. (1990). Prognosis of Down's syndrome with acute leukaemia. *Archives of Disease in Childhood*, *65*(2), 212–216.

Li, Z., Godinho, F. J., Klusmann, J. H., Garriga-Canut, M., Yu, C., & Orkin, S. H. (2005). Developmental stage-selective effect of somatically mutated leukemogenic transcription factor GATA1. *Nature Genetics*, *37*(6), 613–619.

Lie, S. O., Jonmundsson, G., Mellander, L., Siimes, M. A., Yssing, M., & Gustafsson, G. (1996). A population-based study of 272 children with acute myeloid leukaemia treated on two consecutive protocols with different intensity: Best outcome in girls, infants, and children with Down's syndrome. Nordic Society of Paediatric Haematology and Oncology (NOPHO). *British Journal of Haematology*, *94*(1), 82–88.

Lightfoot, J., Hitzler, J., Zipursky, A., Albert, M., & Macgregor, P. (2004). Distinct gene signatures of transient and acute megakaryoblastic leukemia in Down syndrome. *Leukemia*, *18*(10), 1617–1623.

Lorsbach, R. B. (2004). Megakaryoblastic disorders in children. *American Journal of Clinical Pathology*, *122*, *Supplement*, S33–S46.

Ma, X., Renda, M. J., Wang, L., Cheng, E.-c., Niu, C., Morris, S. W., et al. (2007). Rbm15 modulates notch-induced transcriptional activation and affects myeloid differentiation. *Molecular and Cellular Biology*, MCB, *360*(5), 470–480.

Ma, Z., Morris, S. W., Valentine, V., Li, M., Herbrick, J. A., Cui, X., et al. (2001). Fusion of two novel genes, RBM15 and MKL1, in the t(1;22)(p13;q13) of acute megakaryoblastic leukemia. *Nature Genetics*, *28*(3), 220–221.

Malinge, S., Ben-Abdelali, R., Settegrana, C., Radford-Weiss, I., Debre, M., Beldjord, K., et al. (2007). Novel activating JAK2 mutation in a patient with Down syndrome and B-cell precursor acute lymphoblastic leukemia. *Blood*, *109*(5), 2202–2204.

Malinge, S., Izraeli, S., & Crispino, J. D. (2009). Insights into the manifestations, outcomes, and mechanisms of leukemogenesis in Down syndrome. *Blood*, *113*(12), 2619–2628.

Malinge, S., Ragu, C., Della-Valle, V., Pisani, D., Constantinescu, S. N., Perez, C., et al. (2008). Activating mutations in human acute megakaryoblastic leukemia. *Blood*, *112*(10), 4220–4226.

Martin, D. I., Zon, L. I., Mutter, G., & Orkin, S. H. (1990). Expression of an erythroid transcription factor in megakaryocytic and mast cell lineages. *Nature*, *344*(6265), 444–447.

Massey, G. V., Zipursky, A., Chang, M. N., Doyle, J. J., Nasim, S., Taub, J. W., et al. (2006). A prospective study of the natural history of transient leukemia (TL) in neonates with Down syndrome (DS): Children's Oncology Group (COG) study POG-9481. *Blood*, *107*(12), 4606–4613.

McElwaine, S., Mulligan, C., Groet, J., Spinelli, M., Rinaldi, A., Denyer, G., et al. (2004). Microarray transcript profiling distinguishes the transient from the acute type of megakaryoblastic leukaemia (M7) in Down's syndrome, revealing PRAME as a specific discriminating marker. *British Journal of Haematology*, *125*(6), 729–742.

Meissner, B., Borkhardt, A., Dilloo, D., Fuchs, D., Friedrich, W., Handgretinger, R., et al. (2007). Relapse, not regimen-related toxicity, was the major cause of treatment failure in 11 children with Down syndrome undergoing haematopoietic stem cell transplantation for acute leukaemia. *Bone Marrow Transplantation*, *40*(10), 945–949.

Mercher, T., Coniat, M. B., Monni, R., Mauchauffe, M., Khac, F. N., Gressin, L., et al. (2001). Involvement of a human gene related to the Drosophila spen gene in the recurrent t(1;22) translocation of acute megakaryocytic leukemia. *Proceedings of the National Academy of Sciences of the United States of America*, *98*(10), 5776–5779.

Mercher, T., Raffel, G. D., Moore, S. A., Cornejo, M. G., Baudry-Bluteau, D., Cagnard, N., et al. (2009). The OTT-MAL fusion oncogene activates RBPJ-mediated transcription and induces acute megakaryoblastic leukemia in a knockin mouse model. *Journal of Clinical Investigation*, *119*(4), 852–864.

Mullighan, C. G., Collins-Underwood, J. R., Phillips, L. A., Loudin, M. G., Liu, W., Zhang, J., et al. (2009). Rearrangement of CRLF2 in B-progenitor- and Down syndrome-associated acute lymphoblastic leukemia. *Nature Genetics*, *41*(11), 1243–1246.

Mullighan, C. G., Goorha, S., Radtke, I., Miller, C. B., Coustan-Smith, E., Dalton, J. D., et al. (2007). Genome-wide analysis of genetic alterations in acute lymphoblastic leukaemia. *Nature*, *446*, 758–764.

Mullighan, C. G., Su, X., Zhang, J., Radtke, I., Phillips, L. A., Miller, C. B., et al. (2009a). Deletion of IKZF1 and prognosis in acute lymphoblastic leukemia. *New England Journal of Medicine*, *360*, 470–480.

Mullighan, C. G., Zhang, J., Harvey, R. C., Collins-Underwood, J. R., Schulman, B. A., Phillips, L. A., et al. (2009b). JAK mutations in high-risk childhood acute lymphoblastic leukemia. *Proceedings of the National Academy of Sciences of the United States of America*, *106*(23), 9414–9418.

Mundschau, G., Gurbuxani, S., Gamis, A. S., Greene, M. E., Arceci, R. J., & Crispino, J. D. (2003). Mutagenesis of GATA1 is an initiating event in Down syndrome leukemogenesis. *Blood*, *101*(11), 4298–4300.

Muntean, A. G., & Crispino, J. D. (2005). Differential requirements for the activation domain and FOG-interaction surface of GATA-1 in megakaryocyte gene expression and development. *Blood*, *106*(4), 1223–1231.

Norton, A., Fisher, C., Liu, H., Wen, Q., Mundschau, G., Fuster, J. L., et al. (2007). Analysis of JAK3, JAK2, and C-MPL mutations in transient myeloproliferative disorder and myeloid leukemia of Down syndrome blasts in children with Down syndrome. *Blood, 110*(3), 1077–1079.

O'Brien, M. M., Taub, J. W., Chang, M. N., Massey, G. V., Stine, K. C., Raimondi, S. C., et al. (2008). Cardiomyopathy in children with down syndrome treated for acute myeloid leukemia: A report from the Children's Oncology Group Study POG 9421. *Journal of Clinical Oncology, 26*(3), 414–420.

Olson, J. M., Hamilton, A., & Breslow, N. E. (1995). Non-11p constitutional chromosome abnormalities in Wilms' tumor patients. *Medical and Pediatric Oncology, 24*(5), 305–309.

Patja, K., Eero, P., & Iivanainen, M. (2001). Cancer incidence among people with intellectual disability. *Journal of Intellectual Disability Research, 45*(Pt 4), 300–307.

Pine, S. R., Guo, Q., Yin, C., Jayabose, S., Levendoglu-Tugal, O., Ozkaynak, M. F., et al. (2005). GATA1 as a new target to detect minimal residual disease in both transient leukemia and megakaryoblastic leukemia of Down syndrome. *Leukemia Research, 29,* 1353–1356.

Pui, C. H., Raimondi, S. C., Borowitz, M. J., Land, V. J., Behm, F. G., Pullen, D. J., et al. (1993). Immunophenotypes and karyotypes of leukemic cells in children with Down syndrome and acute lymphoblastic leukemia. *Journal of Clinical Oncology, 11*(7), 1361–1367.

Pui, C. H., Relling, M. V., & Downing, J. R. (2004). Acute lymphoblastic leukemia. *New England Journal of Medicine, 350*(15), 1535–1548.

Rabin, K. R., & Whitlock, J. A. (2009). Malignancy in Children with Trisomy 21. *Oncologist, 14*(2), 164–173.

Ragab, A. H., Abdel-Mageed, A., Shuster, J. J., Frankel, L. S., Pullen, J., van Eys, J., et al. (1991). Clinical characteristics and treatment outcome of children with acute lymphocytic leukemia and Down's syndrome. A Pediatric Oncology Group study. *Cancer, 67* (4), 1057–1063.

Rainis, L., Bercovich, D., Strehl, S., Teigler-Schlegel, A., Stark, B., Trka, J., et al. (2003). Mutations in exon 2 of GATA1 are early events in megakaryocytic malignancies associated with trisomy 21. *Blood, 102*(3), 981–986.

Rajantie, J., & Siimes, M. A. (2003). Long-term prognosis of children with Down's syndrome and leukaemia: A 34-year nation-wide experience. *Journal of Intellectual Disability Research, 47*(Pt 8), 617–621.

Rao, A., Hills, R. K., Stiller, C., Gibson, B. E., de Graaf, S. S., Hann, I. M., et al. (2006). Treatment for myeloid leukaemia of Down syndrome: Population-based experience in the UK and results from the Medical Research Council AML 10 and AML 12 trials. *British Journal of Haematology, 132*(5), 576–583.

Ravindranath, Y. (2005). Down syndrome and leukemia: New insights into the epidemiology, pathogenesis, and treatment. *Pediatric Blood & Cancer, 44*(1), 1–7.

Ravindranath, Y., Abella, E., Krischer, J. P., Wiley, J., Inoue, S., Harris, M., et al. (1992). Acute myeloid leukemia (AML) in Down's syndrome is highly responsive to chemotherapy: Experience on Pediatric Oncology Group AML Study 8498 [see comments]. *Blood, 80*(9), 2210–2214.

Reinhardt, K., Blink, M., Sander, A., von Neuhoff, C., Boehmer, K., Kolenova, A., et al. (2009). Is prevention of myeloid leukemia possible? *ASH Annual Meeting Abstracts, 114* (22), 481–.

Robison, L. L., Nesbit, M. E., Jr., Sather, H. N., Level, C., Shahidi, N., Kennedy, A., et al. (1984). Down syndrome and acute leukemia in children: A 10-year retrospective survey from childrens Cancer Study Group. *Journal of Pediatrics, 105*(2), 235–242.

Roizen, N. J., & Patterson, D. (2003). Down's syndrome. *Lancet, 361*(9365), 1281–1289.

Romeo, P. H., Prandini, M. H., Joulin, V., Mignotte, V., Prenant, M., Vainchenker, W., et al. (1990). Megakaryocytic and erythrocytic lineages share specific transcription factors. *Nature, 344*(6265), 447–449.
Rubin, C. M., Mick, R., & Johnson, F. L. (1996). Bone marrow transplantation for the treatment of haematological disorders in Down's syndrome: Toxicity and outcome. *Bone Marrow Transplantation, 18*(3), 533–540.
Russell, L. J., Capasso, M., Vater, I., Akasaka, T., Bernard, O. A., Calasanz, M. J., et al. (2009). Deregulated expression of cytokine receptor gene, CRLF2, is involved in lymphoid transformation in B-cell precursor acute lymphoblastic leukemia. *Blood, 114*(13), 2688–2698.
Ryeom, S., Baek, K. H., & Zaslavsky, A. (2009). Down's syndrome: Protection against cancer and the therapeutic potential of DSCR1. *Future Oncology, 5*(8), 1185–1188.
Ryeom, S., & Folkman, J. (2009). Role of endogenous angiogenesis inhibitors in Down syndrome. *Journal of Craniofacial Surgery, 20*(Suppl. 1), 595–596.
Sandoval, C., Hudson, M. M., Ozkaynak, M. F., Tugal, O., & Jayabose, S. (2000). Down syndrome and Hodgkin disease in childhood. *Medical and Pediatric Oncology, 34*(4), 304–305.
Satge, D., & Rickert, C. H. (2009). A medical enigma: Persons with Down syndrome do not develop medulloblastoma. *Neuroepidemiology, 32*(2), 164.
Satge, D., Sasco, A. J., Carlsen, N.L.T., Stiller, C. A., Rubie, H., Hero, B., et al. (1998a). A Lack of Neuroblastoma in Down Syndrome: A study from 11 European Countries. *Cancer Research, 58*(3), 448–452.
Satge, D., Sommelet, D., Geneix, A., Nishi, M., Malet, P., & Vekemans, M. (1998b). A tumor profile in Down syndrome. *American Journal of Medical Genetics, 78*(3), 207–216.
Shah, N., Al-Ahmari, A., Al-Yamani, A., Dupuis, L., Stephens, D., & Hitzler, J. (2009). Outcome and toxicity of chemotherapy for acute lymphoblastic leukemia in children with Down syndrome. *Pediatric Blood & Cancer, 52*(1), 14–19.
Shivdasani, R. A., Fujiwara, Y., McDevitt, M. A., & Orkin, S. H. (1997). A lineage-selective knockout establishes the critical role of transcription factor GATA-1 in megakaryocyte growth and platelet development. *EMBO Journal, 16*(13), 3965–3973.
Slordahl, S. H., Smeland, E. B., Holte, H., Gronn, M., Lie, S. O., & Seip, M. (1993). Leukemic blasts with markers of four cell lineages in Down's syndrome ("megakaryoblastic leukemia"). *Medical and Pediatric Oncology, 21*(4), 254–258.
Speck, N. A., & Gilliland, D. G. (2002). Core-binding factors in haematopoiesis and leukaemia. *Nature Reviews Cancer, 2*(7), 502–513.
Sullivan, S. G., Hussain, R., Glasson, E. J., & Bittles, A. H. (2007). The profile and incidence of cancer in Down syndrome. *Journal of Intellectual Disability Research, 51*(Pt 3), 228–231.
Sussan, T. E., Yang, A., Li, F., Ostrowski, M. C., & Reeves, R. H. (2008). Trisomy represses Apc(Min)-mediated tumours in mouse models of Down's syndrome. *Nature, 451*(7174), 73–75.
Taub, J. W., & Ge, Y. (2005). Down syndrome, drug metabolism and chromosome 21. *Pediatric Blood & Cancer, 44*(1), 33–39.
Taub, J. W., Huang, X., Matherly, L. H., Stout, M. L., Buck, S. A., Massey, G. V., et al. (1999). Expression of chromosome 21-localized genes in acute myeloid leukemia: Differences between Down syndrome and non-Down syndrome blast cells and relationship to in vitro sensitivity to cytosine arabinoside and daunorubicin. *Blood, 94*(4), 1393–1400.
Taub, J. W., Mundschau, G., Ge, Y., Poulik, J. M., Qureshi, F., Jensen, T., et al. (2004). Prenatal origin of GATA1 mutations may be an initiating step in the development of megakaryocytic leukemia in Down syndrome. *Blood, 104*(5), 1588–1589.
Tchernia, G., Lejeune, F., Boccara, J. F., Denavit, M. F., Dommergues, J. P., & Bernaudin, F. (1996). Erythroblastic and/or megakaryoblastic leukemia in Down syndrome: Treatment with low-dose arabinosyl cytosine. *Journal of Pediatric Hematology/oncology, 18*(1), 59–62.

Tsai, S. F., Martin, D. I., Zon, L. I., D'Andrea, A. D., Wong, G. G., & Orkin, S. H. (1989). Cloning of cDNA for the major DNA-binding protein of the erythroid lineage through expression in mammalian cells. *Nature, 339*(6224), 446–451.

Tunstall-Pedoe, O., Roy, A., Karadimitris, A., de la Fuente, J., Fisk, N. M., Bennett, P., et al. (2008). Abnormalities in the myeloid progenitor compartment in Down syndrome fetal liver precede acquisition of GATA1 mutations. *Blood, 112*(12), 4507–4511.

Ugazio, A. G., Maccario, R., Notarangelo, L. D., & Burgio, G. R. (1990). Immunology of Down syndrome: A review. *American Journal of Medical Genetics Supplement,* 7, 204–212.

Vyas, P., Ault, K., Jackson, C. W., Orkin, S. H., & Shivdasani, R. A. (1999). Consequences of GATA-1 deficiency in megakaryocytes and platelets. *Blood, 93*(9), 2867–2875.

Walters, D. K., Mercher, T., Gu, T. L., O'Hare, T., Tyner, J. W., Loriaux, M., et al. (2006). Activating alleles of JAK3 in acute megakaryoblastic leukemia. *Cancer Cell, 10*(1), 65–75.

Webb, D. K. (2005). Optimizing therapy for myeloid disorders of Down syndrome. *British Journal of Haematology, 131*(1), 3–7.

Wechsler, J., Greene, M., McDevitt, M. A., Anastasi, J., Karp, J. E., Le Beau, M. M., et al. (2002). Acquired mutations in GATA1 in the megakaryoblastic leukemia of Down syndrome. *Nature Genetics, 32*(1), 148–152.

Wheeler, K., Chessells, J. M., Bailey, C. C., & Richards, S. M. (1996). Treatment related deaths during induction and in first remission in acute lymphoblastic leukaemia: MRC UKALL X. *Archives of Disease in Childhood, 74*(2), 101–107.

Whitlock, J. A. (2006). Down syndrome and acute lymphoblastic leukaemia. *British Journal of Haematology, 135*(5), 595–602.

Whitlock, J. A., Sather, H. N., Gaynon, P., Robison, L. L., Wells, R. J., Trigg, M., et al. (2005). Clinical characteristics and outcome of children with Down syndrome and acute lymphoblastic leukemia: A Children's Cancer Group study. *Blood, 106*(13), 4043–4049.

Windham, G. C., Bjerkedal, T., & Langmark, F. (1985). A population-based study of cancer incidence in twins and in children with congenital malformations or low birth weight, Norway, 1967–1980. *American Journal of Epidemiology, 121*(1), 49–56.

Xu, G., Nagano, M., Kanezaki, R., Toki, T., Hayashi, Y., Taketani, T., et al. (2003). Frequent mutations in the GATA-1 gene in the transient myeloproliferative disorder of Down syndrome. *Blood, 102*(8), 2960–2968.

Yoda, A., Yoda, Y., Chiaretti, S., Bar-Natan, M., Mani, K., Rodig, S. J., et al. (2010). Functional screening identifies CRLF2 in precursor B-cell acute lymphoblastic leukemia. *Proceedings of the National Academy of Sciences, 107*(1), 252–257.

Zeller, B., Gustafsson, G., Forestier, E., Abrahamsson, J., Clausen, N., Heldrup, J., et al. (2005). Acute leukaemia in children with Down syndrome: A population-based Nordic study. *British Journal of Haematology, 128*(6), 797–804.

Ziegler, S. F., & Liu, Y. J. (2006). Thymic stromal lymphopoietin in normal and pathogenic T cell development and function. *Nature Immunology,* 7(7), 709–714.

Zipursky, A. (2003). Transient leukaemia—a benign form of leukaemia in newborn infants with trisomy 21. *British Journal of Haematology, 120*(6), 930–938.

Zipursky, A., Brown, E., Christensen, H., Sutherland, R., & Doyle, J. (1997). Leukemia and/or myeloproliferative syndrome in neonates with Down syndrome. *Seminars in Perinatology, 21*, 97–101.

Zon, L. I., Yamaguchi, Y., Yee, K., Albee, E. A., Kimura, A., Bennett, J. C., et al. (1993). Expression of mRNA for the GATA-binding proteins in human eosinophils and basophils: Potential role in gene transcription. *Blood, 81*(12), 3234–3241.

Zorick, T. S., Mustacchi, Z., Bando, S. Y., Zatz, M., Moreira-Filho, C. A., Olsen, B., et al. (2001). High serum endostatin levels in Down syndrome: Implications for improved treatment and prevention of solid tumours. *European Journal of Human Genetics, 9*(11), 811–814.

Zwaan, C. M., Kaspers, G. J., Pieters, R., Hahlen, K., Janka-Schaub, G. E., van Zantwijk, C. H., et al. (2002). Different drug sensitivity profiles of acute myeloid and lymphoblastic leukemia and normal peripheral blood mononuclear cells in children with and without Down syndrome. *Blood*, *99*(1), 245–251.

Zwaan, M. C., Reinhardt, D., Hitzler, J., & Vyas, P. (2008). Acute leukemias in children with Down syndrome. *Pediatric Clinics of North America*, *55*(1), 53–70.

CHAPTER SIX

Cardiovascular Disorders among Persons with Down Syndrome

Jeroen C. Vis,[*,†] Klaartje van Engelen,[*,†,‡] Berto J. Bouma,[*] Catia M. Bilardo,[§] Nico A Blom,[¶] *and* Barbara J.M. Mulder,[*,†]

Contents

[*] Department of Cardiology, Academic Medical Centre, Amsterdam, The Netherlands
[†] Interuniversity Cardiology Institute of the Netherlands, Utrecht, The Netherlands
[‡] Department of Clinical Genetics Academic Medical Centre, Amsterdam, The Netherlands
[§] Department of Obstetrics and Gynaecology, Fetal Medicine Unit Academic Medical Centre, Amsterdam, The Netherlands
[¶] Department of Paediatric Cardiology, Leiden University Medical Center, Leiden, The Netherlands

International Review of Research in Mental Retardation, Volume 39
ISSN 0074-7750, DOI 10.1016/S0074-7750(10)39006-9

Abstract

Down syndrome is the most common chromosomal abnormality among liveborn infants and is the most frequent chromosomal cause of intellectual disability (Frid, Drott, Lundell, Rasmussen, & Anneren, 1999). It is a multisystem disorder, characterized by various congenital defects, organic disorders, dysmorphic features, and other health-related problems (Roizen & Patterson, 2003). The heart is affected frequently and the association between Down syndrome and congenital heart disease was already recognized by Garrod in 1894 (Richards, 1965). Although a critical region on chromosome 21 as well as several candidate genes has been proposed, the genetic basis and pathogenesis of congenital heart defects in Down syndrome remain largely unknown. Cardiovascular disorders related to Down syndrome are numerous. Here, we review prenatal screening, intrauterine interventions, and management of congenital heart defects in early childhood. Moreover, we discuss cardiovascular manifestations in adulthood, in particular pulmonary arterial hypertension and cardiac surgery in adults with Down syndrome.

1. The Unborn Child with Down Syndrome

1.1. The fetal blood circulation

In order to address the cardiovascular problems related to Down syndrome, it is important to understand the basic knowledge of the normal anatomy of the heart and blood circulation and fetal circulation. The development of the heart and blood vessels before birth is a complex and interesting process. At an early stage in pregnancy, after 12 weeks of gestation, the development has already been fully completed. The remaining time before birth will be spent for growth. However, after birth the blood circulation will change dramatically, due to the expansion of the lungs after breathing; pulmonary pressure drops rapidly and blood flows through the lungs. The *ductus arteriosus* closes, left atrial pressure rises above right atrial pressure leading to closure of the *foramen ovale*, the opening between both atria. (see Fig. 6.1)

1.2. Prenatal diagnosis and management of cardiovascular disorders in Down syndrome

In most western countries prenatal screening programs for Down syndrome and structural anomalies are currently available. Since the introduction of first-trimester screening in most countries, the combined test is the screening test of choice for Down syndrome. The combined test includes nuchal translucency (NT) measurement and first-trimester biochemistry (PAPP-A and free Beta-hCG). NT refers to the nuchal fluid accumulation

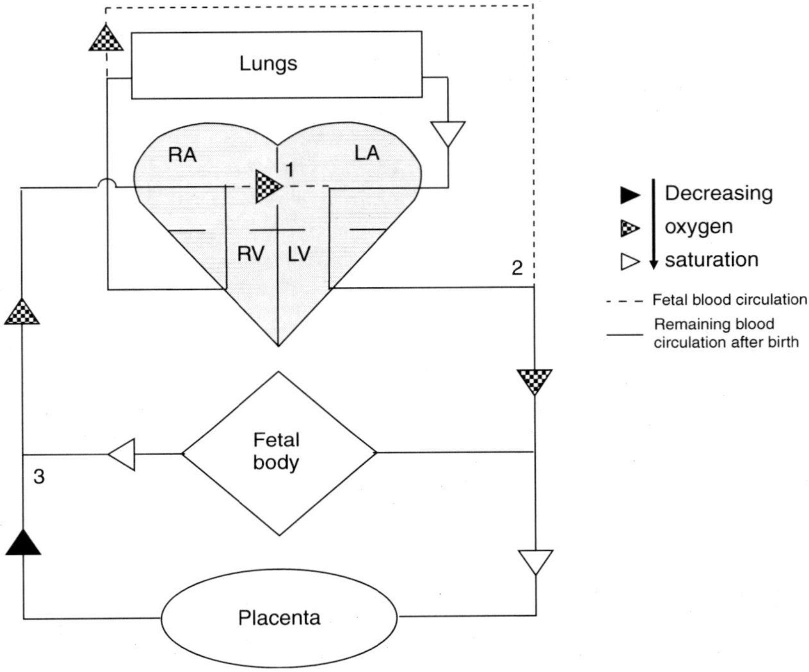

Figure 6.1 Normal fetal blood circulation: LA, left atrium; LV, left ventricle; RA, right atrium; RV, right ventricle. Dotted line represents fetal blood circulation disappearing after birth. Continuous line represents remaining blood circulation after birth; 1, foramen ovale; 2, ductus arteriosus; 3, ductus venosus.

visible in first-trimester fetuses and measurable on ultrasound examination (Nicolaides, Azar, Byrne, Mansur, & Marks, 1992). An enlarged NT entails an increased risk for Down syndrome, but also for congenital heart defects (CHDs) (Clur et al., 2008; Clur, Ottenkamp, & Bilardo, 2009) Therefore, the test preferentially identifies Down syndrome fetuses with a CHD. Mothers of fetuses with an enlarged NT are therefore offered karyotyping and detailed ultrasound examinations for the detection of congenital anomalies already detectable from the late first trimester of pregnancy. Out of 967 fetuses referred to our Fetal Medicine Unit for fetal echocardiography in view of an enlarged NT, 68 (7%) had a CHD. In 13 cases (19%) the cardiac defect (9 atrioventricular septal defect (AVSD), 2 inlet ventricular septal defect, 1 Tetralogy of Fallot, 1 other) was associated with Down syndrome (Clur et al., 2008).

Next to first-trimester screening routine ultrasound screening at 20 weeks is part of standard pregnancy care in most western countries and contributes to the detection of the majority of CHD in the fetus. Diagnostic accuracy and sensitivity of this ultrasound technique varies according to gestational age at diagnosis, characteristics of the equipment used, and experience of the ultrasonographer. Every time a cardiac defect is seen at ultrasound examination mothers are offered karyotyping. Down syndrome is diagnosed in 4–9% of fetuses with cardiac defects (Paladini et al., 2000). In prenatal series more than 50% of Down syndrome fetuses undergoing echocardiography have recognizable cardiac defects (Paladini et al., 2000). All major cardiovascular defects in Down syndrome fetuses are amenable to prenatal diagnosis by fetal echocardiography. The spectrum of CHD is similar to what is seen after birth, AVSD being the most common of the severe defects (44%). Conversely, of all the AVSD diagnosed prenatally by echocardiography, 43% are associated with Down syndrome (Paladini et al., 2000).

In prenatal life the frequency of CHD in Down syndrome fetuses is higher and severe defects are more frequently observed. This is due to the fact that fetuses with severe cardiac defects are more likely to die inutero and mothers may be more inclined to terminate the pregnancy when a severe cardiac defect is seen. Moreover, milder defects such as small ventricular septal defects or subtle variants of endocardial cushion defects may be more frequently missed at fetal echocardiography. Also the prenatal diagnosis of aortic coarctation remains a challenge as the only obvious detectable prenatal feature in this anomaly is ventricular chambers disproportion in the second or third trimester of pregnancy.

One may expect that in view of the increasing availability of prenatal screening the total number of Down syndrome live births and of related CHD should decrease. Interestingly, over the decade 1989–2008 the number of Down syndrome cases diagnosed before or after birth in England and Wales increased by 71%, since mothers are having babies at an older age (Morris & Alberman, 2009). However, owing to the effect of prenatal screening and consequent terminations of pregnancy the number of live births with Down syndrome has fallen by 1%. Overall about 92% of mothers confronted with the diagnosis Down syndrome in England and Wales terminate pregnancy (Morris & Alberman, 2009). In other counties termination rates vary considerably, reflecting prenatal screening participation and women attitudes towards Down syndrome.

When a CHD is diagnosed in a Down syndrome fetus, couples are counselled about the prognosis of the cardiac defect in a baby with a chromosomal anomaly. If they choose for continuation of pregnancy, pregnancy care is organized at a Perinatal Center with a neonatal intensive care unit and experience in the management of delivery and immediate postnatal care of a fetus/neonate with a CHD.

During pregnancy, fetal echocardiography is repeated at regular intervals until birth to check for signs of impending cardiac failure or deterioration of the anomaly (ascites, pericardial effusion, abnormal cardiac rhythm, cardiac chambers dilatation) that may be an indication for earlier delivery.

2. Cardiovascular Disorders in Childhood

2.1. Congenital heart defects in Down syndrome

Down syndrome is associated with multiple malformations and there is an increased risk of leukemia (<1%), hearing loss (75%), gastrointestinal malformations (14%), celiac disease (17%), eye disease (60%), thyroid disease (15%), and CHDs (American Academy of Pediatrics, 2001). In the general population CHDs occur in approximately 8 per 1000 newborns, whereas almost 50% of the neonates with Down syndrome have a CHD (Freeman et al., 1998; Gatzoulis & Webb, 2003). Down syndrome also shows a fixed pattern of CHD, with overrepresentation of septal defects. In patients with a CHD, an AVSD is the most common defect, with a prevalence of 45%, followed by a ventricular septal defect in 35%, and an isolated atrial septal defect in 8% of the cases (see Table 6.1) (Freeman et al., 1998; Frid et al., 1999; van der Velde et al., 2005). Tetralogy of Fallot and a patent arterial duct account for 10% of the cardiac defects in Down syndrome, while other defects are rare. Recent findings suggest that sex and ethnic differences exist in the incidence of AVSDs in Down syndrome, with twice as many females and blacks affected. Hispanics are affected less frequently compared to Caucasians (Freeman et al., 2008).

Septal defects can be classified into three major subgroups based on location of the defect. An atrial septal defect is an opening between the two atria (the upper chambers of the heart). The type of atrial septal defect is classified by the location of the defect in the atrial septum (see Fig. 6.2). A ventricular septal defect is an opening between the two ventricles (the main chambers of the heart). Ventricular septal defects are muscular or membranous and they are located on various locations of the ventricular septum (see Fig. 6.3). Approximately 24% of the small ventricular septal defects close spontaneously by 18 months. Up to 75% are closed by the age of 10. Moderate-to-large ventricular septal defects often become smaller but remain open and allow shunting of blood from one side of the circulation to the other. Because the left (systemic) blood pressure is higher than the right (pulmonary), the shunt is left to right and increased blood is circulated through the lungs. Eventually, the increased flow rates through the pulmonary circulation lead to obliteration of the lung tissue and pulmonary hypertension.

An atrioventricular septal defect, also known as atrioventricular canal defect or endocardial cushion defect, is an opening between the atrial

Table 6.1 Congenital heart defects

	Frid et al. (1999)	Freeman et al. (2008)
	n = 219	*n* = 1469
Percentage with congenital heart defects	48	44
Type of defect[a]		
Atrioventricular septal defect	47	39
Complete	41	29
Partial	6	10
Ventricular septal defect	33	43
Atrial septal defect, type 2	NA	42
Isolated	8	8
Patent arterial duct	8*	NA
Isolated	2*	NA
Aortic coarctation	1	1
Tetralogy of Fallot	2	6
Other	8	3

Values are expressed as %.
[a] among those with any heart defect.
* after one year.
NA; not available.

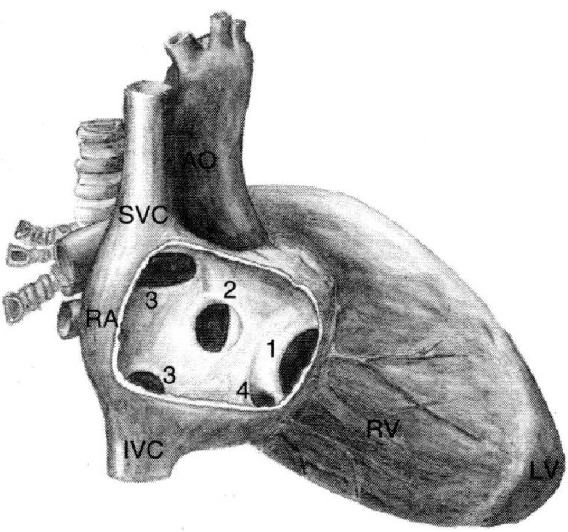

Figure 6.2 Atrial septal defect: RA, right atrium; RV, right ventricle; LV, left ventricle; AO, aorta; VCI, vena cava inferior; VCS; vena cava superior; 1, atrial septal defect type 1; 2, atrial septal defect type 2; 3, sinus venosus defect; 4, sinus coronarius defect.

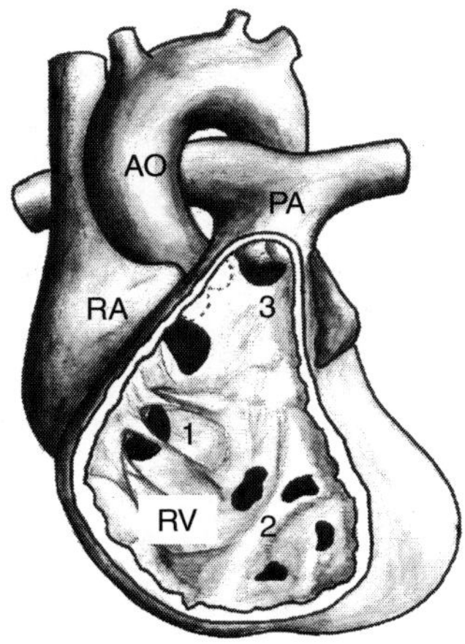

Figure 6.3 Ventricular septal defect: RV, right ventricle; RA, right atrium; AO, aorta; PA, pulmonary artery; 1, perimembranous (inlet) ventricular septal defect; 2, muscular (trabecular) ventricular septal defect; 3, subarterial (outlet) ventricular septal defect.

component of the septum which continues down between the ventricular component of the septum. The primary defect is the failure of formation of the part of the heart that arises from an embryonic structure called the endocardial cushions. The endocardial cushions are responsible for separating the central parts of the heart near the tricuspid and mitral valves (atrioventricular valves), which separate the atria from the ventricles. Two different types of defects can be classified; complete and partial AVSD (see Fig. 6.4). A complete AVSD is one in which there are defects in all structures formed by the endocardial cushions and the atrioventricular valves remain undivided or "common." A partial or incomplete AVSD is one in which the bridging leaflets of the atrioventricular valves are fixed to the ventricular septum, leaving only a (type 1) atrial septal defect, and the atrioventricular valves are divided into two distinct valves. Usually, a ventricular septal defect is absent, but there may be a small, hemodynamically unimportant interventricular communication (Shinebourne & Ho, 2003).

2.2. Presenting symptoms and development

Newborns with a CHD are at risk to develop congestive heart failure. Symptoms are rapid breathing, sweating, and failure to thrive. Frequently, they develop low airway infections and grow slowly or sometimes they even have loss of weight. These symptoms usually develop gradually over the first 1–2 months of life. The turbulence of the increased amount of

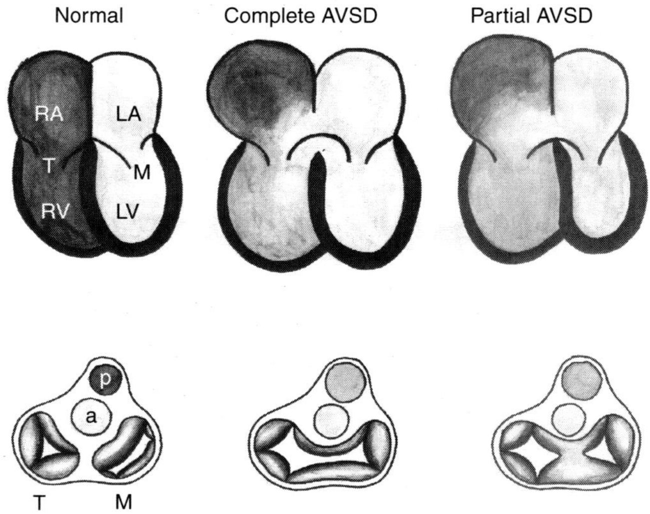

Figure 6.4 Atrioventricular septal defect: RV, right ventricle; RA, right atrium, LA, left atrium; LV, left ventricle; T, tricuspid valve; M, mitral valve; a, aorta; p, pulmonary artery; AVSD, atrioventricular septal defect.

blood being pushed towards the lungs and blood leaking through the pulmonary valve can be heard as a heart murmur.

Down syndrome patients with AVSD are also exposed to persistent left-to-right shunts. The magnitude of the shunt depends on the size of the ventricular septal defect and the ratio of pulmonary to systemic flow. In the healthy newborns without CHDs, pulmonary vascular resistance normalizes from a high fetal value in 7–10 days. However in case of a shunt this mechanism may be delayed for 3–6 weeks, so the onset of pulmonary vascular remodeling causing dyspnea is usually delayed. Particularly in children with Down syndrome the delay in fall of pulmonary vascular resistance may be prolonged or remains high with symptoms of cyanosis and right-to-left shunting occur (Shinebourne & Ho, 2003). Over time, the exposure to increased pulmonary blood flow results in increased shear stress on endothelial cells. Production of nitric oxygen, a potent vasodilator, is impaired and pulmonary arterial hypertension develops.

2.3. Diagnostic procedures

2.3.1. Physical examination

As described above, CHDs are common in Down syndrome. Physical examination alone is insufficient in detection of CHDs (Bhatia, Verma, &

Shrivastava, 1992; Tubman, Shields, Craig, Mulholland, & Nevin, 1991). Therefore, echocardiographic evaluation, shortly after birth, is recommended by the American Academy of Paediatrics (American Academy of Pediatrics, 2001). Tubman et al. (1991) reported that physical examination alone can miss 40–50% of the CHDs (Tubman et al., 1991). The newborn may be asymptomatic and clinical signs such as murmurs may not be evident, due to high pulmonary vascular resistance (Tubman et al., 1991). Nonetheless, physical examination could provide important signs for the presence of a CHD, irrespective of patients with and without Down syndrome. When focused on septal defects the following diagnostic signs should be considered specifically. The pulse, respiratory rate, oxygen saturation, and blood pressure yield important information in a cyanotic infant. Infants with cyanotic CHDs commonly present with cyanosis with mild or absent tachypnea.

2.3.1.1. *Chest radiography*

Chest radiography alone as examination method is insensitive for detecting CHDs in neonates with Down syndrome (Tubman et al., 1991). However, four features of the chest radiograph could provide important information in the evaluation of CHDs: (1) heart size, (2) heart shape, (3) pulmonary vascular markings, and (4) the course of the aortic arch. Patients with left-sided obstructive lesions may have cardiomegaly due to heart failure. Extreme cardiomegaly suggests lesions associated with a dilated right atrium. Characteristic abnormalities of heart shape are associated with specific lesions. Examples are the boot-shape and egg-on-a-string shape in patients with a Tetralogy of Fallot and transposition of the great arteries, respectively. Pulmonary vascular markings are decreased in most cyanotic CHDs and increased in patients with common AVSD as pulmonary vascular resistance falls. An abnormal right descending aortic arch is present in approximately 20% of patients with Tetralogy of Fallot and 30% with truncus arteriosus.

2.3.2. Electrocardiography

In the fetus, the right ventricle has a larger volume load than the left ventricle since there is limited pulmonary flow and thus reduced blood volume in the left heart (see Fig. 6.1). As a result, the normal neonatal electrocardiogram has a right axis and a precordial pattern of right ventricular hypertrophy. In many cyanotic heart lesions, the electrocardiogram is normal in the neonatal period. However, specific markings can indicate that CHDs are present. First-degree heart block is common in AVSD and a superior mean frontal QRS axis (left-axis deviation) is the most common finding on the electrocardiogram (Shinebourne & Ho, 2003). The mechanism responsible for the superior axis is the congenital displacement of the conduction pathways in the ventricles, and thus the superior axis is seen in at least 97% of complete atrioventricular canals at birth (Durrer, Roos, & van Dam, 1966).

2.3.3. Cardiac echocardiography

Because of its non-invasive nature and widespread availability, echocardiography has become the method of choice in the diagnosis of a CHD in neonates with Down syndrome. Two-dimensional echocardiography allows visualization of structural CHDs and valvular abnormalities. Echocardiography, including two-dimensional imaging and pulsed and color flow Doppler interrogation of flow patterns, provides a complete determination of cardiac anatomy and function (see Fig. 6.5). By routine echocardiographic evaluation in the newborn with Down syndrome, definite imaging of AVSDs can be made. An echocardiogram also provides additional information about (1) level and direction of shunting, (2) function of the common or divided atrioventricular valve(s), (3) ventricular function and size, (4) presence of outflow tract obstructions or existence of other anomalies (Shinebourne & Ho, 2003). Echocardiographic images of an adult with Down syndrome and an AVSD are shown in Fig. 6.6. Figure 6.7 highlights the level and direction of shunting by color flow Doppler imaging in a patient with a ventricular septal defect.

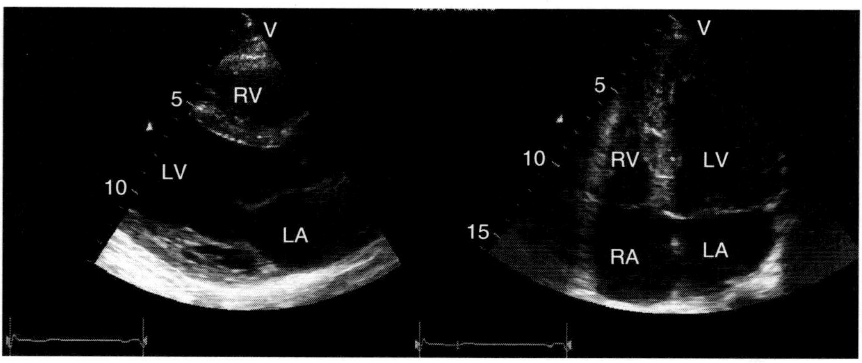

Figure 6.5 Echocardiogram of a normal heart: LA, left atrium; LV, left ventricle; RA, right atrium; RV, right ventricle. (a) On the left panel, a two-chamber parasternal long-axis view of a normal heart. (b) On the right panel, an apical four-chamber view of a normal heart.

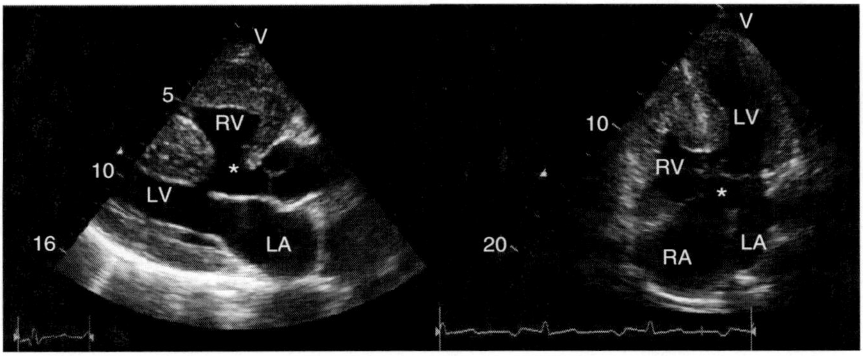

Figure 6.6 Echocardiogram of an adult with Down syndrome and AVSD: AVSD, atrioventricular septal defect; LA, left atrium; LV, left ventricle; RA, right atrium; RV, right ventricle. The asterisk sign shows the defect with interruption of the septum. (a) On the left panel, a two-chamber parasternal long-axis view of a patient with an atrioventricular septal defect and pulmonary arterial hypertension. Note the extremely hypertrophied right ventricle and septum. (b) On the right panel, an apical four-chamber view of a patient with an atrioventricular septal defect and pulmonary arterial hypertension.

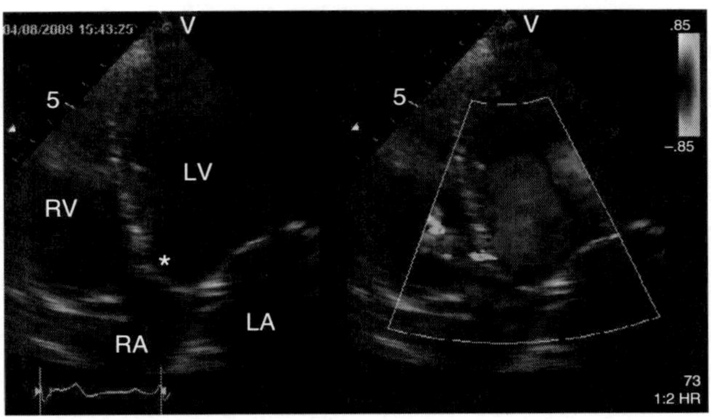

Figure 6.7 Echocardiogram of an adult with Down syndrome and VSD: VSD, ventricular septal defect; LA, left atrium; LV, left ventricle; RA, right atrium; RV, right ventricle. The asterisk sign shows the defect with interruption of the septum. (a) On the left panel, an apical four-chamber view of a patient with a ventricular septal defect. (b) On the right panel, the same apical four-chamber view with Doppler echocardiography. Colors are used to represent the velocity and direction of blood flow. This image shows a left-to-right shunt from left to right ventricle.

2.3.4. Cardiac catheterization

Diagnostic cardiac catheterization in CHD patients have been for the most part replaced by non-invasive imaging techniques such as echocardiography and cardiac Magnetic Resonance Imaging (MRI). However, cardiac catheterization and angiography still remain important to make an anatomic and physiological diagnosis in CHD patients with complex or unusual cardiac anatomy. Meaningful and accurate hemodynamic and anatomical data must be obtained for the preoperative evaluation of CHD patients to guide clinical decision-making. For this reason, the majority of patients with univentricular physiology still undergo diagnostic catheterization before bidirectional Glenn and Fontan surgeries. Also, patients with complex pulmonary atresia and ventricular septal defect usually require catheterization with angiography for optimal visualization of the anatomy of the pulmonary arteries. In older children and adults with large left-to-right shunts, in particular in patients with Down syndrome, precise calculation of pulmonary vascular resistance by catheterization is necessary to assess operability.

2.4. Treatment of congenital heart disease

2.4.1. Catheter interventions

The progress in pediatric interventional cardiology has changed the therapeutic approach for many CHD patients. The balloon atrial septostomy, introduced by Rashkind in 1966, was the first pediatric catheter intervention and is still widely used to create an interatrial communication in cyanotic newborns with transposition of the great arteries. Balloon dilatations and stent placements have become the procedures of choice for pulmonary and aortic valvar stenosis, recoarctation, and branch pulmonary artery stenosis (Cheatham, Coe, Kugler, Fletcher, & Tower, 1998). Lesions with left-to-right shunts, including atrial septal defects, ventricular septal defects, and persistent ductus arteriosus, can now be closed safely and effectively by transcatheter techniques using different devices. These procedures are now considered good alternatives to surgical closure and are the most common transcatheter interventions in patients with Down syndrome. Recently, percutaneous pulmonary valve replacement has become an attractive therapy in CHD patients with pulmonary regurgitation or stenosis delaying the need for open-heart surgery. A heart valve attached to a stent functions as an artificial pulmonary valve for CHD patients, mostly with Tetralogy of Fallot (Hijazi & Awad, 2008).

2.4.2. Cardiac surgery in childhood

Twenty years ago corrective cardiac surgery was often not attempted in children with Down syndrome due to high surgical mortality of up to 60% and short life expectancy (Katlic, Clark, Neill, & Haller, 1977). Since then, techniques of corrective cardiac surgery have produced dramatically improved outcomes. Recent papers have shown that the presence of Down syndrome did not increase operative mortality in children with Down syndrome with ventricular septal defect (Knott-Craig et al., 1995) or Tetralogy of Fallot (Michielon et al., 2006). Interestingly, for patients with AVSD, those with Down syndrome had significantly lower perioperative mortality than those without Down syndrome. Patients with complete AVSDs are operatively corrected usually in the first 6 months of life (Hanley et al., 1993). Moderate ventricular septal defects are generally repaired at the age of 1 if there is associated failure to thrive or recurrent lower respiratory infections. If a moderate ventricular septal defect appears to be getting smaller, one can wait several years (up to age 5 years) to provide an opportunity to avoid surgery. Atrial septal defects that need surgery are typically operated on or after 2 years of age (Shashi, Berry, & Covitz, 2002).

There is paucity of information on surgical outcome in patients with Down syndrome and a single ventricle, due the low incidence of ventricular hypoplasia or unbalanced ventricles in trisomy 21. A study of six children with Down syndrome and single ventricle who underwent surgical palliation showed that single ventricle repair has difficulties due to associated problems in Down syndrome, such as rapidly progressing pulmonary vascular changes and airway obstruction (Wada, Takahashi, Ando, Park, & Sasaki, 2008). Another study showed that mortality after cavopulmonary shunt operations for univentricular hearts was significantly increased in patients with Down syndrome compared to those without (35% vs 10%) (Gupta-Malhotra, Larson, Rosengart, Guo, & Moller, 2010). Down syndrome appeared to be an independent predictor for mortality. Corrective cardiac surgery is not contraindicated in patients with Down syndrome; however, specific surgical procedures are associated with higher mortality rates and patient selection should be done carefully.

2.5. Survival of Down syndrome patients and congenital heart defects

Average life expectancy of all patients with Down syndrome, with and without CHDs, has increased from a mere 12 years in the 1940s to 60 years in present-day populations (Bittles, Bower, Hussain, & Glasson, 2007). In spite of this, neonatal and infant mortality are, respectively, 5 and 8 times higher in patients with Down syndrome compared to the general population, mostly due to the presence of CHDs (Weijerman et al., 2008). In a population-based study of mortality in patients with Down syndrome, almost 18,000 death certificates of persons with Down syndrome in the USA from 1983 to 1997 were analyzed (Yang, Rasmussen, & Friedman, 2002). CHDs and respiratory infections were the most frequently reported medical disorders on death certificates of people with Down's syndrome. A sharply increased median age at death in persons with Down syndrome and additional CHDs was found after 1992, from 0 year of age in 1992 to 18 years of age in 1994. As 50% of the children with Down syndrome have a CHD; this indicates that survival of children with Down syndrome substantially and rapidly improved in the early 1990s (Yang et al., 2002).

3. Cardiovascular Disorders in Adulthood

3.1. Introduction

Acquired cardiovascular disease is common in the general population, affecting the majority of adults past the age of 60 years. Acquired cardiovascular disorders include coronary heart disease (myocardial infarction and heart failure), cerebrovascular disease (stroke, transient ischemic attack), peripheral arterial disease, and atherosclerosis (Lloyd-Jones, Larson, Beiser, & Levy, 1999). Life expectancy has increased over the last few decades; however, the number of cardiovascular deaths in the general population remains high. For persons aged 40 years, the lifetime risk of developing coronary heart disease is 49% in men and 32% in women (Lerner, 1986). Many important risk factors have been identified. These included smoking, dyslipidemia, hypertension, diabetes, abdominal obesity. Beneficial factors are daily consumption of fruits and vegetables, regular alcohol consumption, and regular physical activity (Yusuf et al., 2004).

3.2. Atherosclerosis in Down syndrome

Adults with intellectual disabilities have increased cardiovascular risk factors (Beange, McElduff, & Baker, 1995). A sedentary lifestyle and an unhealthy diet are common, especially in individuals with Down syndrome living in community settings (van den Akker, Maaskant, & van der Meijden, 2006). In patients with Down syndrome, prevalence of overweight and obesity is significantly higher, compared to other patients with intellectual disabilities and to the general population, with a reported prevalence of obesity in adults with Down syndrome between 31 and 47% (Bell & Bhate, 1992; Melville, Cooper, McGrother, Thorp, & Collacott, 2005; Prasher, 1995). Although abnormalities in lipid metabolism, which are associated with high risk of premature atherosclerosis in the general population, are frequently seen in patients with Down syndrome (Dorner, Gaethke, Tolksdorf, Schumann, & Gustmann, 1984), coronary artery disease-related mortality is surprisingly low (Baird & Sadovnick, 1988). Histopathological investigations showed no increase in atherosclerosis, or even a total lack of atherosclerotic changes. Duffels et al. (2010) found a decreased carotid intima media thickness, an accepted valid marker for atherosclerosis, in adult patients with cyanotic congenital heart disease compared to healthy controls. Of the cyanotic patients 35% had Down syndrome (Duffels et al., 2010). The concept of Down syndrome as an atherosclerosis-free model has even been proposed (Murdoch, Rodger, Rao, Fletcher, & Dunnigan, 1977; Yla-Herttuala, Luoma, Nikkari, & Kivimaki, 1989). Both environmental and genetic factors have been suggested to contribute to the low levels of atherosclerosis. Prevalence of smoking and hypertension is low in patients with Down syndrome. Another explanation could be the overexpression, due to triplication of chromosome 21, of atherosclerotic protective factors (Goi, Baquero-Herrera, Licastro, Dogliotti, & Corsi, 2006; Licastro et al., 2007; Nagyova, Sustrova, & Raslova, 2000). Suggested overexpressed protective factors are cystathionine-beta-synthase, leading to decreased level of homocysteine (Ait Yahya-Graison et al., 2007; Boushey, Beresford, Omenn, & Motulsky, 1995; Fallon, Ben-Shlomo, Elwood, Ubbink, & Smith, 2001; Vis et al., 2009) and brain-derived neurotrophic factor (Dogliotti, Galliera, Licastro, & Corsi, 2010). The hypothesis mentioned above is based on the assumption of an overexpression of genes on chromosome 21. However, the assumption of a 50% increase of all genes on chromosome 21 is too simplistic, as some gene products are more sensitive to gene dosage effects than others, caused by negative feedback mechanisms and gene-expression variation among individuals (Ait Yahya-Graison et al., 2007; Prandini et al., 2007).

3.3. Thyroid-related cardiac impairment in Down syndrome

3.3.1. Hypothyroidism

Down syndrome has long been associated with a variety of autoimmune conditions, with the thyroid gland being most frequently affected. Prevalence of thyroid disease in Down syndrome varies between 7 and 50%, depending on the selected population and the diagnostic criteria (Karlsson, Gustafsson, Hedov, Ivarsson, & Anneren, 1998; Karlsson et al., 1998; Rubello et al., 1995). Therefore, the American Academy of Paediatrics recommends routine thyroid screening early in life (American Academy of Pediatrics, 2001). Thyroid disease has an effect on the cardiovascular system and may lead to impairment of ventricular function (Dillmann, 1990). Even subclinical hypothyroidism, with a slight elevation of serum thyrotropin concentrations and normal thyroxin concentrations, is suggested to decrease myocardial contractility and cardiac output (Biondi et al., 1999; Di Bello et al., 2000; Kahaly, 2000). However, these findings were not confirmed by Toscano et al. (2003) who found no increased risk of thyroid-related cardiac impairment in children with Down syndrome and subclinical hypothyroidism, compared to matched euthyroid subjects with Down syndrome.

3.3.2. Hyperthyroidism

Hyperthyroidism occurs less frequently in patients with Down syndrome. Although the reported prevalence varies between 0.8 and 2.5% (Karlsson et al., 1998; Lobo, Khan, & Tew, 1980; Pueschel, Jackson, Giesswein, Dean, & Pezzullo, 1991; Sare, Ruvalcaba, & Kelley, 1978), this could be an underestimation. Firstly, there is low awareness of the association between hyperthyroidism and Down syndrome among physicians. Secondly, symptoms of hyperthyroidism can easily be overshadowed by the intellectual disability. Physicians should be suspicious on thyreotoxicosis, associated tachyarrhythmias, thromboembolism, and heart failure. Moreover, previous reports suggest an association between hyperthyroidism and mild or transient pulmonary hypertension (Marvisi et al., 2006), caused by an increased cardiac output (up to 300%). Hyperthyroidism-related pulmonary hypertension is largely asymptomatic and has good prognosis after restoration of euthyroid state (Siu et al., 2007). Thus, hyperthyroidism can cause potentially serious complications that need prompt recognition and effective management, highlighting the need for routine evaluation of thyroid function in individuals with Down syndrome.

3.4. Pulmonary hypertension

Pulmonary arterial hypertension is a rare syndrome characterized by symptoms of dyspnea, fatigue, chest pain, and syncope. Underlying mechanism is a progressive increase of pulmonary vascular resistance and a sustained elevation of pulmonary arterial pressure (Simonneau et al., 2004). Pulmonary arterial hypertension associated with congenital heart disease is caused by intra-cardiac shunting (most frequently uncorrected AVSD in patients with Down syndrome) and pulmonary blood volume overload (Engelfriet et al., 2007). Patients with Down syndrome and CHDs are at higher risk of developing pulmonary arterial hypertension compared to patients without Down syndrome (Suzuki et al., 2000). Several predisposing factors are recognized to play a role, e.g., a diminished number of alveoli (Cooney & Thurlbeck, 1982), a thinner media of pulmonary arterioles (Yamaki et al., 1993), and an impaired endothelial function in these patients (Cappelli-Bigazzi et al., 2004; Hals, Hagemo, Thaulow, & Sorland, 1993). Most commonly symptoms do not develop until the twenties when evidence of pulmonary vascular disease becomes apparent (Engelfriet, Meijboom, Boersma, Tijssen, & Mulder, 2008). Therefore, early corrective cardiac surgery is warranted to prevent irreversible pulmonary vascular lung damage.

Recent successes have been achieved with the use of therapies targeted against the pathophysiological pathways that underlie pulmonary arterial hypertension. Three main pathways have been detected: prostacyclin (e.g., epoprostenol, iloprost, trepostinil), phosphodiesterase-5-inhibitor (e.g., sildenafil), and endothelin receptor antagonists (e.g., sitaxentan, ambrisentan, bosentan). These advanced therapies have been demonstrated to improve clinical status and life expectancy of patients with pulmonary arterial hypertension (Duffels et al., 2006; van Loon et al., 2007). A recent study showed that the positive effects of these treatment strategies are similar in Eisenmenger patients with Down syndrome, compared to Eisenmenger patients without Down syndrome. Exercise capacity initially improved, and stabilized thereafter (Duffels et al., 2008; 2009).

3.5. Cardiac surgery in adulthood

Nowadays, cardiac surgery at young age is no longer avoided in patients with Down syndrome and CHDs. Thus, the group of adult patients with unrepaired CHDs is declining. However, residual lesions, like residual shunting or residual atrioventricular valve regurgitation require additional reoperations in a substantial group of adult patients. In their single centre retrospective study (40 years follow-up), Majdalany et al. (2010) showed that 27% (4 out of 15) of adult patients with Down syndrome that had been operated in childhood required reoperations. Patients with Down syndrome and uncorrected cardiac defects are also potential candidates for heart–lung transplantation. However, no reports are published on heart–lung transplantation in Down syndrome. Physicians may worry that transplantation is a "bridge too far" for patients with Down syndrome, because of coexisting medical problems, the intellectual disability, and the concerns of immunological abnormalities. Therefore, outcome predictions are hard to make in these patients.

4. Genetics in Congenital Heart Disease in Down Syndrome

Chromosome 21 is among the smallest of human chromosomes, and was originally estimated to contain 225 genes (Hattori et al., 2000) but thus far more than 420 genes have been identified. The function of only a minority of these genes is currently known (http://chr21.egr.vcu.edu:8888/).

Although the phenotypic features of Down syndrome must ultimately be due to the third copy of chromosome 21, the genetic mechanisms by which the phenotype arises are not understood. Two hypotheses exist: one assumes the phenotype is caused by the increased dosage and hence overexpression of one or more genes on chromosome 21; the other states that phenotypic instability due to the extra genetic information leads to the phenotype (Patterson, 2009). Efforts to identify the genes on chromosome 21 involved in the phenotypic features of Down syndrome have been unsuccessful. No single gene has been linked to a specific feature yet. Thus, the genes responsible for the CHDs in Down syndrome are also unknown. Several genes are currently known to be implicated in human CHDs, such as NKX2.5 (Schott et al., 1998), GATA4 (Garg et al., 2003; Joziasse et al., 2008), and NOTCH1 (Garg et al., 2005), but mutations in these genes have been found in only a small proportion of CHD patients, and none of these genes maps to chromosome 21. As the heart defects in Down syndrome typically involve the atrioventricular valve septum, genes expressed in these tissues during heart development may be candidates for the heart defects in Down syndrome. Many of these genes are not located on chromosome 21, however. Although in the past years various candidate genes located on chromosome 21 have been proposed for CHDs in Down syndrome (see below), no gene has been definitively established to be involved in CHDs in Down syndrome.

4.1. Down syndrome–CHD critical region

The existence of rare Down syndrome patients who are trisomic for only a part of chromosome 21 has led to the assumption that only a small region of chromosome 21 may be involved in producing most features of Down syndrome; i.e., that only a small part of chromosome 21 actually needs to be triplicated to cause the Down syndrome phenotype. This chromosomal region was referred to as the so-called 'Down syndrome critical region' (DSCR) (Korenberg et al., 1990; Ronan et al., 2007; Sinet et al., 1994). A relatively large number of patients with partial trisomies has been characterized clinically, cytogenetically, and molecularly to identify the genomic regions responsible for the Down syndrome phenotype (Barlow et al., 2001; Delabar et al., 1993; Korbel et al., 2009; Korenberg, Bradley, & Disteche, 1992; Korenberg et al., 1994; Rahmani et al., 1989). Investigation of additional cases suggested that no DSCR exists which can be said to be totally responsible for the clinical findings in Down syndrome, but that there are multiple critical regions for certain phenotypic features (Korenberg et al., 1994; Korbel et al., 2009; Lyle et al., 2009). It has also been tried to identify a specific critical region for the CHDs in Down syndrome (Down syndrome–CHD critical region), as the identification of such a critical region may guide the search for genes involved in CHDs. Initially, the minimal region believed to be needed to be triplicated to produce CHDs in Down syndrome was 10.5-Mb long and mapped to the chromosomal marker D21S55 region on distal 21q22.2–q22.3 (the telomeric end of chromosome 21q) (Delabar et al., 1993; Korenberg et al., 1990; Korenberg et al., 1992; Korenberg et al., 1994). In the following years, that critical region was narrowed further by analyses of subsequent patients with partial trisomies. Barlow et al. (2001) mapped the Down syndrome–CHD critical region to a 5.5-Mb region between marker

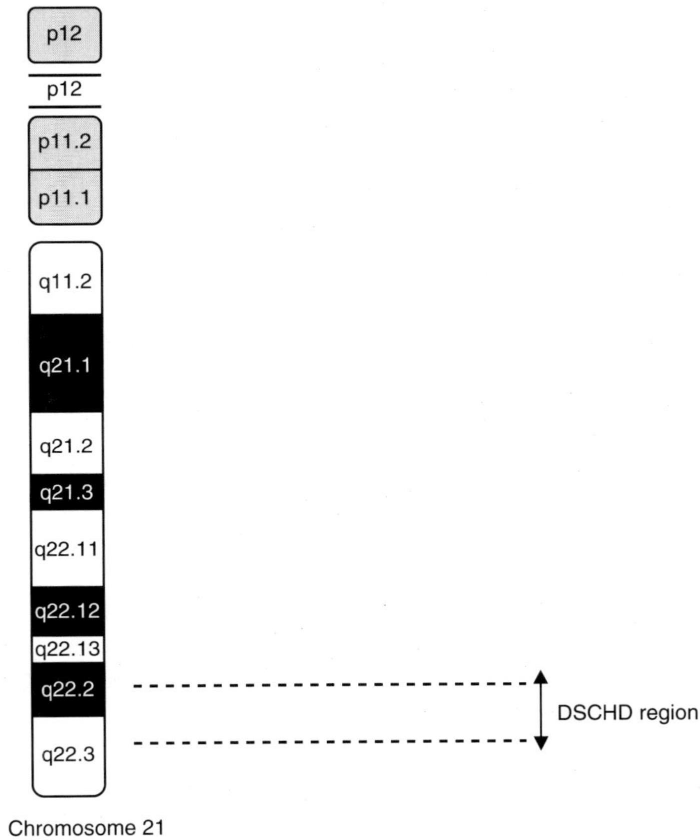

Figure 6.8 Chromosome 21. DSCHD region, Down Syndrome Congenital Heart Defect region, as proposed by Korbel et al. (2009). Figure based on published data of Korbel et al. (2009).

D21S3 and PFKL. Korbel et al. (2009) narrowed this segment to a 2.82-Mb critical region likely involved in defects of the atrioventricular septum. By integrating their data with several other lines of evidence, in particular information from partial trisomic mouse models, the authors proposed a 1.77-Mb Down syndrome–CHD critical region (see Fig. 6.8) containing 10 genes, the Down syndrome cell adhesion molecule (DSCAM) gene defining the centromeric border. The authors suggested DSCAM as a candidate for CHD (Barlow et al., 2001; Korbel et al., 2009). Several other genes previously proposed as having a role in Down syndrome CHD were located outside the mapped region (see below).

Nevertheless, a high degree of phenotypic variability exists in trisomy 21, with more than half of patients with *full* trisomy *not* having CHDs. This suggests that factors other than overexpression of genes on (the critical region of) chromosome 21 must be involved in CHDs and that a possible critical region thus may be described as a susceptibility region (Lyle et al., 2009). The genes on chromosome 21 act together and interact with genes elsewhere in the genome, as well as with environmental and stochastic factors, to produce CHDs and other features of the Down syndrome phenotype (Shapiro, 1999). This makes the CHDs and other features of Down syndrome multifactorial conditions.

4.2. Mouse models and expression studies

Additional approaches for identifying genes and other functional genomic elements contributing to the features of Down syndrome have been the construction of partial trisomic mouse models (Reeves et al., 1995; Sago et al., 1998) and gene and protein expression studies (Lyle, Gehrig, Neergaard-Henrichsen, Deutsch, & Antonarakis, 2004; Mao, Zielke, Zielke, & Pevsner, 2003). A number of trisomy 21 mouse models exhibit heart defects similar to those observed in Down syndrome, suggesting that trisomy of one or more of the genes in these models have a role in heart development (Williams, Mjaatvedt, & Moore, 2008). As theorthologous genes of human chromosome 21 are distributed among three different chromosomes (chromosomes 10, 16 and 17) in the mouse, the development of mouse models of human trisomy 21 has not been easy: the different mouse models are trisomic for genes not located on human chromosome 21, while disomic for genes that would be triplicated in human trisomy 21. This makes translation of results from mouse models to the human situation difficult. More recently, mice trisomic for more precise regions of human chromosome 21 have been produced (Li et al., 2007; O'Doherty et al., 2005), which may aid in identification of genes responsible for CHDs and other features of Down syndrome.

Studies on the spatial and temporal pattern of expression of genes on chromosome 21 also contribute to prioritizing candidate genes (Antonarakis, Lyle, Dermitzakis, Reymond, & Deutsch, 2004). Studies focusing on the level of gene expression found that only part of the genes on chromosome 21 are actually overexpressed in trisomy 21, also in the heart (Conti et al., 2007; Prandini et al., 2007). It was therefore hypothesized that genes showing minimal overlap in expression between Down syndrome and euploid individuals have a primary role in the phenotype of Down syndrome, while the genes having a variable expression might play a role in the phenotypic variability in Down syndrome (Prandini et al., 2007).

4.3. Candidate genes

The study of mouse models and expression studies have led to several genes being proposed as candidates to play a role in CHDs in Down syndrome.

Many of these proposed genes are located outside the latest mapped 'critical region'. A subset of the candidate genes will be discussed here.

Korbel et al. (2009) proposed Down syndrome cell adhesion molecule (DSCAM) as a candidate gene, because of its properties and its location within the critical region that had been identified by the authors. DSCAM encodes a cell adhesion molecule involved in the development of the nervous system, but which is also highly expressed in the heart during cardiac development (Barlow et al., 2001). Located outside their critical region, but also suggested as a candidate gene for CHDs, is the Down syndrome critical region 1 gene (DSCR1, also named Regulator of Calcineurin 1, RCAN1). DSCR1 encodes an inhibitor of calcineurin/NFAT signaling (Fuentes et al., 2000) and is expressed in many tissues including the heart (Lange, Molkentin, & Yutzey, 2004; Rothermel et al., 2000). The NFAT signaling pathway is known to be a critical regulator of vertebrate development and organogenesis (Graef, Chen, & Crabtree, 2001) and was suggested to be critical for CHDs in Down syndrome (Lange et al., 2004). Arron et al. (2006) suggested DSCR1 to act synergistically with another chromosome 21 gene, dual-specificity tyrosine-(Y)-phosphorylation-regulated kinase 1A (DYRK1A), to inhibit the nuclear occupancy of NFAT transcription factors. DYRK1A encodes a nuclear kinase that regulates several transcription factors (Gwack et al., 2006). Increased dosage of these two genes was suggested to produce many of the features of Down syndrome, including heart defects (Arron et al., 2006; Baek et al., 2009).

The genes for the α1 and α2 chains of collagen VI are located on the subtelomeric end of the long arm of chromosome 21. Collagen VI is a microfibrillar component of many extracellular matrices, acting as a bridge between cell surfaces and the surrounding extracellular matrix (Gittenberger-de Groot et al., 2003). Collagen VI has been suggested to play a role in the pathogenesis of atrioventricular canal defects in Down syndrome (Davies et al., 1995; Gittenberger-de Groot et al., 2003). Altered expression of collagen VI was found in endocardial cushions of fetuses with trisomy 21 as compared to normal fetuses (Gittenberger-de Groot et al., 2003). The genes for collagen VI α1 and α2 chains were excluded from the latest Down syndrome–CHD critical region (Barlow et al., 2001; Korbel et al., 2009), because patients with Tetralogy of Fallot or atrial septal defects were observed without a triplication of the collagen VI gene. However, all patients in these studies with defects resulting from abnormal atrioventricular cushion differentiation did have three copies of the collagen VI gene, not excluding a role for collagen VI in these types of CHDs. The gene encoding collagen XVIII is also located on chromosome 21, and collagen XVIII was found to be highly expressed throughout the connective tissue core of the endocardial cushions and forming atrioventricular valve leaflets in mice, suggesting a role in cardiac valve morphogenesis and possibly underlying the CHDs in Down syndrome (Carvalhaes et al., 2006).

The SH3-binding glutamic acid-rich (SH3BGR) gene, encoding a protein containing a highly conserved SH3-binding motif and a glutamic acid-rich domain at the COOH terminal, was also suggested to be involved in CHD in Down syndrome, since it is expressed early in the mouse heart (Egeo et al., 2000; Scartezzini et al., 1997). However, overexpression of SH3BGR was not found to affect heart morphogenesis in mice (Sandri et al., 2004).

In contrast to the above-mentioned genes proposed to have a role in the generation of CHDs, it has also been suggested that overexpression of some chromosome 21 genes may be a protective factor against some types of CHDs, as transposition of the great arteries and atresia of the atrioventricular valves, among others, are virtually absent in patients with Down syndrome (Piacentini et al., 2007).

Although many more candidate genes have been proposed, no gene has definitively been connected to CHD in Down syndrome. Further studies will be required to identify the function of chromosome 21 genes and identify those genes implicated in CHD in Down syndrome.

4.4. Genetics of the atrioventricular septal defect

As AVSD occurs most frequently in the context of Down syndrome, chromosome 21 must harbor at least one gene that increases susceptibility for AVSD. However, AVSD also occurs in other syndromes and chromosomal abnormalities as well as in a non-syndromic fashion, implying genetic heterogeneity. Currently, two loci for non-syndromic AVSD have been identified. The AVSD1 locus is located on chromosome 1p31–p21, but the AVSD1 gene itself is unknown (Sheffield et al., 1997). The AVSD2 locus is on chromosome 3p25 and cysteine-rich with EGF domains 1 (CRELD1) was identified as the responsible gene (Robinson et al., 2003; Rupp et al., 2002). CRELD1 encodes a cell surface protein, that likely functions as a cell adhesion molecule. Missense mutations in CRELD1 are found in a small proportion of patients with non-syndromic AVSD (Robinson et al., 2003; Zatyka et al., 2005). These mutations act in a dominant matter with incomplete penetrance, and therefore CRELD1 is an AVSD susceptibility gene. Maslen et al. (2006) found missense mutations in CRELD1 in two of 39 patients with Down syndrome and complete AVSD, suggesting that defects in CRELD1 may contribute to the pathogenesis of AVSD in the context of trisomy.

Mutations in GATA4, a transcription factor essential for cardiac development, have also been described in a patient with AVSD (Garg et al., 2003), although the main phenotype of GATA4 mutations are secundum atrial septal defects. Other genes that have been suggested to play a role in non-syndromic AVSD are CRELD2, BMP4 (Maslen, 2004), ALK2 (Smith et al., 2009), and CFC1 (Roessler et al., 2008).

4.5. Conclusion

Although a critical region as well as several candidate genes have been proposed, the genetic basis and pathogenesis of CHDs in Down syndrome remain largely unknown. The recent recognition that epigenetic factors such as DNA methylation and micro-RNAs may also be involved in Down syndrome (reviewed in Patterson, 2009) adds to the complexity of the pathogenesis of Down syndrome. A critical aspect of understanding the pathogenesis of CHDs in Down syndrome remains the determination of the function of chromosome 21 genes. Further studies, including continuation of specific mouse model production, expression studies and studies of additional human subjects who are carefully phenotyped, are required to identify genes and other genetically active elements contributing to CHDs. Integration of the many different types of analyses will be required to enlarge our understanding of the pathogenesis underlying the CHDs in Down syndrome.

5. Comment

Down syndrome is a multi-organ disorder, affecting both the structure and function of the heart and vascular. The fixed pattern of congenital heart defects is intriguing, with the atrioventricular septal defect as the most common defect in persons with Down syndrome. Recent papers have shown that operative mortality was not increased in children with Down syndrome and repaired septal defects. This has resulted in a substantially and rapidly improved survival of children with Down syndrome. Although a critical region on chromosome 21 as well as several candidate genes have been proposed, the genetic basis and pathogenesis of congenital heart defects in Down syndrome remain largely unknown. Future molecular studies might give us more insight into cardiac development. Prevalence of thyroid disorders is high and might influence cardiac function. Therefore, routine screening on thyroid dysfunction is warranted in persons with Down syndrome.

Acknowledgments

We would like to thank Dr. J.P.M. Hamer (University Medical Centre Groningen, the Netherlands) for providing his illustrations (Figs. 6.2, 6.3, 6.4) and Mrs. H.A.C.M. de Bruin-Bon, (Academic Medical Centre, the Netherlands) for providing the echocardiographic images (Figs. 6.5, 6.6, 6.7)

REFERENCES

Ait Yahya-Graison, E., Aubert, J., Dauphinot, L., Rivals, I., Prieur, M., Golfier, G. et al. (2007). Classification of human chromosome 21 gene-expression variations in Down syndrome: Impact on disease phenotypes. *American Journal of Human Genetics*, *81*, 475–491.

American Academy of Pediatrics (2001). Health supervision for children with Down syndrome. *Pediatrics*, *107*, 442–449.

Antonarakis, S. E., Lyle, R., Dermitzakis, E. T., Reymond, A., & Deutsch, S. (2004). Chromosome 21 and down syndrome: from genomics to pathophysiology. *Nature Reviews Genetics*, *5*, 725–738.

Arron, J. R., Winslow, M. M., Polleri, A., Chang, C. P., Wu, H., Gao, X. et al. (2006). NFAT dysregulation by increased dosage of DSCR1 and DYRK1A on chromosome 21. *Nature*, *441*, 595–600.

Baek, K. H., Zaslavsky, A., Lynch, R. C., Britt, C., Okada, Y., Siarey, R. J. et al. (2009). Down's syndrome suppression of tumour growth and the role of the calcineurin inhibitor DSCR1. *Nature*, *459*, 1126–1130.

Baird, P. A., & Sadovnick, A. D. (1988). Causes of death to age 30 in Down syndrome. *American Journal of Human Genetics*, *43*, 239–248.

Barlow, G. M., Chen, X. N., Shi, Z. Y., Lyons, G. E., Kurnit, D. M., Celle, L. et al. (2001). Down syndrome congenital heart disease: A narrowed region and a candidate gene. *Genetics in Medicine.*, *3*, 91–101.

Beange, H., McElduff, A., & Baker, W. (1995). Medical disorders of adults with mental retardation: a population study. *American Journal on Mental Retardation*, *99*, 595–604.

Bell, A. J., & Bhate, M. S. (1992). Prevalence of overweight and obesity in Down's syndrome and other mentally handicapped adults living in the community. *Journal of Intellectual Disabilility Research*, *36*, 359–364.

Bhatia, S., Verma, I. C., & Shrivastava, S. (1992). Congenital heart disease in Down syndrome: an echocardiographic study. *Indian Pediatrics*, *29*, 1113–1116.

Biondi, B., Fazio, S., Palmieri, E. A., Carella, C., Panza, N., Cittadini, A. et al. (1999). Left ventricular diastolic dysfunction in patients with subclinical hypothyroidism. *Journal of Clinical Endocrinology & Metabolism*, *84*, 2064–2067.

Bittles, A. H., Bower, C., Hussain, R., & Glasson, E. J. (2007). The four ages of Down syndrome. *European Journal of Public Health*, *17*, 221–225.

Boushey, C. J., Beresford, S. A., Omenn, G. S., & Motulsky, A. G. (1995). A quantitative assessment of plasma homocysteine as a risk factor for vascular disease. Probable benefits of increasing folic acid intakes. *Journal of the American Medical Association*, *274*, 1049–1057.

Cappelli-Bigazzi, M., Santoro, G., Battaglia, C., Palladino, M. T., Carrozza, M., Russo, M. G. et al. (2004). Endothelial cell function in patients with Down's syndrome. *American Journal of Cardiology*, *94*, 392–395.

Carvalhaes, L. S., Gervasio, O. L., Guatimosim, C., Heljasvaara, R., Sormunen, R., Pihlajaniemi, T. et al. (2006). Collagen XVIII/endostatin is associated with the epithelial–mesenchymal transformation in the atrioventricular valves during cardiac development. *Developmental Dynamics*, *235*, 132–142.

Cheatham, J. P., Coe, J. Y., Kugler, J. D., Fletcher, S. E., & Tower, A. J. (1998). Successful transcatheter perforation of the atretic pulmonary valve membrane in a newborn using the new Coe radiofrequency end hole catheter. *Catheterization and Cardiovascular Diagnosis*, *45*, 162–166.

Clur, S. A., Mathijssen, I. B., Pajkrt, E., Cook, A., Laurini, R. N., Ottenkamp, J. et al. (2008). Structural heart defects associated with an increased nuchal translucency: 9 years experience in a referral centre. *Prenatal Diagnosis*, *28*, 347–354.

Clur, S. A., Ottenkamp, J., & Bilardo, C. M. (2009). The nuchal translucency and the fetal heart: a literature review. *Prenatal Diagnosis*, *29*, 739–748.

Conti, A., Fabbrini, F., D'Agostino, P., Negri, R., Greco, D., Genesio, R. et al. (2007). Altered expression of mitochondrial and extracellular matrix genes in the heart of human fetuses with chromosome 21 trisomy. *BMC.Genomics, 8*, 268.

Cooney, T. P., & Thurlbeck, W. M. (1982). Pulmonary hypoplasia in Down's syndrome. *New England Journal of Medicine, 307*, 1170–1173.

Davies, G. E., Howard, C. M., Farrer, M. J., Coleman, M. M., Bennett, L. B., Cullen, L. M. et al. (1995). Genetic variation in the COL6A1 region is associated with congenital heart defects in trisomy 21 (Down's syndrome). *Annals of Human Genetics, 59*, p253–269.

Delabar, J. M., Theophile, D., Rahmani, Z., Chettouh, Z., Blouin, J. L., Prieur, M. et al. (1993). Molecular mapping of twenty-four features of Down syndrome on chromosome 21. *European Journal of Human Genetics, 1*, 114–124.

Di Bello, V., Monzani, F., Giorgi, D., Bertini, A., Caraccio, N., Valenti, G. et al. (2000). Ultrasonic myocardial textural analysis in subclinical hypothyroidism. *Journal of the American Society of Echocardiography, 13*, 832–840.

Dillmann, W. H. (1990). Biochemical basis of thyroid hormone action in the heart. *The American Journal of Medicine, 88*, 626–630.

Dogliotti, G., Galliera, E., Licastro, F., & Corsi, M. M. (2010). Age-related changes in plasma levels of BDNF in Down syndrome patients. *Immunity and Ageing, 7*, 2.

Dorner, K., Gaethke, A. S., Tolksdorf, M., Schumann, K. P., & Gustmann, H. (1984). Cholesterol fractions and triglycerides in children and adults with Down's syndrome. *Clinica Chimica Acta, 142*, 307–311.

Duffels M. G., Berger R. M., Bresser P., de Bruin-Bon H. A., Hoendermis E. S., Bouma B. J. et al. (2006). Applicability of bosentan in Dutch patients with Eisenmenger syndrome: preliminary results on safety and exercise capacity. *Netherlands Heart Journal, 14*, 165–170.

Duffels, M.G., Mulder, K.M., Trip, M.D., de Groot, E., Gort, J., van Dijk, A.P. et al. (2010) Atherosclerosis in patients with cyanotic congenital heart disease. *Circulation Journal, 74*, 1436–1441. Epub 2010 June 4.

Duffels, M. G., Vis, J. C., van Loon, R. E., Berger, R. M., Hoendermis, E. S., van Dijk, A. P. et al. (2008). Down patients with Eisenmenger syndrome: Is bosentan treatment an option? *International Journal of Cardiology, 134*, 378–383.

Duffels, M. G., Vis, J. C., van Loon, R. L., Nieuwkerk, P. T., van Dijk, A. P., Hoendermis, E. S. et al. (2009). Effect of bosentan on exercise capacity and quality of life in adults with pulmonary arterial hypertension associated with congenital heart disease with and without Down's syndrome. *American Journal of Cardiology, 103*, 1309–1315.

Durrer, D., Roos, J. P., & van Dam, R. T. (1966). The genesis of the electrocardiogram of patients with ostium primum defects (ventral atrial septal defects). *American Heart Journal, 71*, 642–650.

Egeo, A., Di, L., Sandri, C., Mazzocco, M., Lapide, M., Schiaffino, S. et al. (2000). Developmental expression of the SH3BGR gene, mapping to the Down syndrome heart critical region. *Mechanisms of Development, 90*, 313–316.

Engelfriet, P., Meijboom, F., Boersma, E., Tijssen, J., & Mulder, B. (2008). Repaired and open atrial septal defects type II in adulthood: an epidemiological study of a large European cohort. *International Journal of Cardiology, 126*, 379–385.

Engelfriet, P. M., Duffels, M. G., Moller, T., Boersma, E., Tijssen, J. G., Thaulow, E. et al. (2007). Pulmonary arterial hypertension in adults born with a heart septal defect: the Euro Heart Survey on adult congenital heart disease. *Heart, 93*, 682–687.

Fallon, U. B., Ben-Shlomo, Y., Elwood, P., Ubbink, J. B., & Smith, G. D. (2001). Homocysteine and coronary heart disease in the Caerphilly cohort: a 10 year follow up. *Heart, 85*, 153–158.

Freeman, S. B., Bean, L. H., Allen, E. G., Tinker, S. W., Locke, A. E., Druschel, C. et al. (2008). Ethnicity, sex, and the incidence of congenital heart defects: a report from the National Down Syndrome Project. *Genetics in Medicine, 10*, 173–180.

Freeman, S. B., Taft, L. F., Dooley, K. J., Allran, K., Sherman, S. L., Hassold, T. J. et al. (1998). Population-based study of congenital heart defects in Down syndrome. *American Journal of Medical Genetics*, *80*, 213–217.
Frid, C., Drott, P., Lundell, B., Rasmussen, F., & Anneren, G. (1999). Mortality in Down's syndrome in relation to congenital malformations. *Journal of Intellectual Disability Research*, *43 (Pt 3)*, 234–241.
Fuentes, J. J., Genesca, L., Kingsbury, T. J., Cunningham, K. W., Perez-Riba, M., Estivill, X. et al. (2000). DSCR1, overexpressed in Down syndrome, is an inhibitor of calcineurin-mediated signaling pathways. *Human Molecular Genetics*, *9*, 1681–1690.
Garg, V., Kathiriya, I. S., Barnes, R., Schluterman, M. K., King, I. N., Butler, C. A. et al. (2003). GATA4 mutations cause human congenital heart defects and reveal an interaction with TBX5. *Nature*, *424*, 443–447.
Garg, V., Muth, A. N., Ransom, J. F., Schluterman, M. K., Barnes, R., King, I. N. et al. (2005). Mutations in NOTCH1 cause aortic valve disease. *Nature*, *437*, 270–274.
Gatzoulis, M., & Webb, G. (2003). Adults With Congenital Heart Disease: A growing Population. In M. Gatzoulis, G. Webb, & P. Daubeney (Eds.), *Diagnosis and management of adult congenital heart disease*, Churchill Livingstone, Spain (2006 ed., pp. 3–5).
Gittenberger-de Groot, A. C., Bartram, U., Oosthoek, P. W., Bartelings, M. M., Hogers, B., Poelmann, R. E. et al. (2003). Collagen type VI expression during cardiac development and in human fetuses with trisomy 21. *The anatomical record.Part A, Discoveries in molecular, cellular, and evolutionary biology*, *275*, 1109–1116.
Goi, G., Baquero-Herrera, C., Licastro, F., Dogliotti, G., & Corsi, M. M. (2006). Advanced oxidation protein products (AOPP) and high-sensitive C-reactive protein (hs-CRP) in an "atheroma-free model": Down's syndrome. *Internal Journal of Cardiology*, *113*, 427–429.
Graef, I. A., Chen, F., & Crabtree, G. R. (2001). NFAT signaling in vertebrate development. *Current Opinion in Genetics and Development*, *11*, 505–512.
Gupta-Malhotra, M., Larson, V. E., Rosengart, R. M., Guo, H., & Moller, J. H. (2010). Mortality after total cavopulmonary connection in children with the down syndrome. *American Journal of Cardiology*, *105*, 865–868.
Gwack, Y., Sharma, S., Nardone, J., Tanasa, B., Iuga, A., Srikanth, S. et al. (2006). A genome-wide Drosophila RNAi screen identifies DYRK-family kinases as regulators of NFAT. *Nature*, *441*, 646–650.
Hals, J., Hagemo, P. S., Thaulow, E., & Sorland, S. J. (1993). Pulmonary vascular resistance in complete atrioventricular septal defect. A comparison between children with and without Down's syndrome. *Acta Paediatrica*, *82*, 595–598.
Hanley, F. L., Fenton, K. N., Jonas, R. A., Mayer, J. E., Cook, N. R., Wernovsky, G. et al. (1993). Surgical repair of complete atrioventricular canal defects in infancy. Twenty-year trends. *Journal of Thoracic and Cardiovascular Surgery*, *106*, 387–394.
Hattori, M., Fujiyama, A., Taylor, T. D., Watanabe, H., Yada, T., Park, H. S. et al. (2000). The DNA sequence of human chromosome 21. *Nature*, *405*, 311–319.
Hijazi, Z. M., & Awad, S. M. (2008). Pediatric cardiac interventions. *Cardiovascular Interventions*, *1*, 603–611.
Joziasse, I. C., van de Smagt, J. J., Smith, K., Bakkers, J., Sieswerda, G. J., Mulder, B. J. et al. (2008). Genes in congenital heart disease: atrioventricular valve formation. *Basic Research in Cardiology*, *103*, 216–227.
Kahaly, G. J. (2000). Cardiovascular and atherogenic aspects of subclinical hypothyroidism. *Thyroid*, *10*, 665–679.
Karlsson, B., Gustafsson, J., Hedov, G., Ivarsson, S. A., & Anneren, G. (1998). Thyroid dysfunction in Down's syndrome: relation to age and thyroid autoimmunity. *Archives of disease in childhood*, *79*, 242–245.
Katlic, M. R., Clark, E. B., Neill, C., & Haller, J. A., Jr. (1977). Surgical management of congenital heart disease in Down's syndrome. *Journal of Thoracic and Cardiovascular Surgery*, *74*, 204–209.

Knott-Craig, C. J., Elkins, R. C., Ramakrishnan, K., Hartnett, D. A., Lane, M. M., Overholt, E. D. et al. (1995). Associated atrial septal defects increase perioperative morbidity after ventricular septal defect repair in infancy. *Annals of Thoracic Surgery, 59*, 573–578.

Korbel, J. O., Tirosh-Wagner, T., Urban, A. E., Chen, X. N., Kasowski, M., Dai, L. et al. (2009). The genetic architecture of Down syndrome phenotypes revealed by high-resolution analysis of human segmental trisomies. *Proceedings of the National Academy of Sciences of the United States of America, 106*, 12031–12036.

Korenberg, J. R., Bradley, C., & Disteche, C. M. (1992). Down syndrome: molecular mapping of the congenital heart disease and duodenal stenosis. *American Journal of Human Genetics, 50*, 294–302.

Korenberg, J. R., Chen, X. N., Schipper, R., Sun, Z., Gonsky, R., Gerwehr, S. et al. (1994). Down syndrome phenotypes: the consequences of chromosomal imbalance. *Proceedings of the National Academy of Sciences of the United States of America, 91*, 4997–5001.

Korenberg, J. R., Kawashima, H., Pulst, S. M., Ikeuchi, T., Ogasawara, N., Yamamoto, K. et al. (1990). Molecular definition of a region of chromosome 21 that causes features of the Down syndrome phenotype. *American Journal of Human Genetics, 47*, 236–246.

Lange, A. W., Molkentin, J. D., & Yutzey, K. E. (2004). DSCR1 gene expression is dependent on NFATc1 during cardiac valve formation and colocalizes with anomalous organ development in trisomy 16 mice. *Developmental Biology, 266*, 346–360.

Lerner, D.J. (1986). Patterns of coronary heart disease morbidity and mortality in the sexes: A 26-year follow-up of the Framingham population.

Li, Z., Yu, T., Morishima, M., Pao, A., LaDuca, J., Conroy, J. et al. (2007). Duplication of the entire 22.9 Mb human chromosome 21 syntenic region on mouse chromosome 16 causes cardiovascular and gastrointestinal abnormalities. *Human Molecular Genetics, 16*, 1359–1366.

Licastro, F., Dogliotti, G., Goi, G., Malavazos, A. E., Chiappelli, M., & Corsi, M. M. (2007). Oxidated low-density lipoproteins (oxLDL) and peroxides in plasma of Down syndrome patients. *Archives of Gerontology and Geriatrics, 44*(Suppl 1), 225–232.

Lloyd-Jones, D. M., Larson, M. G., Beiser, A., & Levy, D. (1999). Lifetime risk of developing coronary heart disease. *Lancet, 353*, 89–92.

Lobo, E. H., Khan, M., & Tew, J. (1980). Community study of hypothyroidism in Down's syndrome. *British Medical Journal, 280*, 1253.

Lyle, R., Bena, F., Gagos, S., Gehrig, C., Lopez, G., Schinzel, A. et al. (2009). Genotype–phenotype correlations in Down syndrome identified by array CGH in 30 cases of partial trisomy and partial monosomy chromosome 21. *European Journal of Human Genetics, 17*, 454–466.

Lyle, R., Gehrig, C., Neergaard-Henrichsen, C., Deutsch, S., & Antonarakis, S. E. (2004). Gene expression from the aneuploid chromosome in a trisomy mouse model of Down syndrome. *Genome Research, 14*, 1268–1274.

Majdalany, D. S., Burkhart, H. M., Connolly, H. M., Abel, M. D., Dearani, J. A., Warnes, C. A. et al. (2010). Adults with Down Syndrome: Safety and Long-term outcome of cardiac operation. *Congenital Heart Disease, 5*, 38–43.

Mao, R., Zielke, C. L., Zielke, H. R., & Pevsner, J. (2003). Global up-regulation of chromosome 21 gene expression in the developing Down syndrome brain. *Genomics,81*, 457–467.

Marvisi, M., Zambrelli, P., Brianti, M., Civardi, G., Lampugnani, R., & Delsignore, R. (2006). Pulmonary hypertension is frequent in hyperthyroidism and normalizes after therapy. *European Journal of Internal Medicine, 17*, 267–271.

Maslen, C. L. (2004). Molecular genetics of atrioventricular septal defects. *Current opinion in cardiology, 19*, 205–210.

Maslen, C. L., Babcock, D., Redig, J. K., Kapeli, K., Akkari, Y. M., & Olson, S. B. (2006). CRELD2: Gene mapping, alternate splicing, and comparative genomic identification of the promoter region. *Gene, 382*, 111–120.

Melville, C. A., Cooper, S. A., McGrother, C. W., Thorp, C. F., & Collacott, R. (2005). Obesity in adults with Down syndrome: a case–control study. *Journal of Intellectual Disabilility Research*, *49*, 125–133.

Michielon, G., Marino, B., Formigari, R., Gargiulo, G., Picchio, F., Digilio, M. C. et al. (2006). Genetic syndromes and outcome after surgical correction of tetralogy of Fallot. *Annals of Thoracic Surgery*, *81*, 968–975.

Morris, J. K., & Alberman, E. (2009). Trends in Down's syndrome live births and antenatal diagnoses in England and Wales from 1989 to 2008: analysis of data from the National Down Syndrome Cytogenetic Register. *British Medical Journal*, *339*, b3794.

Murdoch, J. C., Rodger, J. C., Rao, S. S., Fletcher, C. D., & Dunnigan, M. G. (1977). Down's syndrome: an atheroma-free model? *British Medical Journal*, *2*, 226–228.

Nagyova, A., Sustrova, M., & Raslova, K. (2000). Serum lipid resistance to oxidation and uric acid levels in subjects with Down's syndrome. *Physiological Research*, *49*, 227–231.

Nicolaides, K. H., Azar, G., Byrne, D., Mansur, C., & Marks, K. (1992). Fetal nuchal translucency: ultrasound screening for chromosomal defects in first trimester of pregnancy. *British Medical Journal*, *304*, 867–869.

O'Doherty, A., Ruf, S., Mulligan, C., Hildreth, V., Errington, M. L., Cooke, S. et al. (2005). An aneuploid mouse strain carrying human chromosome 21 with Down syndrome phenotypes. *Science*, *309*, 2033–2037.

Paladini, D., Tartaglione, A., Agangi, A., Teodoro, A., Forleo, F., Borghese, A. et al. (2000). The association between congenital heart disease and Down syndrome in prenatal life. *Ultrasound in Obstetrics and Gynecology*, *15*, 104–108.

Patterson, D. (2009). Molecular genetic analysis of Down syndrome. *Human Genetics*, *126*, 195–214.

Piacentini, G., Digilio, M. C., Sarkozy, A., Placidi, S., Dallapiccola, B., & Marino, B. (2007). Genetics of congenital heart diseases in syndromic and non-syndromic patients: new advances and clinical implications. *Journal of Cardiovascular Medicine (Hagerstown)*, *8*, 7–11.

Prandini, P., Deutsch, S., Lyle, R., Gagnebin, M., Delucinge, V. C., Delorenzi, M. et al. (2007). Natural gene-expression variation in Down syndrome modulates the outcome of gene-dosage imbalance. *American Journal of Human Genetics*, *81*, 252–263.

Prasher, V. P. (1995). Overweight and obesity amongst Down's syndrome adults. *Journal of Intellectual Disability Research*, *39*(Pt 5),437–441.

Pueschel, S. M., Jackson, I. M., Giesswein, P., Dean, M. K., & Pezzullo, J. C. (1991). Thyroid function in Down syndrome. *Research in Developmental Disabilities*, *12*, 287–296.

Rahmani, Z., Blouin, J. L., Creau-Goldberg, N., Watkins, P. C., Mattei, J. F., Poissonnier, M. et al. (1989). Critical role of the D21S55 region on chromosome 21 in the pathogenesis of Down syndrome. *Proceedings of the National Academy of Sciences of the United States of America*, *86*, 5958–5962.

Reeves, R. H., Irving, N. G., Moran, T. H., Wohn, A., Kitt, C., Sisodia, S. S. et al. (1995). A mouse model for Down syndrome exhibits learning and behaviour deficits. *Nature Genetics*, *11*, 177–184.

Richards, B. W. (1965). The diagnosis of Down's syndrome. *Developmental Medicine and Child Neurology*, *7*, 285–288.

Robinson, S. W., Morris, C. D., Goldmuntz, E., Reller, M. D., Jones, M. A., Steiner, R. D. et al. (2003). Missense mutations in CRELD1 are associated with cardiac atrioventricular septal defects. *American Journal of Human Genetics*, *72*, 1047–1052.

Roessler, E., Ouspenskaia, M. V., Karkera, J. D., Velez, J. I., Kantipong, A., Lacbawan, F. et al. (2008). Reduced NODAL signaling strength via mutation of several pathway members including FOXH1 is linked to human heart defects and holoprosencephaly. *American Journal of Human Genetics*, *83*, 18–29.

Roizen, N. J., & Patterson, D. (2003). Down's syndrome. *Lancet*, *361*, 1281–1289.

Ronan, A., Fagan, K., Christie, L., Conroy, J., Nowak, N. J., & Turner, G. (2007). Familial 4.3 Mb duplication of 21q22 sheds new light on the Down syndrome critical region. *Journal of Medical Genetics, 44*, 448–451.

Rothermel, B., Vega, R. B., Yang, J., Wu, H., Bassel-Duby, R., & Williams, R. S. (2000). A protein encoded within the Down syndrome critical region is enriched in striated muscles and inhibits calcineurin signaling. *Journal of Biological Chemistry, 275*, 8719–8725.

Rubello, D., Pozzan, G. B., Casara, D., Girelli, M. E., Boccato, S., Rigon, F. et al. (1995). Natural course of subclinical hypothyroidism in Down's syndrome: Prospective study results and therapeutic considerations. *Journal of Endocrinological Investigation, 18*, 35–40.

Rupp, P. A., Fouad, G. T., Egelston, C. A., Reifsteck, C. A., Olson, S. B., Knosp, W. M. et al. (2002). Identification, genomic organization and mRNA expression of CRELD1, the founding member of a unique family of matricellular proteins. *Gene, 293*, 47–57.

Sago, H., Carlson, E. J., Smith, D. J., Kilbridge, J., Rubin, E. M., Mobley, W. C. et al. (1998). Ts1Cje, a partial trisomy 16 mouse model for Down syndrome, exhibits learning and behavioral abnormalities. *Proceedings of the National Academy of Sciences of the United States of America, 95*, 6256–6261.

Sandri, C., Di, L. R., Picard, A., Argentini, C., Calabria, E., Myklak, K. et al. (2004). Heart morphogenesis is not affected by overexpression of the Sh3bgr gene mapping to the Down syndrome heart critical region. *Human Genetics, 114*, 517–519.

Sare, Z., Ruvalcaba, R. H., & Kelley, V. C. (1978). Prevalence of thyroid disorder in Down syndrome. *Clinical Genitics, 14*, 154–158.

Scartezzini, P., Egeo, A., Colella, S., Fumagalli, P., Arrigo, P., Nizetic, D. et al. (1997). Cloning a new human gene from chromosome 21q22.3 encoding a glutamic acid-rich protein expressed in heart and skeletal muscle. *Human Genetics, 99*, 387–392.

Schott, J. J., Benson, D. W., Basson, C. T., Pease, W., Silberbach, G. M., Moak, J. P. et al. (1998). Congenital heart disease caused by mutations in the transcription factor NKX2–5. *Science, 281*, 108–111.

Shapiro, B. L. (1999). The Down syndrome critical region. *Journal of Neural Transmission. Supplementum, 57*, 41–60.

Shashi, V., Berry, M. N., & Covitz, W. (2002). A combination of physical examination and ECG detects the majority of hemodynamically significant heart defects in neonates with Down syndrome. *American Journal of Medical Genetics, 108*, 205–208.

Sheffield, V. C., Pierpont, M. E., Nishimura, D., Beck, J. S., Burns, T. L., Berg, M. A. et al. (1997). Identification of a complex congenital heart defect susceptibility locus by using DNA pooling and shared segment analysis. *Human Molecular Genetics, 6*, 117–121.

Shinebourne, E. A., & Ho, S. Y. (2003). Atrioventricular septal defect: complete and partial (ostium primum atrial septal defect). In M. A. Gatzoulis, G. D. Webb, & P. E. Daubeney (Eds.), *Diagnosis and management of adult congenital heart disease* (pp. 179–187). London: Elsevier.

Simonneau, G., Galie, N., Rubin, L. J., Langleben, D., Seeger, W., Domenighetti, G. et al. (2004). Clinical classification of pulmonary hypertension. *Journal of the American College of Cardiology, 43*, 5S–12S.

Sinet, P. M., Theophile, D., Rahmani, Z., Chettouh, Z., Blouin, J. L., Prieur, M. et al. (1994). Mapping of the Down syndrome phenotype on chromosome 21 at the molecular level. *Biomedicine and Pharmacotherapy, 48*, 247–252.

Siu, C. W., Zhang, X. H., Yung, C., Kung, A. W., Lau, C. P., & Tse, H. F. (2007). Hemodynamic changes in hyperthyroidism-related pulmonary hypertension: A prospective echocardiographic study. *The Journal of Clinical Endocrinology and Metabolism, 92*, 1736–1742.

Smith, K. A., Joziasse, I. C., Chocron, S., van, D. M., Guryev, V., Verhoeven, M. C. et al. (2009). Dominant-negative ALK2 allele associates with congenital heart defects. *Circulation, 119*, 3062–3069.

Suzuki, K., Yamaki, S., Mimori, S., Murakami, Y., Mori, K., Takahashi, Y. et al. (2000). Pulmonary vascular disease in Down's syndrome with complete atrioventricular septal defect. *American Journal of Cardiology, 86*, 434–437.

Toscano, E., Pacileo, G., Limongelli, G., Verrengia, M., Di, M. O., Di, M. S. et al. (2003). Subclinical hypothyroidism and Down's syndrome; studies on myocardial structure and function. *Archives of disease in childhood, 88*, 1005–1008.

Tubman, T. R., Shields, M. D., Craig, B. G., Mulholland, H. C., & Nevin, N. C. (1991). Congenital heart disease in Down's syndrome: two year prospective early screening study. *British Medical Journal, 302*, 1425–1427.

van den Akker, M., Maaskant, M. A., & van der Meijden, R. J. (2006). Cardiac diseases in people with intellectual disability. *Journal of Intellectual Disabilility Research, 50*, 515–522.

van der Velde, E. T., Vriend, J. W., Mannens, M. M., Uiterwaal, C. S., Brand, R., & Mulder, B. J. (2005). CONCOR, an initiative towards a national registry and DNA-bank of patients with congenital heart disease in the Netherlands: Rationale, design, and first results. *European Journal of Epidemiology, 20*, 549–557.

van Loon, R. L., Hoendermis, E. S., Duffels, M. G., Vonk-Noordegraaf, A., Mulder, B. J., Hillege, H. L. et al. (2007). Long-term effect of bosentan in adults versus children with pulmonary arterial hypertension associated with systemic-to-pulmonary shunt: does the beneficial effect persist? *American Heart Journal, 154*, 776–782.

Vis, J. C., Duffels, M. G., Winter, M. M., Weijerman, M. E., Cobben, J. M., Huisman, S. A. et al. (2009). Down syndrome: A cardiovascular perspective. *Journal of Intellectual Disability Research, 53*, 419–425.

Wada, N., Takahashi, Y., Ando, M., Park, I. S., & Sasaki, T. (2008). Single ventricle repair in children with Down's syndrome. *General Thoracic and Cardiovascular Surgery, 56*, 104–108.

Weijerman, M. E., van Furth, A. M., Vonk, N. A., van Wouwe, J. P., Broers, C. J., & Gemke, R. J. (2008). Prevalence, neonatal characteristics, and first-year mortality of Down syndrome: A national study. *Journal of Pediatrics, 152*, 15–19.

Williams, A. D., Mjaatvedt, C. H., & Moore, C. S. (2008). Characterization of the cardiac phenotype in neonatal Ts65Dn mice. *Developmental Dynamics, 237*, 426–435.

Yamaki, S., Yasui, H., Kado, H., Yonenaga, K., Nakamura, Y., Kikuchi, T. et al. (1993). Pulmonary vascular disease and operative indications in complete atrioventricular canal defect in early infancy. *The Journal of Thoracic and Cardiovascular Surgery, 106*, 398–405.

Yang, Q., Rasmussen, S. A., & Friedman, J. M. (2002). Mortality associated with Down's syndrome in the USA from 1983 to 1997: A population-based study. *Lancet, 359*, 1019–1025.

Yla-Herttuala, S., Luoma, J., Nikkari, T., & Kivimaki, T. (1989). Down's syndrome and atherosclerosis. *Atherosclerosis, 76*, 269–272.

Yusuf, S., Hawken, S., Ounpuu, S., Dans, T., Avezum, A., Lanas, F. et al. (2004). Effect of potentially modifiable risk factors associated with myocardial infarction in 52 countries (the INTERHEART study): Case–control study. *Lancet, 364*, 937–952.

Zatyka, M., Priestley, M., Ladusans, E. J., Fryer, A. E., Mason, J., Latif, F. et al. (2005). Analysis of CRELD1 as a candidate 3p25 atrioventicular septal defect locus (AVSD2). *Clinical Genetics, 67*, 526–528.

CHAPTER SEVEN

Hearing Loss among Persons with Down Syndrome

Heather Porter *and* Anne Marie Tharpe

Contents

Abstract

Communicative interactions provide the foundation for cognitive and social development early in life and continue to impact our behaviors, social patterns, and thoughts throughout our lives. Expressive and receptive exchanges are essential to communication, and hearing is an essential part of all spoken communicative attempts. For individuals who use spoken communication, maximizing auditory ability is imperative. This is especially true for those with Down syndrome as they are susceptible to expressive and receptive communicative difficulties and vulnerable to auditory disorders. Hearing loss can interfere with a child's ability to develop spoken language and influence subsequent academic and psychosocial development. Even children with mild hearing loss can experience greater academic difficulty than their peers with normal hearing. The early effects of hearing loss on academic and social development can remain throughout adulthood. Though individuals with Down syndrome are prone to hearing loss, the effects can be lessened with accurate and early

Department of Hearing & Speech Sciences, Vanderbilt Bill Wilkerson Center, Vanderbilt University, Nashville, Tennessee, USA

International Review of Research in Mental Retardation, Volume 39

ISSN 0074-7750, DOI 10.1016/S0074-7750(10)39007-0

identification when accompanied by appropriate ongoing medical and audiologic management. It is important for all those involved in the lives of children and adults with Down syndrome to recognize the auditory barriers that are likely to exist and to remain diligent in their efforts to seek ongoing otologic and audiologic care. This review discusses typical development of the human auditory system and what is known about the structure and function of the auditory systems of individuals with Down syndrome. In addition, we describe behavioral and physiologic assessments of auditory sensitivity and conclude with a discussion of hearing technology options for individuals with Down syndrome and hearing loss.

1. Introduction

The ability to communicate with others enriches our lives as human beings. Humans use facial expressions, body language, signed language, and spoken language to share ideas, needs, and wants. Communicative interactions are the building blocks of cognitive and social development beginning early in life, and they continue to influence our thoughts, behaviors, and social patterns into senescence. In its most basic form, communicative interaction includes expressive and receptive exchanges. This basic communicative exchange cycles multiple times throughout social, educational, and behavioral interactions and can be as simple as sharing a smile or as complex as the teacher–student interactions in a quantum physics course. The ability to hear the expressive intent of another is an essential part of spoken communicative exchanges.

Individuals with Down syndrome are particularly susceptible to expressive and receptive communication difficulties even in the absence of hearing loss. General hypotonia, motor skill deficits, and increased soft tissue mass in the nasopharyngeal region can confound spoken expressive communication. Furthermore, cognitive delays or deficits can confound receptive communication. Hearing loss can exacerbate preexisting communication barriers for individuals with Down syndrome, increasing expressive and receptive communicative difficulties.

Up to 90% of those with Down syndrome exhibit significant hearing loss compared to about 50% of those with intellectual disabilities without Down syndrome (Mazzoni, Ackley, & Nash, 1994). Hearing loss in individuals with Down syndrome tends to be the direct or indirect result of anatomic characteristics of their peripheral auditory systems. The structure of these systems and consequent functional outcomes are relatively well understood. This chapter begins with a brief review of typical auditory system structure and function. We next discuss what is known about the structure and function of the auditory systems of individuals with Down syndrome. Finally, we describe behavioral and physiologic assessments of auditory sensitivity and conclude with a discussion of hearing technology options for individuals with Down syndrome and hearing loss.

2. Structure and Function of the Auditory System

To understand the structure and function of the auditory system of individuals with Down syndrome, one must first understand the structure and function of the typical auditory system. The auditory system is divided broadly into two main components: (1) the peripheral auditory system and (2) the central auditory system (see Fig. 7.1).

The peripheral auditory system consists of the outer, middle, and inner ears. The outer ear includes the pinna (also called the outer ear), the external auditory canal, and the tympanic membrane (or eardrum). The middle ear includes the bones of the middle ear (or ossicles)—the stapes, incus, and malleus—and the middle ear space. The inner ear includes the cochlear and

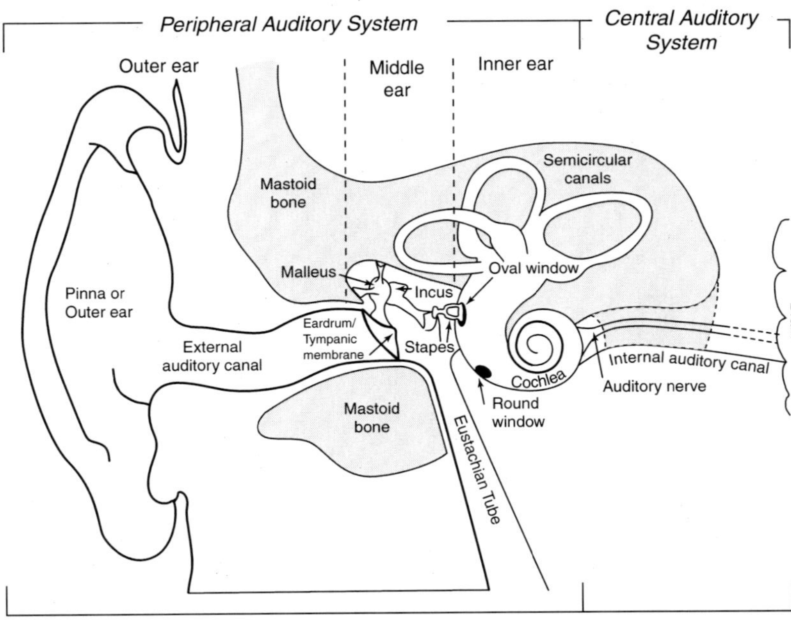

Figure 7.1 Gross anatomic features of the human peripheral and central auditory systems.

vestibular systems. The vestibular system, which is responsible for our balance, is beyond the scope of this discussion. The fluid-filled cochlea is the auditory portion of the inner ear and contains the sensory organ of hearing (organ of Corti). Structures from the auditory nerve (or cranial nerve VIII), intermediate stations of the brainstem, and the primary auditory cortex in the temporal lobe make up the central auditory system.

Sound transduction through the peripheral auditory system requires the coordinated efforts of multiple auditory structures. Sound is collected by the pinna and is then resonated and funneled by the external auditory canal to the tympanic membrane. Sound waves traveling through the air are converted to mechanical energy as the tympanic membrane is set into motion, and this energy is conducted through the middle ear space by the levering motion of the ossicles. A portion of one of the ossicles, the footplate of the stapes, is adjoined to the oval window of the cochlea. This connection allows the ossicles to generate a series of increases and decreases in pressure in the fluid of the cochlea. The motion of the cochlear fluid results in stimulation of the sensory receptors (outer and inner hair cells) of the cochlea. These sensory receptors send messages to the auditory nerve, which in turn transmits these messages along the brainstem to the auditory structures within the brain. The passage of the auditory nerve through the internal auditory canal marks its exit from the peripheral to the central auditory system. Auditory signals are transmitted along the central auditory pathways via synaptic propagation until they reach the auditory cortex and are "heard" by the brain.

Conductive hearing loss is an interruption in the transmission of sound through the outer or middle ear that results in a reduction of sound intensity. Structural anomalies of the outer or middle ear can result in permanent conductive hearing loss. Sound blockages, such as impacted ear wax (or cerumen) or fluid in the middle ear space secondary to an ear infection, can result in temporary conductive hearing loss. Malformations of or damage to the inner ear can result in sensory hearing loss. Individuals with sensory hearing loss not only perceive sounds to be softer than they are, but sounds will also be distorted to a degree that depends on the severity of the hearing loss. Abnormality of the auditory nerve or along the auditory brainstem is referred to as neural hearing loss. When the conduction of sound is not affected but a determination of the origin of the hearing loss beyond the middle ear has not been made, it is commonly referred to as sensorineural. A combination of conductive and sensorineural hearing loss is referred to as mixed hearing loss.

As previously noted, individuals with Down syndrome are more likely to have hearing loss than typically developing persons as a result of anatomical differences within their peripheral and central auditory systems. Studies that have examined the prevalence of hearing loss in individuals with Down syndrome are summarized according to age in Table 7.1.

Table 7.1 Summary of prevalence studies of hearing loss in individuals with Down syndrome by age

Age	N	Prevalence	Degree of hearing loss				Type of hearing loss			Notes	References
			Mild	Moderate	Severe	Profound	Sensorineural	Conductive	Mixed		
<1 year	83	50%						46%		41% had middle ear pathology	(Strome,1981)
2 months–17 years	70	67%	29 cases (unilateral and bilateral)	8 cases bilateral; 10 cases unilateral							(Krecicki et al., 2005)
2 months–60 years	107	78%					13%	65%[a]		40% of conductive or mixed hearing loss could be contributed to middle ear disease	(Balkany et al., 1979)
5 months–6 years	47	96%									(Hassmann, Skotnicka, Midro, & Musiatowicz, 1998)
8 months–22 years	100	62%	36%	21%	4%	1%	4%	58%[a]			(Davies, 1988)
12 months–59 years	78	73%	57%	10%	3%	1%	17%	41%	19%		(Brooks, 1972)
<2 years	48	2.3%	2.3%							Prevalence of hearing loss	(Shott et al., 2001)

Table 7.1 *(Continued)*

			Degree of hearing loss				Type of hearing loss				
Age	*N*	Prevalence	Mild	Moderate	Severe	Profound	Sensorineural	Conductive	Mixed	Notes	References
5–10 years	15									Average hearing thresholds at or better than 20 dB HL	(Buchanan, 1990)
6–20 years	11	73%	60%[b]							Middle ear pathology suspected in at least 30% of cases	(McPherson et al., 2007)
11–20 years	50	Average results show mild hearing loss for high frequencies.									(Buchanan, 1990)
16–37 years	14	85%									(Hassmann et al., 1998)
21–30 years	33	Average results show mild to moderate high-frequency hearing loss									(Buchanan, 1990)

31–40 years	28	Average results show mild sloping to moderately severe hearing loss in high frequencies								(Buchanan, 1990)
50–68 years	20	25%							50% secondary to recurrent middle ear pathology	(Van Allen et al., 1999)
51–60 years	7	Average results show mild sloping to profound hearing loss in high frequencies.								(Buchanan, 1990)
Children and adults (age unspecified)	79	41%	30%	8%		8%	21%	8%		(Fulton, & Lloyd, 1968)

Note. [a] Conductive hearing loss and mixed hearing loss were not differentiated in these studies.
[b] Mild hearing loss and moderate hearing loss were not differentiated in this study.

In general, prevalence estimates of hearing loss in individuals with Down syndrome are high ranging from approximately 40 to 80% (Balkany, Mischke, Downs & Jafek, 1979; Brooks, 1972; Davies, 1988; Keiser, Montague, Wold, Maune, & Pattison, 1981; Mazzoni et al., 1994; Strome, 1981). The majority of hearing loss among those with Down syndrome is conductive although they are also more likely to have sensorineural hearing loss than the general population (Brooks, 1972; Krecicki, Zalesska-Krecicka, Kubiak, & Gawron, 2005; Mazzoni et al., 1994; McPherson, Lai, Leung, & Ng, 2007).

Congenital structural anomalies can result in hearing loss, but hearing loss can also occur after the gestational period. Some individuals with Down syndrome acquire hearing loss after birth or develop progressive hearing loss secondary to other health problems or treatments for such. Risk factors for congenital, progressive, and late-onset hearing loss are outlined in Table 7.2. Those factors that are most likely to affect infants and children with Down syndrome include admission to the neonatal or pediatric intensive care unit and administration of ototoxic medications. In addition, adults with Down syndrome can develop hearing loss secondary to diabetes or acquired pulmonary and vascular issues. Acquired and late-onset hearing losses are the result of changes to the structures and function of the peripheral and/or central auditory systems. The structural differences that translate into various types and degrees of hearing loss hearing loss are discussed in more detail in the following section.

2.1. Peripheral auditory system: Features specific to Down syndrome

2.1.1. Outer ear

The source of entry for sound, the outer ear or pinna, is significantly smaller for infants and children with Down syndrome than for typically developing children. In addition, malformations of the pinna are commonly seen and they are often situated low and rotated backwards relative to the front of the skull (Mazzoni et al., 1994). Figure 7.2 illustrates the outer ear of a typically developing child and a child with Down syndrome.

Children with Down syndrome have ears that are 20% shorter than normal and overall pinna measurements can be two standard deviations below those of their typically developing peers (Aase, Wilson, & Smith, 1973). As such, newborns with Down syndrome are likely to have ear lengths of 3.4 cm or less (Aase et al., 1973).

The pinna is utilized for sound collection and transmits spectral cues that are important for sound localization. We know that typically developing children are not as skilled at localizing sound as adults, in part because of the reduced spectral cues that they get from having smaller pinnae. Therefore, it is reasonable to assume that if individuals with Down syndrome have small

Table 7.2 Risk indicators associated with permanent congenital, delayed-onset, or progressive hearing loss in childhood.

Caregiver concerns regarding hearing, speech, language, or developmental delay
Family history of permanent childhood hearing loss
Neonatal intensive care of more than 5 days or any of the following regardless of length of stay: extracorporeal membrane oxygenation (ECMO), assisted ventilation, exposure to ototoxic medications (gentimycin and tobramycin) or loop diuretics (furosemide/Lasix), and hyperbilirubinemia that requires exchange transfusion[a]
In utero infections, such as cytomegalovirus (CMV), herpes, rubella, syphilis, and toxoplasmosis
Craniofacial anomalies, including those that involve the pinna, ear canal, ear tags, ear pits, and temporal bone anomalies[a]
Physical findings, such as white forelock, that are associated with a syndrome known to include a sensorineural or permanent conductive hearing loss
Syndromes associated with hearing loss or late-onset hearing loss, such as neurofibromatosis, osteopetrosis, and Usher syndrome; other frequently identified syndromes include Waardenburg, Alport, Pendred, and Jervell and Lange-Nielson[a]
Neurodegenerative disorders, such as Hunter syndrome, or sensory motor neuropathies, such as Friedreich ataxia and Charcot-Marie-Tooth syndrome
Culture-positive postnatal infections associated with sensorineural hearing loss, including confirmed bacterial and viral (especially herpes viruses and varicella) meningitis
Head trauma, especially basal skull/temporal bone fracture that requires hospitalization
Chemotherapy

Note. [a]Factors most likely to affect children with Down syndrome.
Source. Adapted from Joint Committee on Infant Hearing (JCIH, 2007).

pinnae, this could negatively affect their localization abilities. Poor sound localization can impact one's safety (e.g., slow down one's ability to determine where a car horn originates). In addition, being able to quickly locate someone talking allows the listener to use his or her vision for speech reading to supplement any deficits in hearing. There are also potential effects of abnormally small pinnae on intervention efforts. When the pinnae are too small or have other structural defects, they might not be able to support hearing technology (e.g., behind-the-ear hearing aids).

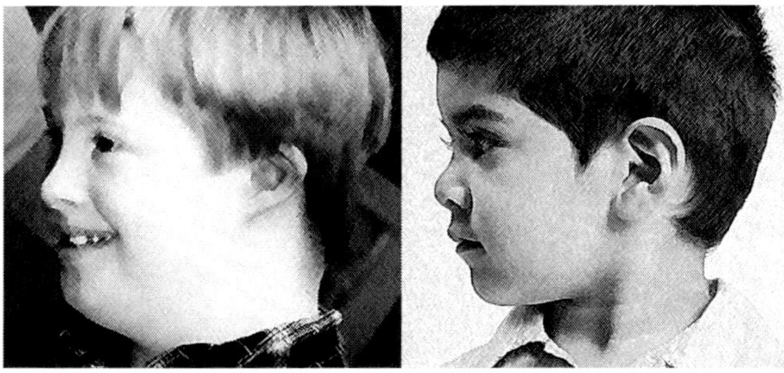

Figure 7.2 The outer ear, or pinna, of a child with Down syndrome (left) and a typically developing child (right).

The next level of sound propagation in the peripheral auditory system, the external auditory canal, is also affected in individuals with Down syndrome. Approximately 40–70% of infants and children with Down syndrome are likely to have stenotic, or narrow, external auditory canals (Satwant, Subramaniam, Prepageran, Raman, & Jalaludin, 2002; Strome, 1981). Consequences of stenotic ear canals can range from complete blockage of the ear canal to frequent blockage of small canals by cerumen and debris. The result of this blockage of sound can be permanent or fluctuating conductive hearing loss. The incidence of cerumen impaction remains high from childhood, throughout adulthood into senescence (Strome & Strome, 1992; Van Buggenhout et al., 1999).

Stenotic ear canals can also impact hearing technology choices. That is, conventional hearing aids input sound into the ear through an earmold that must sit deep in the ear canal. When ear canals are very small, it is difficult to obtain a good earmold fit. Amplified sound can leak from poorly fitting earmolds reducing audibility and affecting the overall quality of the prescriptive fit of the hearing aid. Amplified sound can also be collected by the hearing aid microphone and recycled into the hearing aid amplifier resulting in a squealing noise, or "feedback." This feedback can be irritating to the wearer of the hearing aids as well as others and often results in the volume being turned down or the aids being taken off altogether.

2.1.2. Middle ear

The next stage of sound transmission through the auditory system is the conversion of sound from acoustic to mechanical energy as it passes through the tympanic membrane and is conducted through the middle ear space by the ossicles. Ossicular malformations are common in infants, young children, and adults with Down syndrome (Bilgin, Kasemsuwan, Schachern, Paparella, & Le, 1996; Fulton & Lloyd, 1968; Igarashi, Takahashi, Alford, & Johnson, 1977; Schwartz & Schwartz, 1978). These malformations are often congenital in origin; however, it is likely that ossicular deformations seen in children and adults with Down syndrome are at least partly influenced by chronic ear infections. The incus is most often malformed for individuals with chronic middle ear pathology; however, the stapes and malleus can also be malformed or eroded.

Chronic ear infections afflict approximately 70% of children with Down syndrome (e.g., Mitchell, Call, & Kelly, 2003; Strome, 1981). However, conductive hearing loss due to chronic ear infections is not only found in infants and children with Down syndrome, but approximately 50% of cases of hearing loss in adults with Down syndrome can be secondary to chronic ear infections (Van Allen, Fung, & Jurenka, 1999). Ear infections commonly result in a build-up of fluid in the middle ear, or effusion. The amount of conductive hearing loss experienced as the result of middle ear fluid secondary to ear infections varies relative to amount and viscosity of the effusion (Gravel & Wallace, 2000).

The structure of the nasopharyngeal region and the Eustachian tube are not directly involved in the transmission of sound through the auditory system; however, they serve to maintain appropriate air flow and consequently are essential to the overall health of the middle ear space. The bony confines of the nasopharynx are significantly smaller in children with Down syndrome than in typically developing children; however, the amount of soft tissue is similar between groups (Brown, Lewis, Parker, & Maw, 1989). This relative increase in soft tissue mass confined in the nasopharyngeal region results in decreased airway space for children with Down syndrome. In addition, general hypotonia is speculated to affect the tensor veli palatine muscle and the stapedius muscle, which are responsible for assisting with Eustachian tube and ossicular function. It has been suggested that hypotonicity in combination with decreased nasopharyngeal region can result in Eustachian tube dysfunction for individuals with Down syndrome, which can result in middle ear infections (Schwartz & Schwartz, 1978). In addition to these anatomic contributions, chronic middle ear pathology is exacerbated by the chronic upper respiratory infections and immune deficiencies that are also prevalent in individuals with Down syndrome (Shott, 2006; Shott, Joseph, & Heithaus, 2001).

Chronic middle ear pathology in individuals with Down syndrome should be anticipated, quickly diagnosed, and aggressively treated to avoid permanent residual effects on the overall health of the auditory system. By school age, between 30 and 50% of children with Down syndrome have had pressure-equalizing (PE) tubes surgically placed. PE tubes are inserted into the tympanic membrane to promote healthy air-flow in the middle ear space and to allow drainage of middle ear fluid. This drainage typically results in immediate hearing improvement. However, diligent audiologic and otologic monitoring is required because of the high failure rate of PE tubes in those with Down syndrome. That is, the stenotic canals that are prevalent in these individuals contribute to impaction of the PE tubes with cerumen, drainage, and other debris.

2.1.3. Inner ear

As described previously, sound travels as mechanical energy through the middle ear space and is transmitted to the inner ear by the action of the footplate of the stapes in the oval window of the cochlea. As seen in Fig. 7.1, the cochlea is a spiral-shaped organ that consists of two-and-a-half turns. Recall that the pressure-induced movements of the fluids of the cochlea function to excite the sensory cells that generate signals that travel along the auditory neural pathway.

Multiple congenital malformations of the cochlea and inner ear have been documented for individuals with Down syndrome (Bilgin et al., 1996; Blaser et al., 2006). These structural malformations include portions of the cochlea and a narrower than normal internal auditory canal (Blaser et al., 2006). These structural differences can modify the transmission of acoustic signals, resulting in varying degrees of sensorineural hearing loss. Sensorineural hearing loss can be expected in at least 4–21% of hearing loss in young children with Down syndrome as compared to 1–3% in the general population (Brooks, 1972; Davies, 1988). In general, sensorineural hearing loss occurs more often and is more severe in older individuals with Down syndrome than in children with Down syndrome suggesting the progressive nature of hearing loss in this population (Brooks, 1972; Buchanan, 1990).

This progression in the degree of hearing loss is the result of a number of possible changes within the cochlea and the structures of the inner ear. Bony growth within the cochlea can damage acoustic nerve fibers and lead to the disappearance of the sensory cells within the cochlea that are responsible for relaying information from the cochlea to the auditory nerve (Stern-Padovan & Vukicevi, 1980). This process is typically seen in age-related hearing loss, or presbyacusis. However, progressive bony growth has been shown to occur in children with Down syndrome as young as 7 years of age (Krmpotic-Nemanic, 1970). Results from behavioral studies support histologic findings of early presbyacusis in individuals with Down syndrome (Buchanan, 1990). In a study of 152 participants ranging in age from approximately 5 to 60 years of age, Buchanan (1990) compared data collected from individuals with Down syndrome to data from individuals with intellectual disabilities but no syndromic association. A decrement in high-frequency hearing sensitivity was seen in a group of individuals with Down syndrome as young as 11–20 years of age. In fact, results from the group of individuals with Down syndrome between 11 and 20 years of age were similar to those from the group of individuals with intellectual disabilities between 31 and 40 years of age and to those from typically developing males between 40 and 60 years of age (e.g., Corso, 1963; Spoor, 1967). These results suggest that individuals with Down syndrome appear to experience presbyacusis approximately 20–30 years earlier than other individuals with intellectual disabilities and 30–40 years earlier than typically developing adults.

2.2. Central auditory system: Features specific to Down syndrome

As early as the late nineteenth century, investigators began to consider the characteristics of the neural structures in individuals with Down syndrome (e.g., Wilmarth, 1890). It has been suggested that the brainstem and cerebellum are smaller in individuals with Down syndrome compared to their typically developing peers (Davidoff, 1928; Seidl et al., 1997). In addition, reduced myelin in cortical white matter has been observed for individuals with Down syndrome compared to controls (Banik, Davison, Palo, & Savolainen, 1975). Dendritic branching and total length of dendrites is longer than those of typically developing peers in some regions of the cerebral cortex of infants with Down syndrome (Becker, Armstrong, & Chan, 1986). However, by 2 years of age, the dendritic branches of the cortex are shorter and fewer in number than in typically developing individuals (Chen & Fang, 2005). In addition to these structural distinctions, neurochemical differences contribute to variation in the neural function observed between individuals with Down syndrome and age- and gender- matched peers (Seidl et al., 1997).

Consequences of these central auditory system anomalies are reflected in neural conduction times measured at the level of the brainstem and the cortex. Neural conduction times measured at the brainstem in response to auditory stimuli are shorter (i.e., faster) for individuals with Down syndrome than for typically developing individuals (infancy through adulthood; Folsom, Widen, & Wilson, 1983; Forti et al., 2008; Kittler et al., 2009; Krecicki et al., 2005; Seidl et al., 1997). This might be a reflection of simpler afferent auditory pathways (e.g., shorter and fewer dendritic branches) compared to typically developing peers.

Conversely, conduction times measured at the cortex are longer for some older children and young adults with Down syndrome than their age-matched, typically developing peers (Seidl et al., 1997). These long neural conduction times might suggest general cerebral dysfunction, but could also imply age-related changes or cognitive decline. In addition, these individuals do not experience fast habituation of cortical responses as do their typically developing peers (Seidl et al., 1997). This could suggest deficits in short-term memory and recognition as well as neuropsychological learning such as slower processing or abnormal temporal integration and storage of auditory information. However, the functional implications of shorter or longer neural conduction times are not well understood at this time.

3. Assessment of Auditory Ability

Identification of hearing loss is an important part of medical management in individuals with Down syndrome, particularly for infants and young children who are beginning the process of acquiring spoken language. Adequate descriptions of the type, degree, and causation of hearing loss in individuals with Down syndrome can be affected by multiple factors, including assessment method and technique as well as detection and documentation of co-occurring pathology. For example, if a young child with Down syndrome has an ear infection (which is a common occurrence), diagnosis of permanent hearing loss might be delayed or missed because of attention to the more obvious acute, albeit temporary, condition. Because of the high incidence of middle ear disease in those with intellectual disabilities, especially those who are institutionalized or have Down syndrome, it is most efficient to have otologic examinations prior to audiologic assessments. Otologic examinations can serve to ensure that the external ear canals are free of cerumen and that no active middle ear infection is present.

Early and accurate assessment of hearing sensitivity is essential when considering intervention options for individuals with Down syndrome. Hearing assessments of all children or adults with developmental delays require the use of a test battery that includes behavioral and physiological measures. That is, the determination of hearing status should be made by the converging evidence of several different test results. Once hearing sensitivity has been accurately assessed, appropriate intervention can be determined and implemented. Interventions can result in improved expressive and receptive communication and promote subsequent social and cognitive gains.

The Joint Committee on Infant Hearing (JCIH, 2007) recommends that every infant's hearing be screened by 1 month of age and, if necessary, follow-up diagnostics performed by 3 months of age, and appropriate intervention be initiated by 6 months of age. The American Academy of Pediatrics Committee on Genetics (2001) and the Down Syndrome Medical Interest Group Guidelines (Cohen, 2002) offer protocols for extended management throughout early childhood that include audiologic assessment at birth and then every 6 months up to 3 years of age for infants and toddlers with Down syndrome, after which annual assessments are recommended. Barriers exist to early identification and monitoring efforts. First, health challenges experienced by children with Down syndrome have been described elsewhere and often require continued medical attention (e.g., Mitchell et al., 2003; Roizen & Patterson, 2003). These challenges can take precedence over concerns about hearing loss, which remains a "hidden" disorder. Initial newborn hearing screenings and follow-up testing can be less of a priority in these situations. Second, valid assessment of hearing loss in infants and young children with Down syndrome can be confounded by some of the structural abnormalities previously described, especially the small ear canal size. Stenotic ear canals can prohibit adequate visual inspection of the middle ear. Furthermore, small ear canals can cause sounds to be louder than they would be in a typically sized ear canal and compromise the validity of an assessment of hearing sensitivity. Hearing thresholds could be underestimated by as much as 2–12 dB for infants with Down syndrome if considerations for the size of the ear canal are not made (Taylor, 2008).

Finally, as discussed earlier, children with Down syndrome are at significant risk of recurrent ear infections. These infections often result in the presence of middle ear fluid that adds additional temporary hearing loss (conductive) to any permanent hearing loss the child might have. It is important to note that this fluid can remain long after the infection is cleared. That is, a child might have no signs of an infection (e.g., fever, pain, or lethargy) but still have fluid in the middle ear that causes hearing loss. Therefore, frequent monitoring of hearing health can lead to better management of recurrent ear infections and better auditory outcomes for children with Down syndrome. Shott et al. (2001) aggressively treated children with Down syndrome under the age of 2 years medically and surgically. Treatment included follow-up every 6 months for all children, at least every 3 months for ear cleaning for children with stenotic ear canals, return visits post treatment for acute ear infections, and bi-weekly telephone calls to monitor possible treatment of infections by other medical professionals. Though permanent effects of ear infections are typically common in individuals with Down syndrome, only about 3% of young children in this study had residual hearing loss after treatment intervention was complete.

3.1. Behavioral assessment of auditory ability

Audiometric assessment using behavioral techniques with individuals who have developmental delays poses specific challenges. Behavioral assessments require volitional responses that might not be a true reflection of hearing sensitivity depending on the individual's understanding of the task and motivation to participate. Therefore, the influence of developmental delays must be considered when selecting appropriate assessment tools. The ability to behaviorally assess individuals with Down syndrome, including older children and adults, depends on the individual's cognitive abilities and willingness to participate. The following sections describe two types of behavioral techniques commonly used to assess hearing in children.

3.1.1. Visual reinforcement audiometry

Visual reinforcement audiometry (VRA) involves conditioning a head-turn response to auditory stimuli with a visual reinforcer, such as a lighted toy or a DVD screen. Infants are positioned in a high chair or parent's lap in the center of a sound-proof booth. Older children or adults can be seated in a chair placed in the center of a sound-proof booth. Loudspeakers are typically positioned on either side of the booth at ear level and at 90° degrees azimuth. Visual reinforcers are positioned adjacent to the loudspeakers. The examiner looks for a head turn in response to auditory signals from the loudspeakers. When a head turn is observed, the visual reinforcer is activated for a few seconds. Once under stimulus control, the examiner can raise and lower the intensity of the signals until auditory thresholds are determined for a range of frequencies. For more detailed coverage of behavioral hearing test techniques in children, see Diefendorf and Gravel (1996).

Typically developing children are capable of participating in VRA at about the time they are able to sit unassisted, around 6 months of age. Likewise, when children with developmental delays reach overall developmental ages of about 6 months, regardless of chronological age, they are capable of cooperating for VRA. However, when Greenberg, Wilson, Moore, and Thompson (1978) tested infants and children with Down syndrome using VRA and the Bayley Scales of Infant Development (BSID), they found that children with Down syndrome required a mental age equivalent of 10–12 months before successful VRA testing. Furthermore, infants with Down syndrome have been reported to have extended fixation to visual stimuli and to respond frequently and for extended durations to complex stimuli (Glenn, Cunningham, & Joyce, 1981; Gunn, Berry, & Andrews, 1982; Virji-Babul, Kerns, Zhou, Kapur, & Shiffrar, 2006). These characteristics are advantageous when testing hearing as habituation to the VRA task tends to be less problematic for children with Down syndrome relative to typically developing children.

3.1.2. Conditioned play audiometry

Another behavioral technique for determining hearing sensitivity in children is conditioned play audiometry (CPA). CPA is a traditional operant conditioning procedure (i.e., stimulus → response → reinforcement). CPA uses positive reinforcement (such as social praise) to support response behavior as children engage in a play activity each time they hear a signal. For example, children might drop a block in a bucket or place a brightly colored peg inside a board each time they hear a sound (response), and receive gratuitous praise from a test assistant or the examiner following their response (conditioning).

Children begin to perform CPA around 2 years developmental age. Hypotonia and motor delays can result in slow responses to activities used in CPA. Modifications to test procedures can be made to accommodate individuals with Down syndrome who have significant motor or cognitive delays. For example, individuals can be asked to "high-five" a test assistant or stick out their tongue each time they hear a sound.

3.2. Physiologic assessment of auditory ability

Physiologic assessments do not require active participation of examinees and can be an integral part of the hearing assessment process for individuals with Down syndrome who might not be able to participate in behavioral audiometric assessments. They should be used in combination with results from behavioral testing to accurately determine the status of the auditory system. Commonly used physiologic assessments are described in the following sections.

3.2.1. Tympanometry

Tympanometry is a measure of middle ear function and is used to assess health and function of the outer and middle ear, including the external auditory canal. Measures of external ear canal volume, a part of tympanometric assessment, are used clinically to validate overall tympanometric results and can provide evidence of cerumen impaction, middle ear fluid, or tympanic membrane perforation when thorough visual inspection cannot be performed, a common problem with children who have Down syndrome because of stenotic ear canals. Because of the smaller ear canals of children with Down syndrome, measures of ear canal volume are notably smaller than those of typically developing children. Middle ear pathology, including fluid, can reduce the mobility of the tympanic membrane, another common tympanometric finding for individuals with Down syndrome and cause of reduced hearing.

3.2.2. Otoacoustic emissions

Evoked otoacoustic emissions are produced by healthy ears in response to auditory stimuli introduced into a sealed ear canal. These emissions are measured with the use of a sensitive microphone and provide evidence of cochlear function. Because otoacoustic emissions do not require any behavioral response by the patient, they provide objective information regarding cochlear integrity and make them ideal for screening infants and young children or those unable to cooperative for behavioral tests. Individuals can be awake, but should be quiet during testing to avoid contaminating responses from the cochlea with sounds generated by other means, such as talking, crying, or excessive movement. Otoacoustic emissions are believed to be present in all adults and children whose hearing thresholds are normal to near-normal but, if absent, do not provide information regarding the degree of hearing loss. Therefore, absence of otoacoustic emissions serves as an indication that further evaluation is needed. Otoacoustic emissions can be affected by the presence of ear infections, so their absence must be interpreted in light of other test results such as tympanometry.

3.2.3. Auditory brainstem response

Auditory brainstem responses (ABRs) are very small electrical voltages originating from the auditory nerve, and brainstem. They are recorded from the scalp in response to sounds presented to the ear. Although adults can be tested while they are awake and lying quietly with eyes closed, infants and young children typically must be asleep, or mildly sedated, in order for them to lie quietly. In ABR testing, auditory signals are presented in very quick succession generating multiple neural responses that can be easily measured at the level of the brainstem. Each time a sound is presented to the ear, the auditory system should fire into action resulting in a quick change in the ongoing electroencephalogram (EEG). A computer averages these responses and displays the average waveform.

Waveform amplitudes are greater and more distinct for sounds that are presented at intensities above hearing threshold than those that are presented at or near hearing threshold. ABR testing can be used to estimate hearing sensitivity when behavioral thresholds cannot be obtained because waveform peaks follow a predictable pattern of decreasing amplitude and latency with decreasing presentations of sound intensity.

Each waveform peak reflects responsiveness from one or more areas of the brainstem. Wave I represents processing of auditory stimuli in the peripheral auditory nerve, Wave III is thought to be attributed to the cochlear nuclei in the caudal portion of the auditory pons, and Wave V is attributed to the lateral lemniscus termination at the inferior colliculus in the rostral auditory pons and midbrain (Møller, Jannetta, & Møller, 1981; Møller, Jho, Yokota, & Jannetta, 1995). Wave V is commonly used during ABR testing to estimate hearing sensitivity. The amplitude and latency of Wave V are first observed and recorded at moderately-high intensity levels then subsequently tracked at decreasing intervals of sound intensity (see Fig. 7.3).The softest intensity at which Wave V can be reliably identified provides an estimation of hearing threshold.

In general, ABR latencies are shorter for infants, older children, and adults with Down syndrome as compared to their age-matched, typically developing peers (Folsom et al., 1983; Forti et al., 2008; Kittler et al., 2009;

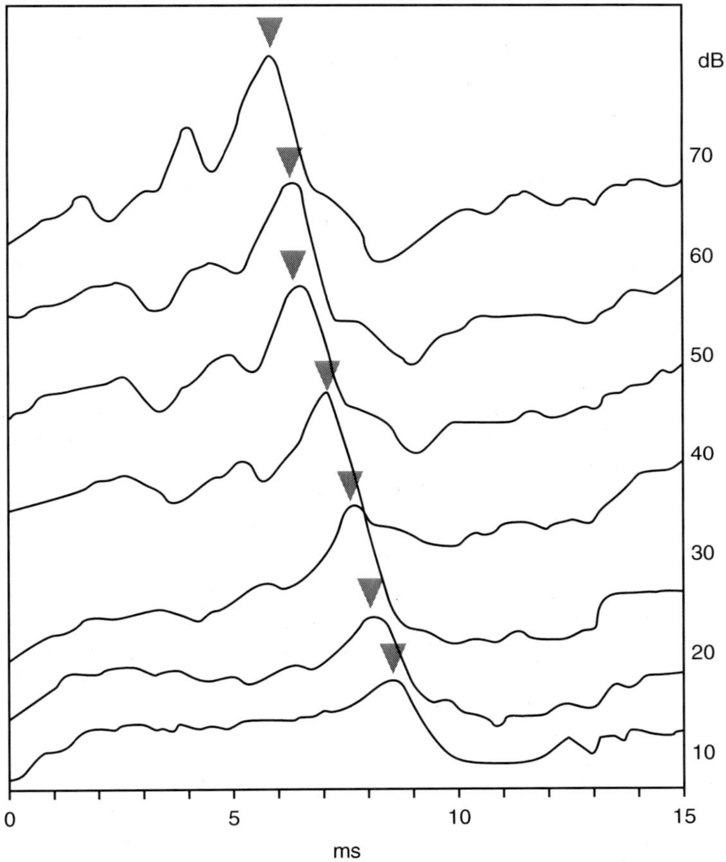

Figure 7.3 Auditory brainstem response (ABR) Wave V at varying intensity levels. Waveforms are larger and more distinct at loud intensities (e.g., 70 dB) compared to soft intensities (e.g., 10 dB).

Krecicki et al., 2005). Figure 7.4 illustrates a sample ABR evoked using moderately-high level stimuli for infants with Down syndrome and typically developing infants.

Recall the size of the ear canal influences sound intensity (i.e., small ear canals result in louder intensities). Calibration techniques were not reported in the literature we reviewed; therefore, their possible influence should not be overlooked. That is, it is possible that the shorter ABR latencies for those with Down syndrome could simply be the result of higher stimulus sound levels relative to normative data. As mentioned earlier, anatomic contributions to decreased latency for individuals with Down syndrome have been suggested including decreased size of the cochlea, central

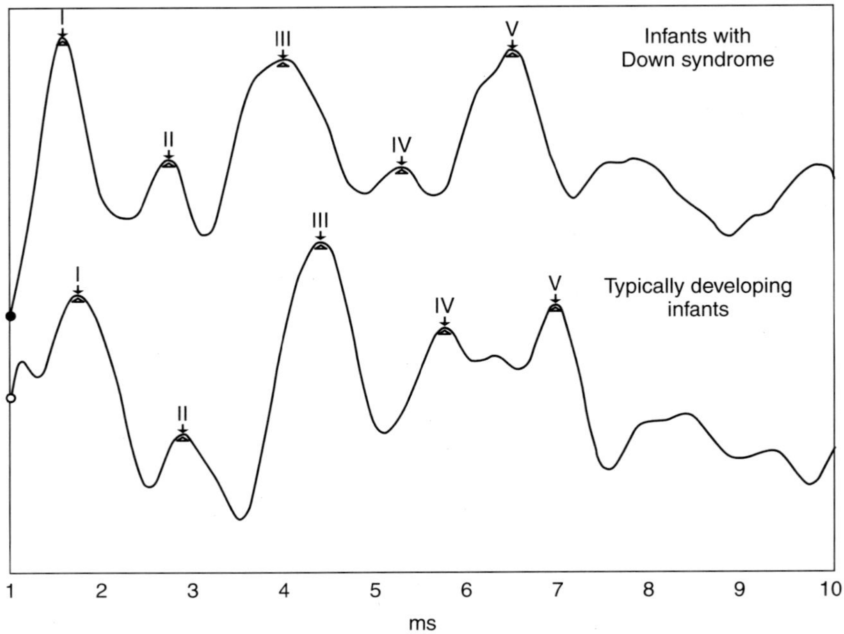

Figure 7.4 Examples of auditory brainstem response (ABR) waveforms to a moderately-high intensity stimuli for healthy infants with Down syndrome and typically developing infants.

auditory pathway, or central cochlear pathway, and shorter neural conduction times (Diaz & Zurron, 1995; Ferri, Gracco, Elia, Musumeci, & Stefanini, 1995; Forti et al., 2008). At least one study examined cognitive ability as a dependent factor in an analysis of ABR latency (Ferri et al., 1995). Significantly longer I–V interpeak intervals have been observed for individuals with Down syndrome who had intelligence quotients (IQ) within the range of 25–39 compared to those with IQs ranging from 40 to 54 (Ferri et al., 1995). As such, extremely low cognitive function could be a contributing factor to ABR results in some instances.

4. Hearing Technology

The primary purpose of early and accurate identification of hearing loss is to initiate early intervention, including the fitting of hearing technology. Those with Down syndrome pose a particular challenge with hearing technology because of possible behavioral issues (e.g., frequent removal of hearing devices), retention issues (e.g., malformed outer ears that cannot hold hearing aids or stenotic canals that cannot maintain earmolds), and chronic ear infections. Ear infections sometimes result in drainage of fluid from the middle ear into the external ear canal. This drainage could be the result of tympanic membrane perforations or PE tube placement. When drainage is present in the external ear canal, ear molds cannot be worn because the ear needs to aerate and one must avoid the fluid getting into the ear mold and hearing aid. The following section reviews the hearing technology options that are commonly considered for those with hearing loss and addresses the specific amplification considerations for those with Down syndrome.

4.1. Hearing aids

When children or adults have hearing loss that cannot be medically treated, they are candidates for various types of hearing technology. Hearing aid options include conventional hearing aids, such as behind-the-ear (BTE) or in-the-ear (ITE) models, and bone-anchored hearing aids (BAHAs). Manual dexterity, size of the outer ear and external auditory canal, cognitive development, and behavioral issues should be considered when deciding on appropriate amplification for individuals with Down syndrome. Most amplification options require some fine motor coordination for insertion, adjustment, and maintenance. Certain styles, such as ITE hearing aids, are prone to be affected by moisture and cerumen build-up in the ear canal and require diligent monitoring and possibly frequent repair. Even traditional BTE hearing aids should be monitored regularly and the ear mold should remain free of debris in order for it to work properly. Because of the size of both ITE and BTE hearing aids, they can be choking hazards—a particular concern with those who are very young or who have intellectual impairments. When retention is an issue, the use of wig tape or other hearing aid retention devices can help them stay in place behind the ears. The use of conventional hearing aids requires no surgery and many manufacturers offer trial periods to determine effectiveness of use for individuals. As such, conventional hearing aids are a viable option for intervention of hearing loss for individuals with Down syndrome.

Some cases of conductive hearing loss are unable to be remedied by medical or surgical intervention of anatomic structures or other blockage of sound. In these cases, sound must bypass the outer and middle ear to reach the cochlea. Sound waves can be transmitted to the cochlea by vibrating the skull directly, rather than traveling through the ear canal, tympanic membrane, and ossicles to reach the inner ear. BAHAs transmit sound directly to the cochlea by using a bone ossicilator that is anchored to the mastoid bone with a surgically implanted titanium abutment. Individuals with Down syndrome can be considered candidates for BAHA surgery and device use if they suffer from conductive hearing loss for which conventional hearing aids cannot be used. A common reason to use BAHAs for individuals with Down syndrome is chronic middle ear disease, but they have also been used for cases of outer ear pathology and ear canal stenosis (McDermott, Williams, Kuo, Reid, & Proops, 2008; Sheehan & Hans, 2006).

4.2. Frequency-modulated (FM) systems

Hearing is important for speech and language development, but also for academic development and general quality of life. Frequency-modulated (FM) systems can be used to improve audibility for individuals with permanent or fluctuating hearing loss, especially in classroom environments where there is considerable background noise. FM systems transmit a signal of interest (e.g., teacher's voice) via a microphone using FM waves directed to a receiver that is coupled to a hearing aid (personal FM system) or to a speaker placed near the listener (sound field FM system). This system amplifies the signal of interest thus reducing the influence of background noise and improving audibility. Personally-worn FM systems can be used in conjunction with conventional hearing aids or alone. Sound field FM systems are ideal for those with fluctuating hearing loss (like that associated with ear infections) because they amplify sound only slightly such that even those with normal hearing can appreciate the enhanced audibility without discomfort. Sound field systems also work well with draining or small ears as there are no components that need to sit in the ear canal or rest on the pinna. Indeed, sound field amplification has been shown to improve the understanding of speech in laboratory and classroom settings for children with Down syndrome (Bennetts & Flynn, 2002; McPherson et al., 2007).

4.3. Cochlear implants

Most children who have hearing loss benefit from some form of amplification. However, in cases of profound hearing loss conventional amplification might not be enough. An alternative to traditional hearing aids for these individuals is the cochlear implant, a surgically implanted device with electrodes that are coiled into the cochlea to stimulate the auditory nerve with electrical current. It is becoming more common to evaluate individuals with developmental delays and other health impairments for cochlear implants. The efficacy of cochlear implantation for children with multiple handicaps, including children with Down syndrome, has been demonstrated (Fukuda et al., 2003; Hans, England, Prowse, Young, & Sheehan, 2009; Wiley, Jahnke, Meinzen-Derr, & Choo, 2005). At one time there were concerns about potential dangers of implantation of children who had recurrent ear infections. Despite concerns about infection spreading from the middle ear into the intracranial space through the channel created by the cochlear implant, there is no evidence to support that fear (Hans et al., 2009).

5. Conclusion

Congenital, progressive, and late-onset hearing losses are significant issues for individuals with Down syndrome. Between 40 and 90% of individuals with Down syndrome have been diagnosed with hearing loss. Although the majority of the hearing losses are conductive, a smaller proportion of individuals with Down syndrome have sensorineural hearing loss. However, the prevalence of both sensorineural and conductive hearing loss is greater than that observed in the general population.

The elevated occurrence of hearing loss for individuals with Down syndrome is not surprising. Every component in the auditory system is potentially adversely affected by the Down syndrome phenotype: (1) the ear canal can be stenotic, (2) the malleus, incus, and stapes can be malformed, (3) the cochlea can be shortened or narrowed, (4) neural transmission rates can be too fast (at the level of the brainstem) and too slow (at the level of the cortex), and (5) the Eustachian tube and surrounding structures combined with diminished immune system functioning can lead to increased middle ear pathology. In addition to these characteristics of the auditory system, individuals with Down syndrome are at risk of adverse birth outcomes that are associated with late-onset or progressive hearing loss such as preterm delivery and low birthweight. These birth conditions lead to exposure to medical procedures and medication during stays in the neonatal and/or pediatric intensive care units, which are risk factors for hearing loss.

Diagnosis of hearing loss can be difficult for infants, children, and adults with Down syndrome. Behavioral test methods might not be appropriate for individuals who have significant intellectual delays. Physiologic procedures that do not require active participant involvement can be used to help determine the presence of hearing loss, but these methods should be used as part of a more comprehensive test battery to determine the cause and verify the severity of the loss.

When hearing loss is identified, some desirable interventions might be problematic. Malformations of the pinnae or ear canals can make the fitting and functioning of BTE hearing aids difficult. Even when aids can be fitted, limited cognitive functioning might make it difficult for individuals to correctly manipulate hearing aids or other types of technology for hearing loss such as personal FM systems or cochlear implants. However, these challenges should not preclude their use. Hearing loss affects speech and language development that then interacts with already compromised cognitive functioning. Management of hearing loss for individuals with Down syndrome might require device modifications or more diligent monitoring of hearing technology, but these efforts can help individuals with Down syndrome maximize their communicative and cognitive potential.

REFERENCES

Aase, J., Wilson, A., & Smith, D. (1973). Small ears in Down's syndrome: A helpful diagnostic aid. The Journal of Pediatrics, *82*(5), 845–847.

American Academy of Pediatrics Committee on Children with Disabilities (2001). Role of pediatrician in family centered early intervention services. *Pediatrics, 107*, 1155–1157.

Balkany, T., Mischke, R., Downs, M., & Jafek, B. (1979). Ossicular abnormalities in Down's syndrome. *Otolaryngology and Head and Neck Surgery, 87*(3), 372.

Banik, N.,Davison, A.,Palo, J., & Savolainen, H. (1975). Biochemical studies on myelin isolated from the brains of patients with Down's syndrome. *Brain: A Journal of Neurology, 98* (2), 213.

Becker, L., Armstrong, D., & Chan, F. (1986). Dendritic atrophy in children with Down's syndrome. *Annals of Neurology, 20* (4), 520–526.

Bennetts, L., & Flynn, M. (2002). Improving the classroom listening skills of children with Down syndrome by using sound-field amplification. *Down Syndrome Research and Practice, 8*(1), 19–24.

Bilgin, H., Kasemsuwan, L., Schachern, P., Paparella, M., & Le, C. (1996). Temporal bone study of Down's syndrome. *Archives of Otolaryngology—Head & Neck Surgery, 122*(3), 271.

Blaser, S., Propst, E., Martin, D., Feigenbaum, A., James, A., Shannon, P., et al. (2006). Inner ear dysplasia is common in children with Down syndrome (trisomy 21). *Laryngoscope, 116*(12), 2113–2119.

Brooks, D. (1972). Hearing loss and middle ear disorders in patients with Down syndrome. *Journal of Mental Deficiency Research, 16*(1), 21–29.

Brown, P., Lewis, G., Parker, A., & Maw, A. (1989). The skull base and nasopharynx in Down's syndrome in relation to hearing impairment. *Clinical Otolaryngology, 14*(3), 241–246.

Buchanan, L. (1990). Early onset of presbyacusis in Down syndrome. *Scandinavian Audiology, 19*(2), 103–110.

Chen, Y., & Fang, P. (2005). Sensory evoked potentials in infants with Down syndrome. *Acta PÞdiatrica, 94*(11), 1615–1618.

Cohen, W.I. (2002). Health care guidelines for individuals with Down syndrome–1999 revision. In W.I. Cohen, L. Nadel, & M.E. Madnick (Eds.), *A Vision for the 21st Century: Down Syndrome* (pp. 237–245). New York, NY: Wiley-Liss.

Corso, J. (1963). Age and sex differences in pure-tone thresholds: Survey of hearing levels from 18 to 65 years. *Archives of Otolaryngology—Head & Neck Surgery*, 77(4), 385.

Davidoff, L. (1928). The brain in mongolian idiocy: A report of ten cases. *Archives of Neurology & Psychiatry, 20*(6), 1229.

Davies, B. (1988). Auditory disorders in Down's syndrome. *Scandinavian Audiology. Supplementum, 30*, 65.

Diaz, F., & Zurron, M. (1995). Auditory evoked potentials in Down's syndrome. *Electroencephalography and Clinical Neurophysiology/Evoked Potentials Section, 96*(6), 526–537.

Diefendorf, A., & Gravel, J. (1996). Behavioral observation and visual reinforcement audiometry. In S. Gerber (Ed.), *Handbook of Pediatric Audiology*, (pp. 55–83). Washington, DC: Gallaudet University Press.

Ferri, R., Gracco, S., Elia, M., Musumeci, S., & Stefanini, M. (1995). Age, sex and mental retardation related changes of brainstem auditory evoked potentials in Down's syndrome. *The Italian Journal of Neurological Sciences, 16*(5), 377–383.

Folsom, R., Widen, J., & Wilson, W. (1983). Auditory brain-stem responses in infants with Down's syndrome. *Archives of Otolaryngology—Head & Neck Surgery, 109*(9), 607.

Forti, S., Amadeo, C., Fagnani, E., Filipponi, E., Pignataro, L., Cesarani, A., et al. (2008). Auditory brainstem responses (ABR) in normal hearing adult subjects with Down's syndrome. *Brain Research, 1233*, 58–62.

Fukuda, S.,Fukushima, K., Maeda, Y., Tsukamura, K., Nagayasu, R., Toida, N., et al. (2003). Language development of a multiply handicapped child after cochlear implantation. *International Journal of Pediatric Otorhinolaryngology, 67*(6), 627–633.

Fulton, R., & Lloyd, L. (1968). Hearing impairment in a population of children with Down's syndrome. *American Journal of Mental Deficiency, 73*(2), 298.

Glenn, S., Cunningham, C., & Joyce, P. (1981). A study of auditory preferences in nonhandicapped infants and infants with Down's syndrome. *Child Development, 52,* 1303–1307.

Gravel, J., & Wallace, I. (2000). Effects of otitis media with effusion on hearing in the first 3 years of life. *Journal of Speech, Language and Hearing Research, 43*(3), 631.

Greenberg, D., Wilson, W., Moore, J., & Thompson, G. (1978). Visual reinforcement audiometry (VRA) with young Down's syndrome children. *Journal of Speech and Hearing Disorders, 43*(4), 448.

Gunn, P., Berry, P., & Andrews, R. (1982). Looking behavior of Down syndrome infants. *American Journal of Mental Deficiency, 87*(3), 344–347.

Hans, P.S., England, R., Prowse, S., Young, E., & Sheehan, P.Z. (2009). UK and Ireland experience of cochlear implants in children with Down Syndrome. *International Journal of Pediatric Otorhinolaryngology, 74*(3), 260–264.

Hassmann, E., Skotnicka, B., Midro, A., & Musiatowicz, M. (1998). Distortion products otoacoustic emissions in diagnosis of hearing loss in Down syndrome. *International Journal of Pediatric Otorhinolaryngology, 45*(3), 199–206.

Igarashi, M., Takahashi, M., Alford, B., & Johnson, P. (1977). Inner ear morphology in Down's syndrome. *Acta Oto-Laryngologica, 83*(1–6), 175–181.

Joint Committee on Infant Hearing (2007). Year 2007 Position Statement: Principles and Guidelines for Early Hearing Detection and Intervention Programs. *Pediatrics, 120*(4), 898–921.

Keiser, H., Montague, J., Wold, D., Maune, S., & Pattison, D. (1981). Hearing loss of Down syndrome adults. *American Journal of Mental Deficiency, 85*(5), 467.

Kittler, P., Phan, H., Gardner, J., Miroshnichenko, I., Gordon, A., & Karmel, B. (2009). Auditory brainstem evoked responses in newborns with Down syndrome. *American Journal on Intellectual and Developmental Disabilities, 114*(6), 393–400.

Krecicki, T., Zalesska-Krecicka, M., Kubiak, K., & \aGawron, W. (2005). Brain auditory evoked potentials in children with Down syndrome. *International Journal of Pediatric Otorhinolaryngology, 69*(5), 615–620.

Krmpotic-Nemanic, J. (1970). Down's syndrome and presbyacousis *The Lancet, 296*(7674), 670–671.

Mazzoni, D., Ackley, R., & Nash, D. (1994). Abnormal pinna type and hearing loss in Down's syndrome. *Journal of Intellectual Disabilities Research, 38*(6), 549–560.

McDermott, A., Williams, J., Kuo, M., Reid, A., & Proops, D. (2008). The role of bone anchored hearing aids in children with Down syndrome. *International Journal of Pediatric Otorhinolaryngology, 72*(6), 751–757.

McPherson, B., Lai, S., Leung, K., & Ng, I. (2007). Hearing loss in Chinese school children with Down syndrome. *International Journal of Pediatric Otorhinolaryngology, 71*(12), 1905–1915.

Mitchell, R., Call, E., & Kelly, J. (2003). Ear, nose and throat disorders in children with Down syndrome. *Laryngoscope, 113,* 259–263.

Møller, A., Jannetta, P., & Møller, M. (1981). Neural generators of brainstem evoked potentials. Results from human intracranial recordings. *The Annals of Otology, Rhinology and Laryngology, 90*(6 Pt 1), 591.

Møller, A., Jho, H., Yokota, M., & Jannetta, P. (1995). Contribution from crossed and uncrossed brainstem structures to the brainstem auditory evoked potentials: A study in humans. *The Laryngoscope, 105*(6), 596–605.

Roizen, N., & Patterson, D. (2003). Down's syndrome. *The Lancet, 361*(9365), 1281–1289.

Satwant, S.,Subramaniam, K.N., Prepageran, N., Raman, R., & Jalaludin, M.A. (2002). Otological disorders in Down's syndrome. *Medical Journal of Malaysia, 57*(3), 278–282.

Schwartz, D., & Schwartz, R. (1978). Acoustic impedance and otoscopic findings in young children with Down's syndrome. *Archives of Otolaryngology—Head & Neck Surgery, 104*(11), 652.

Seidl, R., Hauser, E., Bernert, G., Marx, M., Freilinger, M., & Lubec, G. (1997). Auditory evoked potentials in young patients with Down syndrome. Event-related potentials (P3) and histaminergic system. *Cognitive Brain Research, 5*(4), 301–309.

Sheehan, P., & Hans, P. (2006). UK and Ireland experience of bone anchored hearing aids (BAHAÛ) in individuals with Down syndrome. *International Journal of Pediatric Otorhinolaryngology, 70*(6), 981–986.

Shott, S. (2006). Down syndrome: Common otolaryngologic manifestations. *American Journal of Medical Genetics Part C: Seminars in Medical Genetics, 142C*(3), 131–140.

Shott, S., Joseph, A., & Heithaus, D. (2001). Hearing loss in children with Down syndrome. *International Journal of Pediatric Otorhinolaryngology, \v61*(3), 199–205.

Spoor, A. (1967). Presbycusis values in relation to noise induced hearing loss. *International Journal of Audiology, 6*(1), 48–57.

Stern-Padovan, R., & Vukicevi, S. (1980). Histologic changes in the ageing spiral tract. *The Journal of Laryngology and Otology, 94*(3), 255.

Strome, M. (1981). Down's syndrome: A modern otorhinolaryngological perspective. *The Laryngoscope, \v91*(10), 1581–1594.

Strome, S., & Strome, M. (1992). Down syndrome: An otolaryngologic perspective. *The Journal of Otolaryngology, \v21*(6), 394.

Taylor, J. (2008). *Examination of real-ear-to-coupler difference values in infants with Down syndrome.* Unpublished doctoral dissertation, Central Michigan University, Mount Pleasant, Michigan.

Van Allen, M., Fung, J., & \aJurenka, S. (1999). Health care concerns and guidelines for adults with Down syndrome. *American Journal of Medical Genetics, 89*(2), 100–110.

Van Buggenhout, G., Trommelen, J., Schoenmaker, A., De Bal, C., Verbeek, J., Smeets, D., et al. (1999). Down syndrome in a population of elderly mentally retarded patients: Genetic-diagnostic survey and implications for medical care. *American Journal of Medical Genetics, 85*(4), 376–384.

Virji-Babul, N., Kerns, K., Zhou, E., Kapur, A., & Shiffrar, M. (2006). Perceptual-motor deficits in children with Down syndrome: Implications for intervention. *Down Syndrome Research and Practice, 10*(2), 74–82.

Wiley, S., Jahnke, M., Meinzen-Derr, J., & Choo, D. (2005). Perceived qualitative benefits of cochlear implants in children with multi-handicaps. *International Journal of Pediatric Otorhinolaryngology, 69*(6), 791–798.

Wilmarth, A. (1890). Report on the examination of one hundred brains of feeble-minded children. *Alienist and Neurologist, 11*, 520.

CHAPTER EIGHT

Dementia among Persons with Down Syndrome

Shoumitro Deb* *and* Ryan McHugh†

Contents

Abstract

This chapter aims to review the evidence available for dementia in those with Down syndrome focussing particularly on the diagnosis and screening for dementia in this population.

Down syndrome is the most commonly recognized genetic cause of intellectual disability. As life expectancy for an individual with Down syndrome has increased

* Consultant Psychiatrist & Clinical Professor of Neuropsychiatry & Intellectual Disability, The Barberry-National Centre for Mental Health, Birmingham, University of Birmingham, UK

† Speciality Registrar in Psychiatry for People with Learning Disability, Coventry & Warwickshire Partnership Trust, Brooklands Hospital, Birmingham, UK

International Review of Research in Mental Retardation, Volume 39
ISSN 0074-7750, DOI 10.1016/S0074-7750(10)39008-2

so has the incidence of dementia particularly of Alzheimer's type in this group. The prevalence of dementia in the population with Down syndrome increases with age and has been found to be as high as 75% for those over 65 years. The development of dementia of Alzheimer's type is frequent but not inevitable.

Research has shown that virtually all adults with Down syndrome over 35–40 years have neuropathological changes characteristic of Alzheimer's dementia including β-amyloid plaques and neurofibrillary tangles. The genetic locus for the amyloid precursor protein (APP) has been identified on chromosome 21. As 95% of cases of Down syndrome are caused by trisomy 21, this may explain the vulnerability of people with Down syndrome to developing dementia. Other factors such as apoplipoprotein E (APOE) status and the low cognitive reserve of those with an intellectual disability may be important in the development of dementia.Dementia is more difficult to diagnose in this population as the clinical features may present differently from those without an intellectual disability. Memory loss, loss of function, and behavioral changes are common early features. Symptoms associated with frontal lobe impairment such as apathy, slowness in speech and activities are also early manifestations of dementia in adults with Down syndrome. Ideally individuals with Down syndrome should be screened for signs of dementia from before the age of 35. The development of reliable screening and diagnostic tools has been difficult but there are now a number of valid tools (Dementia Screening Questionnaire for Individuals with Intellectual Disabilities DSQIID, Deb, Hare, Prior, & Bhaumik, 2007b) that can be used. There is also a role for neuropsychological testing and neuroimaging. Important differential diagnoses include hypothyroidism, depression, and sensory impairment.

There is a lack of good evidence for the use of anti-dementia medication in this population with only one small-scale RCT on donepezil showing a non-significant improvement (Prasher, Huxley, & Haque, 2002). There is also a lack of evidence for the use of non-pharmacological interventions such as reminiscence therapy. The management of dementia in this population should be a multidisciplinary approach involving the individual and their caregivers in the process. The aim of management should be to support functioning and prevent further deterioration as long as possible, and provide support for family.

1. Introduction

Down syndrome is the most commonly recognized genetic cause of intellectual disability. Medical advances, particularly in pediatrics, reducing infant mortality and improved living conditions mean that people who have an intellectual disability are living longer (Lubin & Kiely, 1985). Life expectancy for an individual with Down syndrome has increased from 9 years in 1929 to 57 years in 1989 (Steffelaar & Evenhuis, 1989). There has been a concomitant increase in the prevalence of age-associated diseases, most notably dementia.

2. Prevalence of Dementia among People Who Have Down Syndrome

Most prevalence studies of dementia among people over age 65 who have an intellectual disability have tended to focus on people from institutions. This results in a sampling bias, as psychopathology is more prevalent among people who live in institutions than those who are in the community. Even community-based samples include only those people who are in touch with various service providers.

In a two-stage population-based survey, Pate, Goldberg, and Moss (1993) found a prevalence of dementia of 11.4% among 105 adults of age 50 years and over who had an intellectual disability. Cooper (1997) found a rate of dementia of 21.6% in a population-based sample of 134 adults over age 65 who had an intellectual disability, most of whom did not have Down syndrome. In this study, people with dementia tended to be older, female, with more poorly controlled epilepsy, had a larger number of additional physical disorders, were less likely to be smokers, and had a lower adaptive behavior score than did the elderly people without dementia. Cooper hypothesized that the high rate of dementia associated with the intellectual disability may have been related aetiologically with an underlying genetic syndrome, or the lack of brain reserve, or a history of brain damage, all of which are more common among people who have an intellectual disability than in the general population. Between 31 and 78% of adults with an intellectual disability but not Down syndrome show Alzheimer's disease neuropathology (Deb, 2001a).

People who have Down syndrome tend to suffer from accelerated aging with coarsening of skin and thinning of hair. Not only is Alzheimer's dementia much more common, but the age of onset of dementia among people who have Down syndrome is much earlier than in the general population. Since Fraser and Mitchell's early report in the nineteenth century (1876), a series of autopsy studies have shown evidence for the presence of Alzheimer's neuropathology almost universally among adults who have Down syndrome and are over age 40 (Mann, 1988). Jervis (1948) first reported a detailed relationship between Alzheimer's dementia and Down syndrome. The prevalence of clinical dementia among adults who have Down syndrome varies between 0 and 4% under age 30, 2–33% for those 30–39 years of age, 8–55% for 40–49 years of age, 20–55% for 50–59 years of age, and 29–75% for 60–69 years of age (see Deb, 2001b). Coppus et al. (2006) followed 506 people with Down syndrome over 3.3 years. They found the overall prevalence of dementia to be 16.8%. Up to the age of 49 the prevalence was 8.9%, from 50 to 54 years it was 17.7%, and from 55 to 59 it was 32.1%. For those over 60 years it was 25.6% which may be explained by the increased mortality (44%) among those with dementia. This finding argues against the neuropathological findings that suggest all individuals with Down syndrome will develop dementia. This is backed up by Margallo et al. (2007) follow-up of 92 hospitalized adults with Down syndrome for 15 years who concluded that "the development of dementia of Alzheimer's type is frequent but not inevitable, and some people with Down syndrome reach old age without clinical features of dementia".

There has been little research into the prevalence of dementia according to severity of intellectual disability. The cognitive reserve hypothesis if correct should mean that those with more severe intellectual disability should have higher rates of dementia at a younger age. Strydom, Hassiotis, King, and Livingston (2008) looked at the prevalence of dementia according to severity of intellectual disability. They found that the overall prevalence of dementia was 13.1% for those over 60 years and 18.3% for those over 65 years. They found that the prevalence did not differ according to severity of intellectual disability. One possible reason for this is that those with a severe intellectual disability will have increased mortality at a younger age due to additional problems such as epilepsy (Gustavson, Umb-Carlsson, & Sonnander, 2005) and therefore the population that has survived into old age will be relatively healthy. The life expectancy of an adult with an intellectual disability without Down syndrome who reaches 65 years is comparable to that of the general population (Haveman, 2004).

Prevalence studies have also used different methodologies and have included patients in different groups. At the time of inclusion into a study, some individuals may not have been showing clinical expression of dementia, which may have become manifest later in their lives. The difficulty of diagnosing dementia in a person who has an intellectual disability is well known and this also may produce a lower prevalence rate of dementia among people who have Down syndrome. There are differences in the way data were collected in various studies, with some based on information from case notes, some using caregiver interview, and some undertaking direct patient examination. Different instruments have been used to diagnose dementia, with many studies using a screening rather than a diagnostic instrument and different criteria were used to confirm the diagnosis of dementia.

It is worth commenting on the prevalence of other types of mental ill-health in this population. Mantry et al. (2008) looked at a cohort of adults with Down syndrome in order to ascertain rates of all mental ill-health. They found that the point prevalence of mental ill-health of any type, excluding specific phobias varied from 10.8 to 23.7% depending on criteria used. The highest incidence was for depressive episode (5.2%) and dementia/delirium (5.2%) over the 2-year study period. They found that overall the prevalence of mental ill-health is lower in the Down syndrome population compared with other adults with intellectual disability. The findings agreed with previous research that mania and psychosis are uncommon in this population (Collacott, Cooper, & McGrother, 1992; Prasher, 1995a).

3. Neuropathology

Research has shown that virtually all adults with Down syndrome over 35–40 years of age have neuropathological changes characteristic of Alzheimer's dementia including β-amyloid (Aβ) plaques and neurofibrillary tangles (Wisniewski, Wisniewski, & Wen, 1985). This would suggest that all will develop dementia but this has not been shown to be the case (Holland et al., 2000). There are many possible explanations for the apparent discrepancy between the neuropathology findings and the lack of universal clinical manifestations of dementia, even in the age group between 60 and 69 years. Most autopsy studies were carried out among people in long-stay institutions, causing a sampling bias. Also the autopsy studies do not always record the clinical manifestation of dementia prior to death. A study has shown that three adults, aged over 65 years, who died in a Dutch institution and did not show any evidence of dementia when they were alive, did not show any Alzheimer's dementia neuropathology at autopsy (Visser et al., 1997).

Although the cortical distribution of Alzheimer's neuropathology among adults who have Down syndrome is similar to that expected in the general population, it is possible that the quantity of plaques and tangles, the hallmark of the Alzheimer's neuropathology, is not adequate to cause clinical manifestations. It is also possible that the threshold for the neuropathology to manifest clinical dementia is different among people who have Down syndrome than in the general population. Indeed, the plaques and tangles so abundant in the brains of adults who have Down syndrome may be neither the beginning nor the end of the neuropathological cascade in Alzheimer's dementia. Thus their mere presence does not necessarily prove that Alzheimer's dementia has developed.

There is also some suspicion that the plaques and tangles found in the brains of people who have Down syndrome may be qualitatively different from those that are found in the brains of people in the general population who develop Alzheimer's dementia. Wisniewski and Rabe (1986) have suggested that the plaques that are abundant among adults who have Down syndrome in their 30s and 50s (and sometimes older) and who do not show signs of dementia are benign and non-fibrillary in nature. On the other hand, fibrillized plaques that are associated with damage to neurons are also associated with clinical expression of Alzheimer's dementia among people who have Down syndrome. Mann (1993) failed to observe an interaction between neurofibrillary tangles with lectins in brain tissue specimens from people with Down syndrome–a reaction that typically occurs in similarly treated specimens from people with Alzheimer's dementia in the general population.

4. Risk Factors for Dementia among People Who Have Down Syndrome

Increasing age, a positive family history of Alzheimer's dementia, low educational level, inactive lifestyle, history of head trauma and cardiovascular disease have been identified as risk factors for Alzheimer's. The use of non-steroidal anti-inflammatory drugs, antioxidants, and a high educational level may act as protective factors. There are likely to be similarities in the risk factors associated with Alzheimer's dementia among people who have Down syndrome and those who do not. There are also differences in the risk factors between the two groups.

The genetic locus for amyloid precursor protein (APP) has been identified on chromosome 21. As 95% of cases of Down syndrome are caused by a trisomy 21, this may explain the vulnerability of people who have Down syndrome to developing dementia. The overexpression of the APP gene is related to the deposition of amyloid in the brain across the lifespan in Down syndrome and appears to be critical to the development of Alzheimer's dementia in individuals with Down syndrome. The APP gene on chromosome 21 along with Presenilin-1 (PS-1) polymorphism on chromosome 14 and Presenilin-2 (PS-2) on chromosome 1 are responsible for at least half the cases of familiar early-onset Alzheimer's dementia. No significant association was found between a PS-1 intronic polymorphism and dementia in Down's syndrome (Deb et al., 1998). There is evidence that adults with Down syndrome who have atypical karyotypes including translocations, partial trisomies, and mosaicism have an improved survival and decreased rates of Alzheimer's disease (Schupf, 2002). Zigman et al. (2000) found a significantly higher rate of mosaicism in adults with Down syndrome who had survived to 65 years.

The presence of Apolipoprotein E allele 4 (ApoE e4) on chromosome 19 is shown to be a risk factor for Alzheimer's dementia in the general population and there is some evidence that it may act as a risk factor among people who have Down syndrome (Deb et al., 2000). The Apolipoprotein E gene (APOE) is encoded for by three alleles, $\varepsilon 2$, $\varepsilon 3$, and $\varepsilon 4$, is involved in cholesterol transport and lipid metabolism, and is associated with greater accumulation of β-amyloid protein in the brains of the elderly. It is not clear whether the APOE $\varepsilon 2$ allele is protective against Alzheimer's in people who have Down syndrome as it is in the general population. Despite the increased risk associated with the ε4 allele, it is well known that the presence of ε4 allele is neither necessary nor essential for development of dementia (Blacker & Tanzi, 1998).

Some studies (Corder et al., 1993), though not all (Deb et al., 2000), have suggested that ApoE status, the presence of the APOE ε4 allele, affects the age of onset of dementia in people with Down syndrome. It is also suggested that ApoE status may influence the age of death. Hardy et al. (1994) have shown in an autopsy study that the 10 people with Down syndrome who had an ApoE ε4 allele tended to die at a younger age (age of death ranging between 48 and 60 years, with a mean age of 54 years) than the 2 people with Down syndrome who had an ε2 allele (age of death 69 and 76 years) and similar trends have been reported by others (Mann, Pickering-Brown, & Siddons, 1995; Royston, Mann, & Pickering-Brown, 1994), although all are based on small numbers. The APOE ε4 protein may act by accelerating the Alzheimer's disease process, predisposing to greater and earlier accumulation of Aβ. A recent longitudinal prospective study looked at the impact of APOE ε4 on dementia and mortality in those with Down syndrome. They showed a significant long-term effect on the incidence of dementia. When they pooled their data in a meta-analysis they found that the APOE ε4 allele shows a 1.59-fold increase in risk of dementia in persons with Down syndrome (Coppus, Evenhuis, & van Duijn, 2008).

Autopsy findings of people who have Down syndrome show no clear relationship between ApoE status and Alzheimer's disease neuropathology. Wisniewski et al. (1995) reported autopsy findings on 40 subjects with Down syndrome, of whom 15 showed Alzheimer's dementia neuropathology. Only one 21-year-old man had an APOE ε4 allele (ε3ε4 genotype) and his brain did not show Alzheimer's dementia neuropathology. Mann, Pickering-Brown, and Siddons (1995) reported an autopsy study of 20 subjects who had Down syndrome. All these brains showed Alzheimer's neuropathology, but only 7 had an APOE ε4 allele (one with ε2ε4 and six with ε3ε4 genotypes). Similarly, in Hardy et al. (1994) autopsy study of 22 subjects who had Down syndrome, all showed Alzheimer's dementia neuropathology, but only 10 had APOE ε4 allele (all with ε3ε4 genotypes). This apparent discrepancy needs further investigation, perhaps with the use of immunoneuropathological techniques. It is also important to explore the mechanism by which APOE ε4 allele may influence the expression of dementia among those who have Down syndrome.

The cognitive reserve hypothesis has been proposed to explain how adults with similar brain insults may present with different clinical pictures. Stern (2002) proposed that cognitive reserve had two components: passive components such as brain size and synapse count, the "hardware" of the brain. Active components are developed through educational, occupational, and leisure activities that develop the use of different neuronal pathways, the "software" of the brain. The hypothesis proposes that there is a critical threshold of reserve capacity that needs to be breached by pathological processes before symptoms and signs develop. Adults with an intellectual disability will have reduced cognitive reserve due to their underlying decreased cognitive function and the likelihood that they will have had less education and may have resided in environmentally impoverished institutions. The cognitive reserve hypothesis predicts that adults with an intellectual disability should be at risk for dementia and that they will be at risk of developing dementia at a younger age. There is a need for further research into this hypothesis to clearly elucidate its effects on adults with Down syndrome.

5. Diagnosing Dementia in Intellectual Disability

The diagnosis of dementia in this patient group can be problematic. There are a number of important factors that make the diagnosis more difficult than in the adult population without an intellectual disability. An obvious problem is the large variability in cognitive function from those with a mild intellectual disability to those with severe and a profound intellectual disability. There are an ever-growing number of diagnostic tools that can be used from caregiver questionnaires to neuroimaging techniques. Other problems include the difficulty in obtaining reliable baseline levels of cognitive functioning from which to measure change and the difficulty in accurately identifying when the decline began.

Research in the field of dementia in Down syndrome has begun to focus on the practical diagnosis at an early stage. Early and accurate diagnosis is important for the clinical care of those with dementia. The challenge is to develop a reliable method of doing so.

Burt and Aylward (2000) in their working group for the establishment of criteria for the diagnosis of dementia in individuals with an intellectual disability set out a model for best practice in diagnosis. They recommended that a baseline of cognitive functioning is established before the age of 35 years and then reviewed annually. If a decline in functioning is discovered on review then a full investigation should be carried out to gain a diagnosis. They suggested that a person-centered approach should be used to provide appropriate care for the individual and their caregivers.

The principle that the diagnosis of dementia requires evidence of a progressive deterioration in memory other cognitive functions and in daily living skills is the same for individuals with an intellectual disability as it is for the general population.

It is also worth noting that considerable debate exists regarding the overlap of age-related cognitive decline and dementia in the general population as well as in people with an intellectual disability. Studies that have mapped out cognitive decline among adults with an intellectual disability and with and without Down syndrome using prospective design (Carr, 2005; Devenny, Krinsky-Hale, Sersen, & Silverman, 2000) show a trend of relatively greater decline in verbal abilities compared with performance abilities, than has been shown in the general population. However, the exact features associated with normal aging and their overlap with dementia symptoms have never been properly studied among people with an intellectual disability.

6. Clinical Features of Dementia

The main clinical features of dementia in people with an intellectual disability/Down's syndrome are shown in Table 8.1. The features will be modified by the age, level of intellectual disability, personality, physical/mental health, and circumstances of the individual. The level of intellectual disability will tend to modify and mask the early signs and symptoms of dementia. A number of studies have looked at the clinical features of dementia particularly in those with Down syndrome.

Strydom, Livingston, King, & Hassiotis (2007) in the Becoming Older with Learning Disability (BOLD) memory study looked to describe the clinical features and prevalence of dementia and its subtypes. They assessed for diagnosis using the ICD-10 (World Health Organization 1993), DSM-IV (American Psychiatric Association, 2000), and the DCLD (Royal College of Psychiatrists, 2002) criteria. They found that the most common early symptom was a general deterioration in functioning (50% of those with dementia) followed by behavioral/emotional change (15%). They noted that deterioration in memory (7.7%) or other cognitive functions (7.7%) was rarely noted in the early stages. This is supported by Watchman (2007) who conducted a postal survey of caregiver members of Down syndrome Scotland. The first signs of dementia noted by caregivers were change in behavior (80%) and change in living skills (71%). Memory loss was reported in only 29% of cases as an early sign.

Other research has found that there are many similarities with presentation of Alzheimer's Dementia in people without an intellectual disability and those with Down syndrome. Deb, Hare, and Prior (2007a) have looked at the presentation in a qualitative study in the context of developing a caregiver-determined, case-detection instrument for dementia among 27 people who have Down syndrome. They reported that forgetfulness, particularly impairment of recent memory, seems to be a common and

Table 8.1 The main clinical features of dementia among people who have Down syndrome

Forgetfulness
Confusion
Apraxic symptoms: e.g., putting on clothes the wrong way round, doing up buttons the wrong way, etc.
Speech and language problems: e.g., difficulty instigating a conversation, lack of expression and flattening of the tone of voice, repetitive questioning and problems with understanding
Slowness
Loss of skills
Problems with socializing
Lack of confidence
Obsessional behavior
Paranoia/suspiciousness
Sleep problems: early morning waking, wandering at night
Change in appetite, often weight loss
Balance problems: unsteady gait, fearful of kerbs, leaning to one side, shuffling
Emotional problems: crying episodes, easily upset, and frustrated
Shouting and screaming
Agitation/restlessness
Aggression (verbal and physical)
Hallucinations, delusions, and illusions
Loss of interest/apathy
Covering up/confabulating
Seizures

early symptom. However, distant memory (for example, information about the family and where they lived and knowledge of music from the 1960s) remains relatively intact in the early stage. Loss of interest in activities and speech and language problems are also common. General confusion, slowness, loss of pre-existing skills, and emotional and behavioral problems often occur early in dementia in people with Down syndrome, but tend to occur later in people with Alzheimer's disease in the general population. Illusions (for example, thinking a cat is rubbing against them, while the cat is sitting still), visual agnosia (for example, picking things out of the air), and tactile hallucinations (for example, feeling of touch sensation that is not there) are reported but not frequently.

Lack of motivation, apathy, inability to socialize, general slowness, and lack of interest in life in general may be a manifestation of early frontal lobe dysfunction. Non-demented people who have Down syndrome tend to have structurally abnormal frontal lobes (Deb, 1997) and this may predispose them to manifest symptoms of "frontal lobe" dysfunction early in the process of Alzheimer's dementia. Change in personality is rarely manifested in the form of aggression but as apathy and social withdrawal.

Many adults with Down syndrome exhibit problems in following more than one instruction at one given time at an early stage of dementia. An example of such problem is that a person would pick up all the knives or all the forks when he was asked to pick up a knife and a fork from a drawer in the next room. Similarly, when a person with Down syndrome would be able to drink from a cup when asked, the same person would not be able to go upstairs, open a wardrobe in his room, and bring his clothes downstairs. This example shows that the person is still able to follow simple instruction but not complex instructions.

An early symptom of dementia in people with Down syndrome is evidence of slowness that affect almost all aspect of their functioning including walking slowly, eating slowly, speaking slowly, particularly failing to initiate conversations, and slowness in the overall body movement. This slowness is manifested at times in the way of stopping in the middle of a task such as eating or drinking etc.

Many adults with Down syndrome at early stage of dementia show speech and language problems in the form of tardiness in instigating a conversation, lack of expression and flattening of the tone of voice, and repetitive questioning (which was not present previously). Other examples include speech becoming slow and difficult to understand (which was not the case before), and problem with their own comprehension, which was manifested in the inability to follow simple instructions.

Sleep problems in the form of early morning wakening and wandering at night may be prominent features of dementia in adults with Down syndrome. Some show evidence of catnapping during the day at the expense of less and less sleep at night. One unusual example of sleep problem may be switching the bed light on and off continuously during the night, not sleeping at all during the night and instead speaking to themselves all night long.

Loss of self-help skills could be an early symptom of dementia among adults with Down syndrome. In the beginning the caregivers often report that the person with Down syndrome needs more and more prompts to carry out simple self-help chores such as wiping face with a flannel or brushing teeth or drinking from a cup. Eventually people lose these skills altogether and cannot carry them out even with a lot of prompts.

Many adults with Down syndrome show lack of socialization and withdraw from other people around them and also do not show interest in activities that they used to enjoy before. Another prominent feature of dementia in people with Down syndrome is unsteady gait. Some people tend to lean to one side while walking while others take a big step over a crack on the surface or an uneven surface, including kerbs and uneven patterns in the carpet. One reported unusual symptom associated with dementia in people with Down syndrome is "pica" (eating/mouthing inedible substances).

We believe that there are two possible explanations for finding prominent features of "frontal lobe" dysfunction early in dementia among adults with Down syndrome. First, people with Down syndrome show structural abnormalities in the frontal and the temporal lobes (Deb, 1997), and are therefore vulnerable to loss of frontal and temporal lobe functions early because of any brain insult. Second, it is often not possible to detect dementia in its early stage among adults who have an intellectual disability. Therefore, dementia tends only to be diagnosed in these people when the disease has already progressed to its middle or late stage. This is also evident from the shorter period of time that is clinically observed between making the diagnosis of dementia and death among adults with Down syndrome compared with people without an intellectual disability. The features of "frontal lobe" dysfunction are not uncommon in the later-stage dementia in the general population; therefore, it is not surprising to detect these features fairly early in the diagnosis among adults with an intellectual disability, given that these people are probably already in an advanced stage of dementia by the time a diagnosis is made.

Symptoms associated with confusion such as putting two legs in one trousers' leg may be the manifestation of disorientation or memory problem or dressing dyspraxia. Similarly, slowness of speech and failure to initiate conversation may be explained by either language problems or apathy symptoms, which are associated with the frontal lobe dysfunction. Obsessive tendencies may reflect the development of true obsession or may have been caused by loss of memory for which the person needs to check everything several times or may be the part of overall slowness in information processing or perseveration caused by frontal lobe dysfunction. Similarly, failure to carry out more than one instruction at a time may have been caused by the loss of procedural memory or language difficulty such as comprehension problems or slowness in information processing, which again is associated with frontal lobe dysfunction.

Deb et al. (2007a) found differential manifestation of early symptoms of dementia depending on the severity of intellectual disability. For example, among people with severe intellectual disability early manifestation may be gradual loss of self-help skills, whereas early symptoms of dementia among adults with a mild intellectual disability may be similar to that of people who do not have an intellectual disability, for example impaired recent memory. In Deb et al. (2007a) study spatial disorientation was a frequent symptom and was present in both those with a moderate and a severe intellectual disability. Epilepsy and urinary incontinence were more commonly present at diagnosis of dementia in the severely intellectually disabled group than in the moderately intellectually disabled group but apathy symptoms were more common among adult females with a moderate than a severe intellectual disability. None of these differences were statistically significant though.

It is interesting to note that most early and primary symptoms of dementia among adults with Down syndrome in Deb et al. (2007a) study were similar to those found in adults without an intellectual disability. For example, the loss of recent memory in the absence of loss of distant memory was the early prominent symptom in most cases of adults with Down syndrome. This trend was particularly noticeable among adults with a mild-to-moderate degree of intellectual disability. This is also the case for people without an intellectual disability. However, these symptoms may be difficult to detect, particularly in the early stage of dementia among adults who have a severe and a profound intellectual disability. In these people loss of skills and some behavioral problems seem to be the early indicators of dementia. Caregivers often report these early symptoms. However, caregiver's memory may not be totally accurate in this context as they describe events retrospectively. Therefore, a true account of the order of appearance of different symptoms could only be determined from a prospective assessment.

Seizures can be a feature of dementia in those with Down syndrome. There is a bimodal distribution of epilepsy in the Down syndrome population; an early-onset epilepsy occurring in about 10% and a late-onset epilepsy associated with dementia. The seizures are most frequently generalized tonic–clonic seizures, although they may be accompanied by partial complex and myoclonic seizures in about 10% of cases. They are a poor prognostic feature being associated with death within 3–5 years (Berney, 2009).

Strydom et al. (2007) attempted to diagnose the different subtypes of dementia that occur in the general population in those with an intellectual disability. They found that they were able to diagnose cases of vascular dementia, Lewy body dementia, and frontotemporal dementia as well as Alzheimer's type. Alzheimer's was the most common form as it is in the general population. They noted that the vascular dementia prevalence was lower than expected and was less common than the Lewy body and frontotemporal dementia types.

In Prasher's (1995a) study common early symptoms of dementia among adults with Down syndrome included mental deterioration, slowing, confusion, reduced output of speech, and deterioration in gait and personality change. Evenhuis (1990) on the other hand described apathy and withdrawal symptoms as the most common early features of dementia among people with both a moderate and a severe intellectual disability. As per Prasher (1995b) the late features of dementia among adults with an intellectual disability include severe intellectual deterioration, marked change in personality and mood, loss of sphincter control, onset of epileptic seizures, loss of mobility with increased muscle tone, and eventual complete loss of all self-help skills.

Many studies have highlighted the similarities in clinical presentation of Alzheimer's dementia in the general population who do not have an intellectual disability and in people with Down syndrome using both cross-sectional design (Roeden & Zitman, 1995) and prospective design (Lai & Williams, 1989). Holland et al. (2000) and Ball et al. (2006) highlighted the importance of caregiver reporting of symptoms of dementia among adults with Down syndrome. Holland et al. (2000) found in an 18-month follow-up study that in the initial assessment caregivers reported changes predominantly in behavior and personality among adults with Down syndrome who later developed dementia. In Holland et al. (2000), study the frontal lobe-like dementia was more prevalent particularly among the younger groups. On the basis of their findings the authors hypothesized that the frontal lobe functions are the first to be compromised with the progressive development of Alzheimer-like neuropathology in people with Down syndrome. Crayton, Oliver, Holland, Bradbury, & Hall (1998) in another 4-year follow-up study found that those adults with Down syndrome who developed dementia at the follow-up showed evidence of impaired orientation and visuospatial memory at the beginning of the study but language function and praxis deteriorated later.

7. Differential Diagnosis of Dementia among People Who Have Down Syndrome

Sensory impairments, such as difficulty in hearing and vision, are not uncommon among people who have Down syndrome and they develop symptoms that may mimic dementia. Some authors have reported a higher prevalence of depression among people who have Down syndrome, compared with adults who have an intellectual disability but not Down syndrome (Collacott et al., 1992), whilst others have not confirmed this (Haveman et al., 1994). The clinical expression of depression can be confused with dementia, but the distinction is important, as most cases of depression are treatable. Subclinical hypothyroidism (high basal level of TSH and low total or free T4) is present in approximately one-third of adults who have Down syndrome (Deb, 2001c) and antithyroid antibodies are present in 18% of people who have Down syndrome, compared with 6% of matched healthy control subjects (Rubello, Pozzan, & Casara, 1995). The presence of antithyroid antibodies makes people who have Down syndrome vulnerable to develop clinical hypothyroidism and this must be differentiated from other causes of dementia.

Table 8.2 Differential diagnosis of dementia/decline in function

Depression
Decline secondary to sensory impairment (visual and hearing)
Endocrine disorders such as hypothyroidism
Delirium
Vascular disease: multi-infarct dementia
Physical brain damage: tumor, head injury, epilepsy
High-dose antipsychotics, medications with anti-cholinergic adverse effects, antiepileptic drugs, and multiple medications
Degenerative disorders: Parkinson's disease
Infections: Encephalitis, meningitis, Creutzfeldt–Jakob disease
Anaemia, chronic infection, nutritional deficiency: Vitamin B12, folate
Impact of life events (bereavement, change in environment, move from home, loss of day activities, etc.)
Physical and emotional abuse (Dodd et al., 2009)

There are a wide variety of potential causes for decline in function in the aging population with an intellectual disability (Table 8.2).

8. Diagnostic or Screening Instruments

Two main approaches have been taken for screening or making a diagnosis of dementia in people who have an intellectual disability: completion by caregivers of observer-rated behavior questionnaire or face-to-face neuropsychological tests (Table 8.3).

9. Observer-Rated Scales

Some of the early symptoms of dementia may be subtle or may present as an exacerbation of the existing behavioral traits or manifest differently in people with Down syndrome than they do in people who do not have an intellectually disability. Only caregivers will notice these early and, sometimes, unusual changes in the person's behavior and only by asking caregivers can we ensure that such symptoms are included in any case detection instrument. Therefore, an informant-rated instrument is ideal for screening or diagnostic purposes among adults with an intellectual disability.

Table 8.3 Instruments used for assessing dementia among adults who have an intellectual disability/Down syndrome

Observer-rated questionnaires
Dementia questionnaire for people with Learning Disabilities (DLD)–formerly known as the DMR (Evenhuis et al., 2007)
DSDS (Gedye, 1995)
MOSES (Dalton & Fedor, 1997)
Early Signs of Dementia Checklist (Visser et al., 1997)
Adaptive Behavior Scale (Nihara et al., 1974)
Modified CAMDEX-DS informant interview (Roth et al., 1998; Ball et al., 2006)
DSQIID (Deb, 2007)
Adaptive Behavior Dementia Questionnaire (ABDQ) (Prasher et.al., 2004)
Neuropsychological tests
Modified MMSE (Folstein et al., 1975)
Modified Boston Naming Test (Kaplan et al., 1978)
McCarthy Verbal Fluency (McCarthy, 1972)
Modified Fuld (Altman, 1977)
Modified Purdue Pegboard (Tiffin & Asher, 1948)
Brief Praxis Test (Dalton, 1992)
Spatial Recognition Span (Moss et al.,1986)
Test for Severe Impairment (TSI) (Albert & Cohen, 1992)
Severe Impairment Battery (SIB) (Saxton, McGonigle, Swihart, & Boller, 1993)
Neuropsychological Assessment of dementia in adults with Intellectual Disabilities (NAID) (Crayton et al., 1998)
CAMCOG-DS (Ball et al., 2006) is the neuropsychological assessment part of CAMDEX-DS

The Dementia Scale for Down Syndrome (DSDS, Gedye, 1995), the Dementia Questionnaire for people with Learning Disabilities (DLD, Evenhuis, Kengen, & Eurlings, 2007), formerly the DMR (Evenhuis, 1996), and the Dementia Screening Questionnaire for Individuals with Intellectual Disabilities (DSQIID) (Deb et al., 2007b) are the most widely used observer-rated scales.

The DSDS was adapted from a document produced by the Canadian Association for the Mentally Retarded. This listed possible symptoms of dementia in early, middle, and late stages of the condition and provided caregivers with guidelines on management of symptoms at every stage. There are 60 questions (20 for each stage of dementia) and each behavior is rated as "present", "absent", "not applicable", or "typical of that individual". Only those that are "present" are scored for early, middle, and late stages of dementia. There are some problems with use of this scale, as two informants have to be interviewed by a trained chartered psychologist and the terminologies used and scoring system are very complicated. The scale has not been published in any peer-reviewed journal.

The DLD/DMR has 50 questions, under the categories of "short-term memory", "long-term memory", "spatial and temporal orientation" (making up the sum of cognitive scores) "speech", "practical skills", "mood", "activity and interest" and behavioral disturbance (making up the sum of social skills score). Each of the behaviors is rated as present either "normally yes" (0), "sometimes" (1), or "normally no" (2). The overall score is calculated under two headings, namely the "sum of cognitive scores" (SCS) and the "sum of social scores" (SOS). The cut-off scores for screening positive for dementia are different for people who have mild, moderate, or severe intellectual disability. This scale has shown low reliability when completed by caregivers. Further, professionals may find it difficult to work out the severity of a person's intellectual disability, which is required to determine cut-off scores for dementia.

Visser et al. (1997) followed up adults who had Down syndrome in a Dutch Institution with the Early Signs of Dementia Checklist (ESDC), and Dalton and Fedor (1997) have used the Multi-dimensional Observation Scale for Elderly Subjects (MOSES). Neither has been properly validated for use in people with an intellectual disability. Some studies have used the Adaptive Behavior Scale (Nihira et al., 1974) to estimate the rate of decline in adaptive behaviors in adults who have Down syndrome over a period of time (Collacott et al., 1992). The Adaptive Behavior Dementia Questionnaire (ABDQ) is a 15-item questionnaire used to detect changes in adaptive behavior and can be used as a screening tool (Prasher, Farooq, & Holder, 2004).

Deb et al. (2007b) developed the Dementia Screening Questionnaire for Individuals with Intellectual Disabilities (DSQIID). Their aim was to develop a user-friendly observer-rated dementia screening questionnaire with strong psychometric properties for adults with intellectual disabilities. A "bottom-up" approach incorporating the views of caregivers regarding the symptoms of dementia was adopted. They used qualitative methods to gather information from caregivers of people with Down syndrome about the symptoms of dementia. They then used these results to develop the screening questionnaire. The DSQIID is completed by a professional taking information from caregivers that have known the individual for some time. The DSQIID is divided into three parts; the first asks about the "best" ability the person has or has had. The second part contains 43 questions (Table 8.4) about behavior or symptoms that are usually associated with dementia in adults with Down syndrome. Each item is scored on a 4-point scale: (a) Always has been the case, (b) Always, but worse, (c) New symptoms, and (d) Does not apply. Items with a response of "does not

Table 8.4 DSQIID items (adapted from Deb, 2007)

1. Can't wash/bathe without help
2. Can't dress without help
3. Dresses inappropriately
4. Undresses inappropriately
5. Needs help eating
6. Needs help using bathroom
7. Incontinence including accidents
8. Does not initiate conversation
9. Can't find words
10. Can't follow simple instructions
11. Can't follow more than one instruction
12. Stops in the middle of a task
13. Can't read
14. Can't write
15. Changed sleep pattern
16. Wakes at night
17. Confused at night
18. Sleeps during the day
19. Wanders at night
20. Can't find way in familiar surroundings
21. Wanders
22. Loses track of time
23. Not confident to walk over small cracks
24. Unsteady walk/loses balance
25. Can't walk unaided
26. Can't recognize familiar persons
27. Can't remember names of persons
28. Can't remember recent events
29. Withdraws from social activities
30. Withdraws from persons
31. Loss of interest in hobbies/activities
32. Seems to go into own world
33. Obsessive or repetitive behavior
34. Hides or hoards objects
35. Loses objects
36. Puts familiar things into wrong places
37. Does not know what to do with objects
38. Appears insecure
39. Appears anxious or nervous
40. Appears depressed
41. Shows aggression
42. Fits/epilepsy
43. Talks to self

apply" or "always been the case" are scored 0, those with "always but worse" or "new symptom" are scored 1. This scoring system was adapted to overcome the floor effect of the existing dementia screening scales which do not score changes in behavior. The third part of the DSQIID contains 10 questions, all of which are comparative; for example, "seems generally more tired" and "speaks (signs) less". A response of "yes" is scored 1 and a response of "no" is scored 0.

The DSQIID was then administered to the caregivers of 193 adults with Down syndrome, 117 of whom were examined by clinicians and a diagnosis of dementia was made in 49 cases. They asked the caregivers to identify any other caregivers who knew the individuals with Down syndrome and sent the second caregiver the DSQIID in order to test inter-rater reliability. They also asked caregivers to repeat the DSQIID immediately after receiving the first completed questionnaire in order to test test–retest reliability. DSQIID has shown very good score on test re-test and inter-rater reliability. DSQIID has also shown good factor structure. The results showed that a cut-off score of 20 has sensitivity of 0.92 and a specificity of 0.97. They concluded that the DSQIID is a valid, reliable, and user-friendly questionnaire for dementia screening among adults with Down syndrome.

There were some adults with Down syndrome who scored above 20 but did not receive a clinical diagnosis of dementia and similarly there were some people who scored below 20 but had a clinical diagnosis of dementia. Therefore, the score should be used as a rough guide. DSQIID is a screening instrument and not a diagnostic instrument and should be used as such. This instrument is best scored by a professional who should gather information by interviewing a caregiver who knows the person with the intellectual disability well. In a clinical setting the DSQIID is best used to explore each item with the caregiver in more detail in order to build up a clinical picture. DSQIID should be used in a prospective manner; however, certain items may show floor effect as dementia progresses thus giving a lower total score as time progresses. Also it is worth keeping in mind that there are certain physical and psychological conditions that may affect scoring of certain items. For example, stroke will affect scoring on items on "walking and gait".

10. Neuropsychological Tests

Matthews et al. (1974) was one of the first researchers who attempted to design a neuropsychological test for use with individuals with an intellectual disability. He adapted subtests from the Halstead–Reitan battery. Since then more research has been focused on how to diagnose dementia earlier in individuals with an intellectual disability. Most diagnostic tests in the adult population with dementia are based on the premise that individuals tested have an IQ of at least 100 (Prasher et al., 2004).

When testing adults who have an intellectual disability, adult versions of neuropsychological tests are usually amended, or children's versions are used. For example, the original "Mini-Mental State Examination" (MMSE, Folstein, Folstein, & McHugh, 1975) has been modified to offer a "multiple choice" answer for some questions such as "which day of the week is it today?" (Wisniewski & Hill, 1985). The "Test for Severe Impairment" (Albert & Cohen, 1992) is a downward extension of the MMSE that tries to negate the floor effect in the later stages of dementia. The "Fuld Object-Memory Evaluation" (Altman, 1977) is a modified version (Seltzer, 1997) of Buschke's original "Selective reminding test" (Buschke, 1973). Ten easy-to-identify objects, such as a ball, a key, a button etc. are taken out of a bag and presented to the subject for memorizing. This test assesses registration, retention, and retrieval from memory after a delay. The "Spatial Recognition Span" (Moss, Albert, Butters, & Payne, 1986) is a test of non-verbal memory without delay in which a board is used with 30 "locations" in a 5 × 6 grid. The subject is asked to remember the position of a new disk every time they are placed on the board.

The "McCarthy Verbal Fluency" test (McCarthy, 1972), designed originally for children with normal cognitive function, has also been used among adults who have an intellectual disability. This test requires the subject to name as many words as possible within four specific categories, namely "food", "animals", "things to wear", and "things to ride". The initial simpler items of the "Boston Naming Test" (Kaplan, Goodglass, & Weubtraub, 1978) can also be used to test language. The "Purdue Pegboard modified" (Tiffin & Asher, 1948) tests constructional and psychomotor skills and requires the individual to place as many round pegs in round holes as is possible in 30 seconds. The "Brief Praxis Test" was developed by Dalton (1992) specifically to screen for early features of dementia in adults who have an intellectual disability. In this test the individual is asked to carry out simple motor tasks such as raising an arm, shaking hands, unscrewing the top of a jar etc.

Ball et al. (2004) looked at the reliability and validity of a modified version of the Cambridge Examination for Mental Disorders of the Elderly (CAMDEX) informant interview, for use when assessing individuals with Down syndrome suspected as having dementia. The original CAMDEX was developed by Roth et al. (1986) and revised in 1998 (Roth, Huppert, Mountjoy, & Tym, 1998). The full schedule includes an informant interview, an interview with the participant, an objective examination of cognitive function (CAMCOG), and a physical examination and information on laboratory investigations. It was modified for use with individuals with an intellectual disability for the study. They found that the modified CAMDEX informant interview was a valid and reliable tool. They found that the point estimates for sensitivity and specificity were high (0.88 and 0.94 respectively) and comparable with the levels found by Deb and Braganza (1999) for the DMR and the DSDS. They did find that the difficulty level of the CAMCOG led to exclusion of participants and limits the degree to which the results can be generalized to the Down syndrome population as a whole. Beacher et al. (2009) found the CAMCOG to be an appropriate test for assessing function in people with an intellectual disability and that the subtests with a small number of exceptions did not produce ceiling or floor effects.

Despite the use of all the above tests, their validity for use among adults who have an intellectual disability still remains questionable. Perhaps an important strategy is to use these tests alongside an observer-rated behavior questionnaire on a prospective basis. If used repeatedly, these tests should be able to detect both the onset of dementia, but also any age-related decline in cognitive function that may not always lead to a dementing process (Devenny et al., 1996).

There are two primary problems with using direct neuropsychological tests in this population. Firstly, the tests used for general population screening show floor effects in people who have an intellectual disability, as these people often have cognitive deficits that pre-date the onset of dementia. Secondly, people with an intellectual disability have a very varied range of ability and cognitive function (from profoundly impaired at one end to mild intellectual disability at the other). Therefore, it will not be possible to determine a cut-off score for screening of dementia that can be applied to people with all degrees of severity of intellectual disability. Deb and Braganza (1999) have highlighted these problems in their study. They compared clinicians' diagnosis of dementia with DSDS, DMR, and MMSE scores among 36 adults who have Down syndrome but no dementia and 26 adults with Down syndrome and dementia. DSDS and DMR correlated with each other and also with the clinicians' diagnosis (possibly because the same clinicians rated DSDS and DMR, and also have made the clinical diagnosis). It was only possible to administer the MMSE to 34 of the 62 (55%) subjects. Thirty of these 34 adults (95%) had a score below 24 (the usual cut-off score for possible dementia diagnosis), but 23 of these had no diagnosis of dementia according to either DSDS or DMR or the clinician's diagnosis.

11. Diagnostic Criteria

Strydom et al. (2007) in the Becoming Older with Learning Disability (BOLD) memory study assessed for diagnosis using the ICD-10 (World Health Organization, 1993), DSM-IV (American Psychiatric Association,

2000), and the DC-LD (Royal College of Psychiatrists, 2001) criteria. They found that generally correlations between the criteria were good but that there were important differences. They noted that the ICD-10 criteria were more specific but less sensitive than the DSM-IV criteria. The ICD-10 criteria are more demanding to apply because they are more dependent on reliable information from informants. The ICD-10 and DC-LD criteria require behavioral and emotional changes to make the diagnosis but the DSM-IV does not. Strydom et al. (2007) note that these symptoms were not good at discriminating between those with and without dementia and therefore limit the number diagnosed. They concluded that the DSM-IV was the preferred option in this population and that its use may enable earlier diagnosis of dementia in larger numbers of adults with intellectual disability. This could lead to earlier interventions.

12. Practical Diagnosis

As discussed above there are a wide variety and ever-expanding number of tests available but it would be hugely impractical to use them all or even most of them. The assessment of an individual with an intellectual disability suspected of dementia should start with a history from the individual and their caregivers. A mental state and physical examination of the person with an intellectual disability is imperative in order to make a diagnosis. Physical examination includes assessment of all bodily systems including neurological examination for focal neurological signs and cardiovascular system including high blood pressure. Standard laboratory tests should include vitamin B12 and folate levels, thyroid function test, full blood count (FBC), serum glucose, lipid profile, urea and electrolytes, renal function test, and liver function test.

There are differing views on the usefulness of neuroimaging in the work-up of the individual. Structural neuroimaging is widely considered to be useful to exclude space occupying mass lesions and it may also have a role in early diagnosis. Beacher et al. (2009) found that there were reliable "biomarkers" (medial temporal and striatal volume reductions) for the presence of Alzheimer's dementia on MRI. Functional neuroimaging is not widely available and therefore not recommended by many (Feldman et al., 2008; Nieuwenhuis-Mark, 2009) although advances are being made in SPECT (Deb et al., 1992) and PET (Haier, Head, Head, & Lott, 2008). An electroencephalograph (EEG) will be useful in those who have seizures. Neuroimaging requires informed consent which will require adapted information to be given to the patient and also possibly an assessment of capacity to consent to the procedure. The procedures are often long and complex requiring the co-operation of the patient and this is often difficult in this population. The recent report by the Royal College of Psychiatrists UK (Dodd et al., 2009) concluded that neuroimaging was not an essential investigation but that it may be of value where other brain lesions or vascular dementia are suspected.

An observer-rated scale such as the DSQIID should be used at baseline and then for follow-up to identify changes. More detailed neuropsychological tests such as the CAMDEX-DS (Ball et al., 2004) should only be used if decline is noted or if the diagnosis is unclear. An assessment of environmental factors is also mandatory.

13. Challenging Behavior

The non-cognitive symptom such as aggression is one of the common causes of burden for care in the general population as reported by caregivers of people with dementia (Donaldson, Tarrier, & Burns, 1997). However, in general a lower rate of aggression is reported among people with Down syndrome both with but also without dementia (Collacott, Cooper, Branford, & McGrother, 1998). In a study of 128 adults with Down syndrome, 29 of whom had dementia, Cosgrave, Tyrell, McCarron, Gill, & Lawlor (1999) found that the presence of dementia was not predictive of aggression. Prasher and Filer (1995) also recorded a low prevalence of significant maladaptive behavior in people with dementia and Down syndrome. In a study of 19 adults with Down syndrome and dementia, and 26 adults with other causes of an intellectual disability and dementia, Cooper and Prasher (1998) found that aggression occurred with greater frequency in those subjects with an intellectual disability due to other causes but low mood, restlessness/excessive overactivity, disturbed sleep, uncooperativeness, and auditory hallucinations were more common among adults with Down syndrome and dementia. Huxley, Van-Schaik, and Witts (2005) found a higher rate of challenging behaviors among 15 adults with Down syndrome and dementia compared with 19 adults with Down syndrome who did not have dementia. However, in their study, challenging behavior did not include aggression but included behaviors such as irritability, hyperactivity, stereotypy, and lethargy.

The family caregivers in Deb et al. (2007a) study did not report severe behavioral problems, although they were not altogether absent. As this study analyzed data based on caregiver's report, it is possible that the caregivers may have underreported the behavioral symptoms. It is possible that some of the cognitive deficits such as language problems or inability to follow instructions may have indirectly caused behavior problems through frustration. The lack of initiative that may sometimes be interpreted as sheer "laziness" may cause frustration and lead to aggression. Similarly, if someone has lost interest in activities and has become socially withdrawn, any demand placed on that person in order to comply with social activities are likely to cause further friction, which may lead to aggression. It is therefore of utmost importance to try to find an explanation and an underlying cause for aggression in a person who has developed dementia in order to minimize unnecessary use of medication.

Bird (2002) points out that challenging behavior has been a known feature of dementia, which has been largely ignored by research. This has led to behaviors such as aggression and screaming being managed with medication often inappropriately. Urv, Zigman, and Silverman (2003) study of maladaptive behaviors related to adaptive decline in 529 adults with a learning disability (202 of whom had Down syndrome) found that the occurrence or increasing frequency of some maladaptive behaviors were early indicators for dementia.

Huxley et al. (2005) looked at the occurrence of challenging behavior in a group of individuals with Down syndrome and dementia as compared with its occurrence in a group with Down syndrome without dementia. They used the Aberrant Behavior Checklist-Community Version (Aman & Singh, 1986) and the DSDS to look at problem behaviors and cognitive function. They found a significant difference between the groups for lethargy and hyperactivity and close to significance for stereotypy and irritability. They concluded that challenging behavior is a behavioral symptom of dementia and not solely attributable to normal aging. This research has relevance for the practical management of individuals with dementia as well as planning for future services. It also adds more evidence that change in behavior early may indicate an onset of dementia.

14. Treatment

The treatment may include both pharmacological and non-pharmacological management. The pharmacological treatment may be required to treat (a) cognitive impairment associated with dementia, (b) non-cognitive psychological and behavioral symptoms, and (c) co-existing physical health problems. The mainstay of treatment for cognitive impairment is the acetylcholinesterase inhibitors (donepezil, galantamine, and rivastigmine). The other type of treatment includes memantine, which is an NMDA (*N*-methyl-D-aspartate) antagonist. There is equivocal evidence to support the effectiveness of donepezil in people with an intellectual disability, and no RCT-based published data on the effectiveness on any other anti-dementia drugs for this special population are available yet. In the UK, the National Institute for Clinical Excellence (NICE; www.nice.org) has developed guideline for the drug treatment of dementia. The outcome measure according to NICE depends on the score based on the Mini Mental State Examination (MMSE), which is totally irrelevant as for use among people with an intellectual disability (see discussion above). The NICE guideline allows use of suitable measures other than MMSE to assess outcome among people with an intellectual disability.

There has been one major study looking at pharmacological treatment in this population (Prasher et al., 2002). They carried out a 24-week double-blind, placebo-controlled trial involving 30 patients with Down syndrome and Alzheimer's dementia treated with donepezil. The authors used the Dementia Scale for Mentally Retarded Persons (DMR) by Evenhuis (1996) as the primary outcome measure. They found that the treatment group had a non-significant reduction in deterioration in global functioning, adaptive behavior, and cognitive functions. They continued the study to an open-label phase (Prasher et al., 2003) for 104 weeks. They concluded that the treatment group showed significant reduction in deterioration after this period of time. This was the only study included in the Cochrane intervention review of donepezil for dementia in people with Down syndrome (Mohan, Bennett, & Carpenter, 2009b). The review concluded that the available literature does not support the use of donepezil in this group and that further larger randomized controlled studies with longer-term follow-up are required. The Cochrane reviews on rivastigmine and galantamine found no studies suitable for inclusion (Mohan, Bennett, & Carpenter, 2009c, d). In the general population with dementia, memantine is shown to be an effective treatment for dementia (McShane, Sastre, & Minakaran, 2006). The Cochrane intervention review for memantine in Down syndrome found no studies suitable for inclusion (Mohan, Bennett, & Carpenter, 2009a). It is clear that more research is required to assess the efficacy of the anti-dementia medication in this population group.

In an open-label trial of patients with Down syndrome and dementia comparing 9 patients treated with donepezil with 9 untreated matched patients, Lott Osann, Doran, and Nelson (2002) reported significant improvement in the treated group over a 3–5-month period ($p = 0.03$). Prasher, Fung, and Adams (2005) compared 17 patients with Down syndrome and Alzheimer disease treated with rivastigmine with 13 patients treated with placebo. The rate of decline was less in the rivastigmine-treated group although both groups of patients deteriorated over a 24-week period. A meta-analysis of studies carried out by Zana, Janka, and Kalman (2007) pointed towards either insufficient evidence or lack of positive evidence of cognitive improvement from antioxidants, Gingko Biloba, piracetam, and vitamins among adults with Down syndrome.

A baseline electrocardiogram should be carried out before starting anti-dementia drugs. This is necessary to exclude cardiac dysrhythmias such as supraventricual tachycardia, sick sinus syndrome, etc. Caution should also be used in persons who have a history of epilepsy, peptic ulcer, chronic upper respiratory disorders, bronchial asthma, etc.

Ballard et al. (2008) reviewed the evidence on the use of antipsychotics for treatment of behavioral and psychological symptoms among adults with dementia who did not have a pre-existing learning disability. All antipsychotics increase the vulnerability for cerebrovascular disorders among patients with dementia. Although no studies exist to guide practice among people with Down syndrome or an intellectual disability, the same caution should be exercised when using antipsychotics among these patients. In any case non-medication-based management is preferred over medication-based treatment in order to manage problem behaviors among people with an intellectual disability (see Deb, Clarke, & Unwin, 2006).

Other medications that are used to treat non-cognitive symptoms of dementia among the general population who do not have an intellectual disability include cholinesterase inhibitors, anti-epileptic medications such as carbamazepine, sodium valproate (including valproic acid + semisodium valproate), and gabapentin, beta blockers, benzodiazepine, hormonal therapy, etc. (Sadavoy, Lanctôt, & Deb, 2008). Not much RCT-based evidence is available for these medications. However, no literature-based evidence is available for the efficacy of these medications in the treatment of non-cognitive symptoms of dementia in people with an intellectual disability. Deb, Sohanpal, Soni, Unwin, & Lenôtre (2007c), Deb et al. (2008) and Sohanpal et al. (2007) have reported systematic reviews on the efficacy of antipsychotics, antidepressants, and mood stabilizers for the management of problem behaviors among adults with an intellectual disability.

Sadavoy et al. (2008) reviewed the efficacy of different non-pharmacological management of non-cognitive psychological and behavioral symptoms of dementia in the general population of people who do not have an intellectual disability. Non-pharmacological management techniques include reminiscence therapy, group psychotherapy, validation therapy, pet therapy, bright light therapy, etc. Other specific non-pharmacological interventions include sensory therapy, activities therapy, modified activities of daily living routines based on patient needs, environmental modifications, behavioral theory treatments, social contact intervention, etc. (Sadavoy et al., 2008). Currently no such evidence base exists either to support or to refute the use of non-pharmacological interventions for the non-cognitive symptoms of dementia among adults with an intellectual disability. However Hassiotis and Hall (2009) carried out a recent Cochrane review on the use of non-pharmacological management of problem behaviors among people with an intellectual disability who do not have dementia. Similar reviews were carried out in the past by Scotti, Evans, Mayer, & Walker (1991), Didden, Duker, and Korzilius (1997), Carr, Horner, and Turnbull (1999) (cited in Deb, 2007).

Other important areas of assessment and management include physical health including management of pain, incontinence, mobility issues, eating/ feeding/ swallowing issues, self-help skills issues (modelling, guiding, prompting, pacing; providing appropriate support to maintain self-help and domestic skills, and adaptation of the environment to aid daily living), orientation and confusion problems (reminiscence, life story work), communication problems (use of communication passport, pictures, symbols, and images), occupational activities (sensory stimulation, aromatherapy, music therapy, other appropriate activities), and also anxiety management and relaxation therapy for some psychological symptoms (Dodd et al., 2009).

15. Service Needs

A case could be made to make caregivers aware of the main themes of expression of dementia in people who have an intellectual disability so that the caregivers could raise suspicion at an early stage about the condition and an appropriate referral could be made to specialist services for the confirmation of the diagnosis. Caring for a person who has an intellectual disability causes extra burden, which is exacerbated when the same person also develops dementia. Therefore, a multidisciplinary approach to assessment and service provision in which GPs, Psychiatrists, Neurologists, Nurses, Psychologists, Physiotherapists, and Occupational Therapists are involved, is vital in order to lessen the burden of care. In the UK people who have an intellectual disability and develop dementia are likely to be known to the local Community Learning Disability Support teams, who are likely to co-ordinate services for these people and their caregivers. Watchman (2007) suggests a need for increased awareness and training for GPs, who are likely to have no more than five people with Down syndrome registered on their list at any one time. She also suggests that one individual should take responsibility for sharing the diagnosis with the individual and their caregivers.

Good practice guidance from the Foundation for People with a Learning Disability (Turk, Dodd, & Christmas, 2001) recommended that every service for people with intellectual disability should set up a register of adults with Down syndrome. A baseline assessment of cognitive and adaptive functioning should be carried out before that age of 30 years. McBrien, Whitwham, Oliverman, and Masters (2005) propose a two-yearly screen for people in their 40s and an annual screen for those in their 50s or older. Turk et al. (2001) advise that each service should develop specialist skills in this area and offer training to other professionals, frontline staff and caregivers. This is echoed in a study by Adams et al. (2008) who examined the behavioral characteristics of those referred for assessment. They concluded that caregivers and health professionals need more information on behavioral and cognitive changes in early dementia so that an earlier and more effective referral can be made. In terms of accommodation, best practice is to facilitate aging and caring in the same home they have lived in if possible to do so. Moving home at the time of increased confusion may be detrimental and hasten their decline. In the late stage of the disease a co-ordinated service from Health, Social, Voluntary, and Private sector may be required because in majority of cases patients may have to be transferred away from their home settings and looked after within one of the above-mentioned services.

16. Conclusion

There are many similarities and some differences in the clinical expression of dementia in people who have an intellectual disability/ Down syndrome. Many symptoms, including features of "frontal lobe dysfunction" that tend to appear late in the dementing process in the general population may appear early among people who have Down's syndrome. An important early sign is any change in behavior or functioning and dementia must always be considered as a possible cause for the change. Both clinical dementia and the presence of Alzheimer's neuropathology are more common among adults who have Down syndrome than the general population and they are particularly vulnerable to develop Alzheimer's neuropathology from the age of 40 years onwards. However, the clinical expression of dementia is observed in only a proportion of these subjects.

There are difficulties in making an early and accurate diagnosis of dementia, and the screening instruments such as the MMSE that are used in the general population often show floor effects when used for people who have an intellectual disability because of the pre-existing cognitive deficits that are present in this population. Both observer-rated and direct neuropsychological tests have been used for the case detection of dementia among people who have an intellectual disability. However, the validity of most of the neuropsychological tests in this population has not been properly established, although there is a growing amount of research into developing better tools or adapting those existing tools to better serve this population.

Because of the risks of acquiring dementia in Down syndrome adults, consideration needs to be given to the viability of screening over the age of 30 years. A longitudinal approach to diagnosis would be desirable, where the intervals between assessments decrease in proportion to increase in age and subsequent amplification of risk. This should be part of an integrated approach to the management of those with dementia who also have Down syndrome/intellectual disability. Work into developing guidelines and policies is ongoing such as the recent report from the Royal College of Psychiatrists (Dodd et al., 2009). The use of anti-dementia medication in this population requires further research to help assess efficacy so that guidelines for its use can be developed.

ACKNOWLEDGEMENT

This chapter is adapted from the following two publications.

Deb. (2003). Dementia in people who have an intellectual disability. *Reviews in Clinical Gerontology, 13*, 137–144.

Kannabiran, M. & Deb. (2010). Diseases of the nervous system II: Neurodegenerative diseases including dementias. In J. O'Hara, J. McCarthy, & N. Bouras (Eds.) Intellectual disability and ill health—A review of evidence (pp. 203–213). Cambridge: Cambridge University Press.

REFERENCES

Adams, D., Oliver, C., Kalsy, S., Peters, S., Broquard, M., Basra, T., Konstandinidi, E., & McQuillan, S. (2008). Behavioural characteristics associated with dementia assessment referrals in adults with Down syndrome. *Journal of Intellectual Disability Research, 52* (4), 358–368.

Albert, M., & Cohen, C. (1992). The Test for Severe Impairment: an instrument for the assessment of patients with severe cognitive dysfunction. *Journal of the American Geriatric Society. 40*, 449–453.

Altman, P. (1977). *Fuld Object-Memory Evaluation: Instruction manual*. Wheat Dale, IL, USA: Stoelting.

Aman, M. G., & Singh, N. N. (1986). *The aberrant behaviour checklist-community version*. Slosson: East Aurora, NY.

Ball, S. L., Holland, A. J., Huppert, F. A., Treppner, P., Watson, P., & Hon, J. (2004). The modified CAMDEX informant interview is a valid and reliable tool for use in the diagnosis of dementia in adults with Down's syndrome. *Journal of Intellectual Disability Research, 48*, 611–620.

Ball, S. L., Holland, A. J., Hon, J., Huppert, F. A., Treppner, P., & Watson, P. C. (2006). Personality and behaviour changes mark the early stages of Alzheimer's disease in adults with Down's syndrome: findings from a prospective population-based study. *International Journal of Geriatric Psychiatry, 21*, 661–673.

Ballard, C., Hanney, M. L., Theodoulou, M., et al. (2008). A randomised blinded, placebo-controlled trial in dementia patients continuing or stopping neuroleptics (the DART-AD trail). *PloS Medicine, 15*, 4, 587–599.

Beacher, F., Daly, E., Simmons, A., Prasher, V., Morris, R., Robinson, C., Lovestone, S., Murphy, K., & Murphy, D.G.M. (2009). Alzheimer's disease and Down's syndrome: an *in vivo* MRI study. *Psychological Medicine, 39*, 675–684.

Berney, T. (2009). Ageing in Down syndrome. In G. O'Brien, & L. Rosenbloom (Eds.). *Developmental disability and ageing*. London: Mac Keith Press.

Bird, M. (2002). Psychology and the older person. *Australian Psychology, 34*, 144–148.

Blacker, D., & Tanzi, R. E. (1998). The genetics of Alzhiemer's disease. *Archives of Neurology, 55*, 294–296.

Burt, D. B., & Aylward, E. H. (2000). Test battery for the diagnosis of dementia in individuals with intellectual disability. Working Group for the Establishment of Criteria for the Diagnosis of Dementia in Individuals with Intellectual Disability. *Journal of Intellectual Disability Research, 44*, 175–180.

Buschke, H. (1973). Selective reminding for analysis of memory and learning. *Journal of Learning and Verbal Behaviour. 12*, 543–550.

Carr, E. G., Horner, R. H., & Turnbull, A. P. (1999). *Positive behaviour support for people with developmental disabilities: a research synthesis*. Washington, DC: American Association on Mental Retardation.

Carr, J. (2005). Stability and change in cognitive ability over the life span: a comparison of populations with and without Down's syndrome. *Journal of Intellectual Disability Research, 49*, 915–928.

Collacott, R. A., Cooper, S. A., & McGrother C. (1992). Differential rates of psychiatric disorders in adults with Down's syndrome compared with other mentally handicapped adults. *British Journal of Psychiatry. 161*, 671–4.

Collacott, R. A., Cooper, S. A., Branford, D., & McGrother C. (1998). Behaviour phenotype for Down's syndrome. *British Journal of Psychiatry. 172*, 85–89.

Cooper, S.-A. (1997). High prevalence of dementia among people with learning disabilities not attributable to Down's syndrome. *Psychological Medicine. 27*, 609–616.

Cooper, S.-A., & Prasher, V. P. (1998). Maladaptive behaviours and symptoms of dementia in adults with Down's syndrome compared with adults with intellectual disability of other aetiologies. *Journal of Intellectual Disability Research. 42*(4), 293–300.

Coppus, A., Evenhuis, H., Verberne, G.-J., Visser, F., van Gool, P., Eikelenboom, P., & van Duijin, C. (2006). Dementia and mortality in persons with Down's syndrome. *Journal of Intellectual Disability Research, 50*(10), 768–777.

Coppus, A. M., Evenhuis, H. M., & van Duijn, C. M. (2008). The impact of apolipoprotein E on dementia in persons with Down's syndrome. *Neurobiology of ageing, 29*(6), 828–835.

Corder, E. H., Saunders, A. M., Strittmater, W. J. et al. (1993). Gene dose of apolipoprotein E-type 4 allele and the risk of Alzhiemer's disease in late onset families. *Science, 261*, 921–922.

Cosgrave, M. P., Tyrell, J., McCarron, M., Gill, M., & Lawlor, B. A. (1999). Determinants of aggression, and adaptive and maladaptive behaviour in older people with Down's syndrome with and without dementia. *Journal of Intellectual Disability Research, 43*(5), 393–9.

Crayton, L., Oliver, O., Holland, A., Bradbury, J., & Hall, S. (1998). The Neuropsychological assessment of age-related cognitive deficits in adults with Down's syndrome. *Journal of Applied Research in Intellectual Disabilities, 11*, 255–272.

Dalton, A. J. (1992). Dementia in Down syndrome: methods of evaluation. In L. Nadel & C. J. Epstein (Eds.) '*Alzheimer's disease and Down syndrome*' (pp. 51–76). New York, NY, USA: Wiley Liss.

Dalton, A. J., & Fedor, B. L. (1997). The Multi-dimensional Observation Scale for Elderly Subjects applied for persons with Down syndrome. In '*Proceedings of the International Congress III on the dually diagnosed*' (pp. 173–178). National Association for the Dually Diagnosed, Washington DC, USA.

DCLD [Diagnostic criteria for psychiatric disorders for use with adults with learning disabilities/mental retardation] (2002). *Royal College of Psychiatrists Occasional Paper OP48*. Gaskell, London.

Diagnostic and Statistical Manual of Mental Disorders—fourth edition (2000), Text revision. Washington DC: American Psychiatric Association.
Deb, S., de Silva, P. N., Gemmell, H. G., Besson, J. A., Smith, F. W., & Ebmeier, K. P. (1992). Alzheimer's disease in adults with Down's syndrome: the relationship between regional cerebral blood flow equivalents and dementia. *Acta Psychiatrica Scandinavica, 86* (5), 240–345.
Deb, S. (1997). Structural neuroimaging in mental retardation. *British Journal of Psychiatry, 171*, 417–419.
Deb, S., Braganza, J., Owen, M., Kehoe, P., Williams, H., & Norton, N. (1998). No significant association between a PS-1 intronic polymorphism and dementia in Down's syndrome. *Alzheimer's Reports, 1*(6), 365–368.
Deb, S., & Braganza, J. (1999). Comparison of rating scales for the diagnosis of dementia in adults with Down's syndrome. *Journal of Intellectual Disability Research, 43*, 400–407.
Deb, S., Braganza, J., Norton, N., Williams, H., Kehoe, P., Williams, J., & Owen, M. J. (2000). ApoE e4 influence the manifestation of Alzhiemer's dementia in adults with Down's syndrome. *British Journal of Psychiatry. 176*, 468–472.
Deb, S. (2001a). Epidemiology of psychiatric illness in adults with intellectual disability. In L. Hamilton-Kirkwood et al. (Eds.), *Health evidence bulletins Wales: Learning disabilities* (pp. 14–17). Cardiff: NHS Wales. http://hebw.uwcm.ac.uk.
Deb, S. (2001b). Dementia in Down's syndrome. In L. Hamilton-Kirkwood et al. (Eds.), *Health evidence bulletins Wales: Learning disabilities* (pp. 56–57). Cardiff: NHS Wales. http://hebw.uwcm.ac.uk
Deb, S. (2001c). Medical conditions in people with intellectual disability. In L. Hamilton-Kirkwood et al. (Eds.), *Health evidence bulletins Wales: Learning disabilities* (pp. 48–55). Cardiff: NHS Wales. http://hebw.uwcm.ac.uk.
Deb, S., Clarke, D., & Unwin, G. (2006). Using medication to manage behaviour problems among adults with a learning disability: Quick Reference Guide (QRG). University of Birmingham, MENCAP, *The Royal College of Psychiatrists*, London, UK. ISBN: 0855370947. www.ld-medication.bham.ac.uk
Deb, S. (2007). The role of medication in the management of behaviour problems in people with learning disabilities. *Advances in Mental Health and Learning Disabilities, 1*(2), 26–31.
Deb, S, Hare, M., & Prior, L. (2007a). Symptoms of dementia among adults with Down's syndrome: a qualitative study. *Journal of Intellectual Disability Research, 51*, 726–739.
Deb, S., Hare, M., Prior, L., & Bhaumik, S (2007b). Dementia Screening Questionnaire for Individuals with Intellectual Disabilities. *British Journal of Psychiatry. 190*, 440–444.
Deb, S., Sohanpal, S. K., Soni, R., Unwin, G., & Lenôtre, L. (2007c). The effectiveness of antipsychotic medication in the management of behaviour problems in adults with intellectual disabilities. *Journal of Intellectual Disability Research, 51*, 10, 766–777.
Deb, S., Chaplin, R., Sohanpal, S., Unwin, G. Soni, R., & Lenôtre, L. (2008). The effectiveness of mood stabilisers and antiepileptic medication for the management of behaviour problems in adults with intellectual disability: a systematic review. *Journal of Intellectual Disability Research, 52* (2), 107–113.
Devenny, D. A., Silverman, W. P., Hill, A. L., Jenkins, E., Sersen, E. A., & Wisnieski, K. E. (1996). Normal ageing in adults with Down's syndrome: a longitudinal study. *Journal of Intellectual Disability Research. 40*, 208–221.
Devenny, D. A., Krinsky-Hale S. J., Sersen G., & Silverman W. P. (2000). Sequence of cognitive decline in adults with Down's syndrome. *Journal of Intellectual Disability Research 44*, 654–665.
Dodd, K., Bhaumik, S., Benbow, S. M., Black, S., Bush, A., Finnamore, A., Holland, T., Gangadharan, S. K., McBrien, J. Turk, V. (2009). Dementia and people with learning disabilities: Guidance on the assessment, diagnosis, treatment and support of people with

learning disabilities who develop dementia. Royal College of Psychiatrists & The British Psychological Society. Council Report (CR) 155, September 2009.
Donaldson, C., Tarrier, N., & Burns, A. (1997). The impact of the symptoms of dementia on caregivers. *British Journal of Psychiatry, 170,* 62–68.
Didden, R., Duker, P. C., & Korzilius, H. (1997). Meta-analytic study on treatment effectiveness for problem behaviors with individuals who have mental retardation. *American Journal on Mental Retardation, 101*(4), 387–399.
Evenhuis, H. M, (1990). The natural history of dementia in Down's syndrome. *Archives of Neurology, 47*(3), 263–267.
Evenhuis, H. M. (1996). Further evaluation of the Dementia questionnaire for persons with Mental Retardation (DMR). *Journal of Intellectual Disability Research. 40,* 369–373.
Evenhuis, H. M., Kengen, M. M. F., & Eurlings, H. A. L. (2007). *Dementia Questionnaire for People with Learning Disabilities (DLD).* UK adaptation. Harcourt Assessment.
Feldman, H., Jacova, C., Robilliard, A., Garcia, A., Chow, T., Borrie, M. et al. (2008). Diagnosis and treatment of dementia: 2. Diagnosis. *Canadian Medical Association Journal, 178,* 825–836.
Folstein, M. F., Folstein, S. E., McHugh, P. R. (1975). 'Mini-Mental State'. A practical method for grading the cognitive state of patients for the clinician. *Journal of Psychiatry Research. 12,* 189–198.
Fraser, J., Mitchell, A. (1876). Kalmuc idiocy: Report of a case with autopsy, with notes on sixty-two cases. *The Journal of Mental Sciences, 22,* 169–79.
Gedye, A. (1995). *Dementia Scale for Down Syndrome.* Vancouver BC, Canada: Manual Gedye Research Consulting.
Gustavson, K. H., Umb-Carlsson, O., & Sonnander, K. (2005). A follow-up study of mortality, health conditions and associated disabilities of people with intellectual disabilities in a Swedish county. *Journal of Intellectual Disabilities Research, 49*(12), 905–914.
Haier, R. J., Head, K., Head, E., & Lott, I. T. (2008). Neuroimaging of individuals with Down's syndrome at-risk for dementia: Evidence for possible compensatory events. *Neuroimage, 39*(3), 1324–1332.
Hardy, J., Crook, R., Perry, R. et al. (1994). ApoE genotype and Down's syndrome. *Lancet. 343,* 979–980.
Hassiotis, A. A., Hall, I. (2008). Behavioural and cognitive-behavioural interventions for outwardly-directed aggressive behaviour in people with learning disabilities. *Cochrane Database of Systematic Reviews,* Issue 3. Art. No.: CD003406. DOI: 10.1002/14651858. CD003406.pub3.
Haveman, M. J., Maaskant, M. A., van Schrojenstein, H. M., Urlings, H. F. K., & Kessels, A.G.H. (1994). Mental health problems in elderly people with and without Down's syndrome. *Journal of Intellectual Disability Research. 38*(3), 341–355.
Haveman, M. J. (2004). Disease epidemiology and ageing people with intellectual disabilities. *Journal of Policy and Practice in Intellectual Disabilities 1,* 16–23.
Holland, A. J., Hon, J., Huppert, F. A., et al. (2000). Incidence and course of dementia in people with Down's syndrome: findings from a population based study. *Journal of Intellectual Disability Research, 44*(2), 138–146.
Huxley, A., Van-Schaik, P. & Witts, P. (2005). A comparison of challenging behaviour in an adult group with Down's syndrome and dementia compared with an adult Down's syndrome group without dementia. *British Journal of Learning Disabilities, 33,* 188–193.
The ICD-10 Classification of Mental and Behavioural Disorders, tenth edition. Geneva. *World Health Organization,* 1992.
Jervis, G. A. (1948). Early senile dementia in mongoloid idiocy. *American Journal of Psychiatry. 105,* 102–106.
Kaplan, E., Goodglass, H., & Weubtraub, S. (1978). *The Boston Naming Test.* Philadelphia, PA, USA: Lea & Febiger.

Lai, F. & Williams, R. S. (1989). A prospective study of Alzheimer disease in Down syndrome. *Archives Neurology, 46*(8), 849–853.

Lott, I. T., Osann, K., Doran, E., & Nelson, L. (2002). Down Syndrome and Alzheimer's disease: Response to donepezil. *Archives Neurology, 59*(7), 1133–1136.

Lubin, R. A., & Kiely, M. (1985). Epidemiology of aging in developmental disabilities. In M. P. Janicki, & H. M. Wisniewski (Eds.) *Aging and developmental disabilities: Issues and approaches* (pp. 95–113). Baltimore: P.H. Brooks.

Mann, D. M. A. (1988). Alzheimer's disease and Down's syndrome. *Histopathology. 13*, 125–137.

Mann, D. M. A. (1993). Association between Alzheimer's disease and Down syndrome: Neuropathological observations. In J. M. Berg, Karilnsky & A. J. Hilland (Eds.) *Alzheimer's disease, Down syndrome and their relationship* (pp. 71–92). Oxford: Oxford University Press.

Mann, D. M. A., Pickering-Brown, S. M., & Siddons, M. A. et al., (1995). The extent of amyloid deposits in brain in patients with Down's syndrome does not depend upon the apolipoprotein E genotype. *Neuroscience Letters. 196*, 105–108.

Mantry, D., Cooper, S.-.A., Smiley, E., Morrison, J., Allan, L., Williamson, A., Finlayson, J., & Jackson, A. (2008). The prevalence and incidence of mental ill-health in adults with Down syndrome. *Journal of Intellectual Disability Research. 52*(2), 141–155.

Margallo-Lana, M. L., Moore, P. B., Kay, D. W. K., Perry, R. H., Reid, B. E., Berney, T., & Tyrer, S. P. (2007). Fifteen-year follow-up of 92 hospitalized adults with Down's syndrome: Incidence of cognitive decline, its relationship to age and neuropathology. *Journal of intellectual Disability Research, 51*(6), 463–477.

Matthews, C. G. (1974). Applications of neuropsychological test methods in mentally retarded adults. In R. M. Reitan, & L. A. Davidson (Eds.). *Clinical neuropsychology: Current status and applications* (pp. 267–287). Wiley, New York.

McBrien, J. A., Whitwham, S., Oliverman, K., & Masters, S. (2005). Screening adults with Down's syndrome for early signs of Alzheimer's disease. *Tizard Learning Disability Review, 10*(4), 23–32.

McCarthy, D. (1972). *Manual for the McCarthy Scales of Children's Ability*. San Antonio, TX, USA: The Psychological Corporation.

McShane, R., Sastre, A. A., & Minakaran, N. (2006). Memantine for dementia. *Cochrane Database of Systematic Reviews*. Issue 2. Art. No.: CD003154. DOI: 10.1002/14651858. CD003154.pub5.

Mohan, M., Bennett, C. & Carpenter, P. K. (2009a). Memantine for dementia in people with Down syndrome. *Cochrane Database of Systematic Reviews*. Issue 1. Art. No.:CD007657. DOI: 10.1002/14651858.CD007657.

Mohan, M., Bennett, C., & Carpenter, P. K. (2009b). Donepezil for dementia in people with Down syndrome. *Cochrane Database of Systematic Reviews*. Issue 1. Art No: CD007178. DOI: 10.1002/14651858.CD007178.pub2.

Mohan, M., Bennett, C., & Carpenter, P. K. (2009c). Rivastigmine for dementia in people with Down syndrome. *Cochrane Database of Systematic Reviews*. Issue 1. Art No: CD007658. DOI: 10.1002/14651858.CD007658.

Mohan, M., Bennett, C., & Carpenter, P. K. (2009d). Galantamine for dementia in people with Down syndrome. *Cochrane Database of Systematic Reviews*. Issue 1. Art No: CD007656. DOI: 10.1002/14651858.CD007656.

Moss, M. B., M. S., Butters, N., & Payne, M. (1986). Differential patterns of memory loss among patients with Alzhiemer's disease, Huntington's disease, and alcoholic Korsakoff's syndrome. *Archives of Neurology. 43*, 239–246.

Nieuwenhuis-Mark, R. E. (2009). Diagnosing Alzheimer's dementia in Down syndrome: problems and possible solutions. *Research in Developmental Disabilities, 30*, 827–838.

Nihira, K., Foster, R., Shellhaas, M., et al. (1974). *Adaptive Behaviour Scale*. Washington DC, USA: American Association on Mental Retardation.

Patel, P., Goldberg, D., & Moss, S. (1993). Psychiatric morbidity in older people with moderate and severe learning disability (mental retardation). Part II: The prevalence study. *British Journal of Psychiatry*. *163*, 481–491.

Prasher, V. (1995a). Age-specific prevalence, thyroid dysfunction and depressive symptomatology in adults with Down's syndrome and dementia. *International Journal of Geriatric Psychiatry*, *10*, 25–31.

Prasher, V. P. (1995b). End-stage dementia in adults with Down's syndrome. *International Journal of Geriatric Psychiatry* *10*, 1067–1069.

Prasher, V., & Filer, A. (1995). Behavioural disturbance in people with Down's syndrome and dementia. *Journal of Intellectual Disability Research* *39*, 432–446.

Prasher, V. P., Huxley, A., & Haque, M. S. (2002). A 24-week, double-blind, placebo-controlled trial of donepezil in patients with Down syndrome and Alzheimer's disease–Pilot study. *International Journal of Geriatric Psychiatry*, *17*, 270–278.

Prasher, V. P., Adams, C., & Holder, R. and The Down Syndrome Research Group (2003). Long term safety and efficacy of donepezil in the treatment of dementia in Alzheimer's disease in adults with Down syndrome: open label study. *International Journal of Geriatric Psychiatry*, *18*, 549–551.

Prasher, V., Farooq, A., & Holder, R. (2004). The Adaptive Behaviour Dementia Questionnaire (ABDQ): Screening questionnaire for dementia in Alzheimer's disease in adults with Down Syndrome. *Research in Developmental Disabilities*, *25*, 385–397.

Prasher, V., Fung, N., & Adams, C. (2005). Rivastigmine in the treatment of Dementia in Alzheimer's disease in Adults with Down Syndrome. *International Journal of Geriatric Psychiatry*, *20*(5), 496–497.

Roeden, J. M., & Zitman, F. G. (1995). Ageing in adults with Down's syndrome in institutionally based and community based residences. *Journal of Intellectual Disability Research*, *39*(5), 399–407.

Roth, M., Tym, E., Mountjoy, C., Huppert, F., Hendrie, H., Verma, S., & Goddard, R. (1986). CAMDEX—a standardised instrument for the diagnosis of mental disorder in the elderly with special reference to the early detection of dementia. *British Journal of Psychiatry*, *149*, 698–709.

Roth, M., Huppert, F., Mountjoy, C., & Tym, E. (1998). *CAMDEX-R: The Cambridge Examination for Mental Disorder of the Elderly (Revised Edition)*. Cambridge: Cambridge University Press.

Royston, M. C., Mann, D., Pickering-Brown, S. M. et al. (1994). Apolipoprotein E e2 allele promotes longevity and protects patients with Down's syndrome from dementia. *Neuroreport*. *5*, 2583–2585.

Rubello, D., Pozzan, G. B., Casara, D. et al. (1995). Natural course of subclinical hypothyroidism in Down's syndrome: prospective study results and therapeutic considerations. *Journal of Endocrinological Investigation*. *17*, 35–40.

Sadavoy, J., Lanctôt, K. L., & Deb, S. (2008). Management of behavioural and psychological symptoms of dementia and acquired brain injury. In P. Tyrer, & K. R. Silk (Eds.) *Cambridge Textbook of Effective Treatments in Psychiatry* (pp. 187–216). Cambridge: Cambridge University Press.

Saxton, J., McGonigle, K. L., Swihart, A. A., & Boller, F. (1993). *The Severe Impairment Battery*. San Antonio, TX: Pearson.

Schupf, N. (2002). Genetic and host factors for dementia in Down's syndrome. *British Journal of Psychiatry*. *180*, 405–410.

Scotti, J. R., Evans, I. M., Mayer, L. H., & Walker, P. (1991). A meta analysis of intervention research with problem behaviour: treatment validity and standards of practice. *American Journal on Mental Retardation*, *96*, 233–256.

Seltzer, G. B. (1997). *Modified Fuld object memory evaluation*. Madison, WI, USA: Waisman Center, University of Wisconsin Madison.

Sohanpal, S. K., Deb, S., Thomas, C., Soni, R., Lenôtre, L., & Unwin, G. (2007). The effectiveness of antidepressant medication in the management of behaviour problems in adults with intellectual disabilities: A systematic review. *Journal of Intellectual Disability Research 51*, (10), 750–765.

Steffelaar, J., & Evenhuis, H. (1989). Life expectancy, Down syndrome and dementia. *Lancet 1*, 492–493.

Stern, Y. (2002). What is cognitive reserve? Theory and research application of the reserve concept. *Journal of the International Neuropsychological Society. 8*, 448–460.

Strydom, A., Livingston, G., King, M., & Hassiotis, A. (2007). Prevalence of dementia in intellectual disability using different diagnostic criteria. *British Journal of Psychiatry, 191*, 150–157.

Strydom, A., Hassiotis, A., King, M., & Livingston, G. (2008). The relationship of dementia prevalence in older adults with intellectual disability (ID) to age and severity of ID. *Psychological Medicine, 39*, 13–21.

Tiffin, J., & Asher, E. J. (1948). The Purdue Pegboard: Norms and studies of reliability and validity. *Journal of Applied Psychology. 32*, 234–247.

Turk, V., Dodd, K., & Christmas, M. (2001). *Down's syndrome and dementia: Briefing for commissioners*. London: Mental Health Foundation.

Urv, T. K., Zigman, W. B., & Silverman, W. (2003). Maladapted behaviours related to adapted decline in ageing adults with mental retardation. *American Journal of Mental Retardation, 108*, 327–329.

Visser, F. E., Aldenkamp, A. P., van Huffelen, A. C., Kuilman, M., Overweg, J., & van Wijk, J. (1997). Prospective study of the prevalence of Alzheimer-type dementia in institutionalised individuals with Down syndrome. *American Journal of Mental Retardation. 101*, 404–412.

Watchman, K. (2007). Dementia and Down syndrome the Diagnosis and Support Needed. *Learning Disability Practice, 10*(2), 10–14.

Wisniewski, K. E., Wisniewski, H. M., & Wen, G. Y. (1985). Occurrence of neuropathological changes and dementia of Alzheimer's disease in Down's syndrome. *Annals Neurology, 17*, 278–282.

Wisniewski, H., & Hill, L. (1985). Clinical aspects of dementia in mental retardation and developmental disabilities. In H. Wisniewski, & M. Janicki (Eds.) *Aging and developmental disabilities* (pp. 195–210). Baltimore, USA: Brookes.

Wisniewski, H. M., & Rabe, S. (1986). Discrepancy between Alzheimer-type neuropathology and dementia in persons with Down syndrome. *Annals of the New York Academy of Sciences. 477*, 247–260.

Wisniewski, T., Morelli, L., Wegiel, J. et al. (1995). The influence of apolipoprotein E isotopes on Alzheimer's disease pathology in 40 cases of Down's syndrome. *Annals of Neurology. 37*, 136–138.

Zana, M., Janka, Z., & Kalman, J. (2007). Oxidative stress: A bridge between Down's syndrome and Alzheimer's disease. *Neurobiology of Aging, 28*(5), 648–676.

Zigman, W., Jenkins, E., Mehta, P. et al. (2000). Alzheimer's disease, survival, and genetics in the 'oldest old' with Down syndrome. *Down syndrome Research Foundation (Canada)/(National Down Syndrome Society (US) New Directions in Down Syndrome Research Conference*, Toronto, Canada.

CHAPTER NINE

Sociodemographic Characteristics of Families of Children with Down Syndrome and the Economic Impacts of Child Disability on Families

Scott D. Grosse

Contents

Abstract

This chapter reviews the research examining the demographic and socioeconomic characteristics of families of children with Down syndrome as well as how Down syndrome and other disabilities impact the economic situations of families. Two consistent demographic patterns are found. First, parents of children with Down syndrome on average are older than parents of other children. Second, families of children with Down syndrome are more likely to have social advantages in terms of parental education, income, and race/ethnicity status relative to families of children with other intellectual or developmental disabilities, consistent with a "Down syndrome advantage." In

National Center on Birth Defects and Developmental Disabilities, Centers for Disease Control and Prevention, Atlanta, Georgia, USA

International Review of Research in Mental Retardation, Volume 39
ISSN 0074-7750, DOI 10.1016/S0074-7750(10)39009-4

addition, most US studies find that live-born infants with Down syndrome are more likely to be born to Hispanic parents and less likely to have a Black or African American parent than other infants. Financial impacts on families with a child with disabilities such as Down syndrome can result from high out-of-pocket expenditures and reduced parental employment and earnings. Studies differ in terms of specific results as to whether employment effects of child disability are greater among two-parent or one-parent families and whether fewer mothers of children with disabilities are in the paid work force or part-time employment is substituted for full-time employment. Reductions in maternal employment appear to be a function of the severity of the medical condition or disability and the time requirements for care. As children age, the effect of child disability on current maternal employment appears to decline, but a permanent reduction in earnings capacity and household savings can result from altered career trajectories. Many families of children with disabilities experience financial stress, in part as a result of underinsurance. Public programs, notably Supplemental Security Income (SSI) benefits, can help to buffer the financial impact of caring for a child with a serious disability.

1. Introduction

Researchers have long described a "Down syndrome advantage" (Corrice & Glidden, 2009) among families of children with Down syndrome that refers to psychosocial aspects, notably less parental stress and increased psychological well-being and family cohesion, relative to other families with children with intellectual and developmental disabilities (Hodapp, Ly, Fidler, & Ricci, 2001; Rasmussen, Whitehead, Collier, & Frías, 2008). This "advantage" has been reported to persist past childhood (Seltzer, Krauss, & Tsunematsu, 1993). Not coincidentally, children with Down syndrome are also reported to be more likely to live in families that have social advantages due to race/ethnicity, parental education, and family income (Hodapp & Urbano, 2008). This is particularly the case for families of children with Down syndrome relative to families of children with mild to moderate intellectual disability, who are more likely to be low-status groups and live in poverty (Drews, Yeargin-Allsopp, Decouflé, & Murphy, 1995; Fujiura, 1998). The apparent advantage in family psychosocial measures for parents of children with Down syndrome relative to parents of children with other disabilities appears to be largely attributable to better child functioning and more advantageous family income and marital status (Cahill & Glidden, 1996).

Down syndrome cannot be equated with intellectual disability. Approximately 70% of children with Down syndrome meet the epidemiologic case definition for intellectual disability based on IQ scores (Decouflé, Boyle, Paulozzi, & Lary, 2001), although behavioral measures are better indicators of disability or functioning in people with Down syndrome (Rasmussen et al., 2008). Critically, people with Down syndrome also experience a range of medical conditions (Schieve, Boulet, Boyle, Rasmussen, & Schendel, 2009), the most common of which is congenital heart defects, which occur in 40–50% of infants with Down syndrome (Freeman et al., 2008).

Regardless of socioeconomic status prior to their birth, families of children with disabilities or chronic health conditions such as Down syndrome are likely to experience some degree of economic disadvantage as a result of having an affected child (Emerson, 2007). This might occur for either of two reasons. First, caring for a child with chronic health conditions or disabilities can negatively affect family finances resulting from increased out-of-pocket costs associated with increased need for medical and developmental services. Second, caring for an affected child can lead to reduced family income if one or both parents reduce the amount of time they spend working in order to provide caregiving services. For some families with children with complex health care needs, the increased need for income to pay out-of-pocket costs may dominate and result in either no change in employment or an increase in paid employment and earnings. Also, time spent caring for a child with a disability may come at the expense of sleep, personal care, recreation, or social participation rather than paid work. Even if parents do not reduce hours of paid employment, they may still feel financial pressure as a result of out-of-pocket expenses related to their child's condition and increased use of purchased services (e.g. prepared meals) due to less availability of time.

The overall association between family socioeconomic status and having a child with Down syndrome is a priori indeterminate. Socioeconomic status may have both positive and negative effects on having a child with Down syndrome, which can operate through one or more of three pathways: (1) the risk of a conception with a chromosome abnormality, (2) the likelihood of an affected fetus being carried to term, and (3) the probability of postnatal survival. In addition, as discussed above, causation can run in the opposite direction, because having a child with Down syndrome can affect family income. Finally, having an affected child and family income may be jointly determined by a third variable, notably parental age. Although older maternal age is the leading risk factor for trisomy 21, which comprises about 95% of cases of Down syndrome, it is often not realized that two-thirds of children with Down syndrome are born to women under 35 years of age (Hodapp & Urbano, 2008).

Families of children with Down syndrome may differ from families of unaffected children in terms of a number of sociodemographic characteristics, most notably parental age. The second most studied characteristic is race/ethnicity. Differentials in prevalence across population groups may reflect differences in the distribution by maternal age at birth or the use of prenatal diagnostic services. Measures of socioeconomic status, including parental education level, family income, and average income by area of residence, may also differ between families with Down syndrome-affected children and those with only unaffected children.

This chapter addresses both the sociodemographic characteristics of families of children with Down syndrome, particularly newborn infants with Down syndrome, and the potential economic impact on families of having a child with Down syndrome or other disability, given a lack of data specific to Down syndrome. Large, representative samples of children with Down syndrome can be obtained from three types of data: household surveys, vital statistics (e.g., birth certificates), and special data collections, which include both administrative data (e.g., hospital discharge records) and surveillance systems or registries (Hodapp & Urbano, 2009). Most published population-based research studies on Down syndrome have used the second or third of these, with information on the characteristics of the family generally available only at the time of birth. Household surveys can collect information on the characteristics of families reported to have a child with Down syndrome. For each source of data, though, it is important to consider the validity of the diagnosis or report of Down syndrome.

The first part of this chapter reviews what is known about the sociodemographic characteristics of children with Down syndrome, their parents, and their families in the United States. The focus is on race/ethnicity and socioeconomic status, including parental education, family income, and community-level economic measures, because of the availability of published studies that have used these measures. This review focuses primarily on studies using representative, population-based samples using the first three types of data sources listed above. Some of those studies examined characteristics associated with having either a fetus or a live birth with Down syndrome; the practice of prenatal diagnosis often drives a wedge between the two. In addition, findings are presented on the characteristics of families of children with Down syndrome from the analysis of data from a national survey of US households in which parents were asked if they had a surviving child with Down syndrome (Schieve et al., 2009).

The second part of the chapter reviews the published literature on the economic impacts of having a child with disability on families. Few studies have collected information on employment and earnings for parents of children with Down syndrome, and only one with a representative, population-based sample of children with validated diagnoses of Down syndrome, a study from Sweden (Hedov, Annerén, & Wikblad, 2002; Hedov, Wikblad, & Annerén, 2006). Published studies of families of children with Down syndrome have generally been conducted using convenience samples of families recruited through clinics or family support organizations, which are not necessarily representative of families of children with Down syndrome. Consequently, to get at the economic impact of Down syndrome on families, the broader literature on the economic consequences of having a child with a disability is reviewed. Two types of economic impacts are assessed: (1) participation in the paid labor force and loss of work time and earned income due to caregiving demands, and (2) measures of financial burden, including out-of-pocket expenditures associated with the child's condition, both in absolute terms and relative to family income. Finally, financial burden is assessed using reported perceptions of adequacy of income and health insurance to meet needs for health care and developmental or other therapeutic services.

2. Epidemiologic Studies on Down Syndrome

2.1. Newborns and fetuses

The primary source of epidemiologic data on Down syndrome among newborns comes from birth defects surveillance systems. These systems ascertain cases of structural malformations and chromosome abnormalities through a variety of means. Certain programs, generally characterized as passive birth defects surveillance, rely largely on information reported through vital records, including birth, fetal death, and infant death records, and hospital discharge records. Other programs, characterized as active birth defects surveillance, complement those two sources of data with reviews by abstractors of medical charts from birthing centers to identify additional cases for which ICD-9 codes were not recorded and to verify that reported cases met actual clinical case definitions. Many active surveillance programs also canvas prenatal diagnostic and other genetics services for information on recognized pregnancies with a malformation or chromosome abnormality. That is crucial for accurate and complete information on the incidence of birth defects because many abnormalities do not result in a live birth. However, because such surveillance programs operate in only certain places, no complete data are available at the national level. Prenatal diagnostic clinics account for a substantial fraction of all cases of Down syndrome (Siffel, Correa, Cragan, & Alverson, 2004). In addition, active surveillance systems typically use the results of cytogenetic testing to confirm or exclude cases of Down syndrome, with some 5–6% of cases recorded on birth certificates classified as false positives after careful review (Huether et al., 1998).

Comparisons of cases identified through different sources provide valuable information on the completeness and accuracy of each data source. Several epidemiologic studies have used birth records alone to ascertain Down syndrome cases among live births. The advantage is that such data are readily available in public use datasets for all states across many years.

The disadvantage is that birth records miss a large fraction of cases of Down syndrome. A study from Tennessee which linked birth and hospital discharge records for the years 1996–2002 found that barely half of cases identified through the presence of an ICD-9-CM code of 758.0x for Down syndrome in hospital discharge records had the diagnosis of Down syndrome recorded on birth records, whereas all the latter were also identified in hospital discharge records (Hodapp & Urbano, 2008; Urbano & Hodapp, 2007). Those authors presumed that hospital discharge diagnoses of Down syndrome were accurate, which is not necessarily the case. Overall, 54% of major birth defects identified in hospital discharge records in Minnesota were confirmed by reviews of medical records through birth defects surveillance (Frohnert et al., 2005).

2.1.1. Parental age

Whether one uses birth defects surveillance data or birth records, older maternal age is strongly associated with Down syndrome due to trisomy 21. The dominant hypothesis for this association is that the quality of a woman's oocyte pool decreases with increasing age (Sherman, Allen, Bean, & Freeman, 2007). In particular, the risk of Down syndrome increases rapidly after about age 30. A cut point of age 35 years is used in many studies, which reflects the traditional convention that prenatal testing for Down syndrome and other chromosome abnormalities is offered routinely only to women aged 35 years or above. However, there is a continuum of risk, both above and below any arbitrary age cutoff. Because women with advanced maternal age are more likely to be offered prenatal screening and diagnosis of Down syndrome, along with termination of affected fetuses, the association of maternal age with Down syndrome is less pronounced among live-born infants than among fetuses.

Both paternal age and parity are positively associated with higher maternal age and also with Down syndrome through their association with maternal age. Whether these variables have independent associations with Down syndrome controlling for maternal age is uncertain. One study found no independent association of paternal age with risk of Down syndrome live birth in California, controlling for maternal age, but did find a residual association in the Czech Republic (Dzurova & Pikhart, 2005). A study that used birth certificate data from Washington State reported an independent effect of higher parity (Doria-Rose, Kim, Augustine, & Edwards, 2003). Although it is unlikely that parity affects the conception of a fetus with trisomy, heterogeneity among women in probability of fetal survival could account for such an association if women with more births also have a higher probability of carrying a fetus with Down syndrome to term.

2.1.2. Race/ethnicity

Epidemiologic studies often report that race/ethnicity of the mother is associated with risk of Down syndrome (Sherman et al., 2007). In some populations this reflects differences in maternal age at delivery. Ethnic differences in Down syndrome prevalence are often attenuated and not statistically significant after adjustment for maternal age (Forrester & Merz, 2002). In metropolitan Atlanta, for example, differences between Black and White mothers in Down syndrome prevalence in one study were significantly different, but not after adjustment for maternal age 35 years or greater (Siffel et al., 2004).

It is important to distinguish Down syndrome-affected pregnancies that end in termination from those that result in live births, which many epidemiologic studies do not (e.g., Canfield et al., 2006). One US study created a population-based sample of linked birth records and hospital discharge records from Tennessee for the years 1990–2002 (Hodapp & Urbano, 2008; Hodapp, Urbano, & Rosenbloom, 2008; Urbano & Hodapp, 2007). The investigators identified a total of 918 live births with Down syndrome. The composition of Down syndrome births classified by maternal race was 82.8% White, 15.8% Black, and 1.4% Other (Hodapp et al., 2008). The distribution of all births by race in Tennessee during that period was 76.5% White, 21.9% Black, and 1.6% Other. Thus, Tennessee mothers who were Black were two-thirds as likely to have an infant with Down syndrome as White mothers, not controlling for maternal age at birth or Hispanic ethnicity.

Racial/ethnic differences in Down syndrome birth prevalence may vary depending on the region, time period, and inclusion of prenatal terminations. In metropolitan Atlanta, no racial difference in the birth prevalence of Down syndrome among live births or recognized pregnancies was observed during 1990–1993, but the Black–White prevalence ratio during 1994–1999 was 0.87 for live births and 0.64 for recognized pregnancies (Siffel et al., 2004). The difference between the two ratios reflected more use of prenatal services among White women. A study that used national birth certificate data found that the availability of publicly funded abortions in a state was associated with a 40% reduction in births with Down syndrome among non-Hispanic Whites and an insignificant reduction among Blacks (Khoshnood, Pryde, Blondel, & Lee, 2003).

Differential use of prenatal services can affect relative rates of Down syndrome births, and Hispanics tend to be both less likely to use prenatal testing and more likely to have a live birth with Down syndrome (Kuppermann et al., 2006). For example, in California during 1990–1991 the prevalence of Down syndrome among live births was higher among Hispanics (1.44 per 1000 live births) than among non-Hispanic Whites (0.93 per 1000 births), whereas the prevalence of Down syndrome among all recognized pregnancies was higher among non-Hispanic Whites than among Hispanics (Bishop, Huether, Torfs, Lorey, & Deddens, 1997). Controlling for maternal age, the risk of a live-born infant with Down syndrome was 20% higher among California mothers of Mexican or Central American origin (Hook, Carothers, & Hecht, 1999).

The most up-to-date national-level data on Down syndrome in different racial/ethnic groups which used validated diagnoses based on birth defects surveillance was reported for 10 areas of the country for the years 1999–2003 with information on 5,579,947 live births, excluding terminations and stillbirths (Shin et al., 2009). The highest prevalence was among Hispanics, 13.5 per 10,000, and the lowest among non-Hispanic Blacks, 9.0 per 10,000. Both groups differed significantly in prevalence from the non-Hispanic White group, which was 11.7 per 10,000 births after adjustment for maternal age.

2.1.3. Socioeconomic status

Socioeconomic status has been examined in fewer Down syndrome studies, particularly in the United States. The most readily available measure of socioeconomic status is parental education; in the United Kingdom, paternal occupational status is frequently used as a measure of socioeconomic status. A smaller number of birth defects studies have collected data on family income, which generally requires that parents be surveyed. Case–control studies of birth defects collect measures of family socioeconomic status but typically exclude chromosome abnormalities; one exception is a study from California (Torfs & Christianson, 2003). An alternative approach to controlling for income levels is to use geocoded data to link census data on median family income in a defined area to data with confirmed cases of Down syndrome.

Findings on the association of socioeconomic status with Down syndrome are mixed. Several epidemiologic studies have reported that higher-status families or residential districts are significantly more likely to have children with Down syndrome, not controlling for maternal age (Gath & Gumley, 1986; Hodapp et al., 2008; Shepperdson, 1985; Vrijheid et al., 2000). Two cohort studies from the United Kingdom reported that the distribution of paternal occupations was similar to that of a comparison group but with a small excess of higher-status occupations in the Down syndrome group along with older parental age (Carr & Hewett, 1982; Cunningham, 1996). Some other studies have reported no significant difference in socioeconomic characteristics of families with infants with Down syndrome and families of other infants, including studies from Sweden using a national birth register that included measures of family income and housing quality (Ericson, Eriksson, & Zetterstrom, 1984), birth defects surveillance data in the Czech Republic (Dzurova & Pikhart, 2005), and a case–control study of live births in Italy (Rosano, Del Bufalo, & Burgio, 2008). Other studies have reported an inverse association, with higher socioeconomic status families having a lower probability of having a child with Down syndrome (Dzurova & Pikhart, 2005; Khoshnood et al., 2006; Knox & Lancashire, 1991; Torfs & Christianson, 2003). Ecological studies in the United Kingdom found no association between local measures of socioeconomic status and the prevalence of Down syndrome (Lopez, Stone, & Gilmour, 1995).

Torfs and Christianson (2003) tested the hypothesis that social and economic disadvantage experienced by a woman throughout her lifetime increases her risk of having a fetus with Down syndrome. The data come from a survey of families of children with birth defects collected during 1991–1993 by the California Birth Defects Monitoring Program (CBDMP), in which parents were interviewed regarding potential risk factors. The authors constructed a scale based on five measures of low socioeconomic status over a woman's lifespan up to time of conception—mothers' education less than high school, mother's low-status occupation, father's education less than high school, father's low-status occupation, and current family income less than $20,000. The scale had a linear association with Down syndrome, with a positive response on each item associated with an 18% higher risk of Down syndrome. The authors reported adjusted odds ratios ranging from 1.2 for one risk factor up to 1.9 for four or more socioeconomic status risk factors, controlling for maternal age and Hispanic ethnicity. When the association was restricted to live births, the association with low socioeconomic status was stronger for older women.

A second study from California also reported an inverse association of socioeconomic status with risk of Down syndrome, using a single socioeconomic status measure, maternal education, and outcomes restricted to live births (Dzurova & Pikhart, 2005). The investigators used routinely collected CBDMP data on live births from 1996 to 1997, with mother's education level used as a proxy for socioeconomic status. After adjusting for maternal and paternal age, mothers with only a secondary education were roughly twice as likely and primary-educated mothers almost three times as likely as university-educated mothers to have a live-born infant with Down syndrome. No such association was observed in a parallel analysis of data from the Czech Republic. The authors suggested that the gradient of Down syndrome risk with education in California likely reflected differential use of prenatal diagnosis and termination by more highly educated couples, unlike the situation in the Czech Republic.

One US study used both maternal education and average family income in a locality as measures of socioeconomic status. Hodapp et al. (2008) reported that significantly fewer mothers of children with Down syndrome in Tennessee did not graduate from high school, 17.3% vs. 22.7% for mothers in general. However, very young mothers, who are less likely to have completed high school, are unlikely to have a Down syndrome-affected birth. Unless one adjusts for maternal age, incomplete education may not be a useful indicator of socioeconomic status. The authors also reported that the median family income based on maternal zip code of residence at time of birth was 3.7% higher ($38,584 vs. $37,218) for mothers of children with Down syndrome compared to mothers of unaffected children in Tennessee. That tabulation did not adjust for differences in maternal age or race.

Researchers in Europe have reported varying associations of socioeconomic status with Down syndrome. UK studies found that ecologic measures of both socioeconomic status and occupational status were positively associated with Down syndrome, which reflects differences in maternal age at birth (Gath & Gumley, 1986; Lopez et al., 1995; Shepperdson 1985; Vrijheid et al., 2000). A study from France found that maternal socioeconomic status, as proxied by her occupation, was inversely associated with Down syndrome live birth as a result of low socioeconomic status mothers being more likely to bring a Down syndrome fetus to term (Khoshnood et al., 2006), similar to the pattern observed in California.

2.2. Children of all ages

The characteristics of children with Down syndrome can be influenced by differential postnatal survival as well as risk factors for conception or prenatal survival (Besser, Shin, Kucik, & Correa, 2007). Survival among US children with Down syndrome differs by race/ethnicity, with higher rates of mortality among Blacks with Down syndrome than among Whites (Rasmussen, Wong, Correa, Gambrell, & Friedman, 2006; Yang, Rasmussen, & Friedman, 2002). Linking MACDP data with the National Death Index, the Black–White prevalence ratio was estimated to be 0.87 at birth and 0.65 at ages 0–19 (Besser et al., 2007) due to differences in survival. Shin et al. (2009) calculated pooled estimates of prevalence from 10 active birth defects surveillance systems in the United States using the same method. The Black–White prevalence ratio for the national sample, restricted to those not of Hispanic ethnicity, was estimated to be 0.77 at birth and 0.71 among children of all ages, a smaller difference relative to the analysis by Besser et al. (2007).

Relative to families with children with intellectual and developmental disabilities, families of children with Down syndrome typically appear socially and economically advantaged. As reviewed above, relative to the general population of children, families of children with Down syndrome typically have similar socioeconomic status after adjusting for parental age. By contrast, families of children with intellectual and developmental disabilities are typically disadvantaged relative to families of normally developing children (Croen, Grether, & Selvin, 2001; Drews et al., 1995). Therefore, families of children with Down syndrome are likely to have more economic resources than families of children with intellectual disability. One US study reported that mean family income was 50% higher for a convenience sample of 25 families of children with Down syndrome than for a matched group of 49 families of children with developmental delays of mixed etiologies who had approximately the same racial/ethnic composition (Most, Fidler, Booth-LaForce, & Kelly, 2006).

Confirmation of a "Down syndrome advantage" relative to other developmental disabilities comes from a recent study of national survey data. Schieve et al. (2009) used data from the 1997 to 2005 Child Sample Core in the National Health Interview Survey (NHIS) on one child <18 years of age selected randomly from each family with children in the NHIS, an annual, multistage, probability-sample, household survey of the US civilian noninstitutionalized population. Among 96,345 children 3–17 years of age, 146 children were reported to have Down syndrome and 604 other children had intellectual disability ("mental retardation" in the survey) without Down syndrome. Children with Down syndrome were as likely to be living below the poverty level as children without intellectual disability (16.5 and 16.3%), and only half as likely as children with intellectual disability (32.5%). Likewise, children with Down syndrome were similar in racial classification to children without intellectual disability and only half as likely as other children with intellectual disability to be classified as Black 13.1 and 26.0%, respectively. Children with Down syndrome resembled children with intellectual disability with regard to maternal education beyond high school, 43.4 and 43.5%, respectively, compared with 55.3% of mothers of typically developing children.

It should be noted that the estimated Down syndrome prevalence of 14.3 per 10,000 children aged 3–17 years based on parental reports in the NHIS data is high relative to the estimated prevalence of Down syndrome 10.3 per 10,000 among US children and adolescents from 10 surveillance systems located throughout the United States (Shin et al., 2009). The accuracy of parental characterizations of children's medical diagnoses in the NHIS and other household surveys is not well established. Data from one birth defects case–control study suggest that the accuracy of parental reports of having a child with Down syndrome is extremely high (Rasmussen, Mulinare, Khoury, & Maloney, 1990). That study reported that there were no cases of false negatives for Down syndrome or any other birth defect other than a limb defect. In epidemiologic terms, the specificity of parental reports of Down syndrome in that study was 100% as confirmed by birth defects surveillance, which in turn was based on abstraction of hospital or medical records.

One study called into question the accuracy of parental reports of children's diagnoses. Miller, Gaboda and Davis (2001) analyzed data on approximately 6200 children who participated in the 1991 Longitudinal Follow-up to the 1988 National Maternal and Infant Health Survey. The investigators contacted physician practices to review medical records for children reported to have conditions (not including Down syndrome). The investigators obtained physician confirmation for 18–50% of cases of congenital heart conditions, spina bifida, or cerebral palsy reported by mothers, compared with 100% for the same conditions reported by Rasmussen et al. (1990). The difference in findings could relate to the difference in the age of the children, the focus of one study on birth defects, and the incompleteness of medical records.

2.3. Summary

Race/ethnicity is the sociodemographic variable which, after parental age, is most commonly reported to be associated with Down syndrome. Among US live births, the prevalence of Down syndrome is highest for Hispanics and lowest for non-Hispanic Blacks. Among Black and White mothers, the relative ratio of having a Down syndrome live birth varies from 0.67 (Hodapp et al., 2008) to 0.87 (Besser et al., 2007; Siffel et al., 2004). Using data pooled from 10 regions of the country, the prevalence of Down syndrome among non-Hispanic Black children, after adjusting for survival, is 29% lower and that for Hispanics is 21% greater compared to that of non-Hispanic whites (Shin et al., 2009). In NHIS data, the prevalence of Down syndrome among Blacks is 16% lower than for Whites, based on small numbers (Schieve et al., 2009). More importantly for the "Down syndrome advantage," the NHIS data confirm that US children with Down syndrome are much less likely to be classified as Black or African American than are other children with intellectual disability.

The association between socioeconomic status and Down syndrome is less consistent. Some studies suggested that more educated and higher-income families were more likely to have a child with Down syndrome (Hodapp et al., 2008), whereas others suggested the opposite to be true after adjusting for maternal age (Dzurova & Pikhart, 2005; Torfs & Christianson, 2003). In general, though, Down syndrome families appear to have socioeconomic status similar to that of families of normally developing children but more advantaged status than families of children with intellectual disability, as indicated by nationally representative NHIS data for federal poverty status and race/ethnicity, although not for maternal education without adjustment for maternal age (Schieve et al., 2009).

3. Economic Impacts of Child Disability on Families

The economic impacts of illness or disability can be calculated in financial terms, relative to the net impact on family finances, or more broadly in terms of well-being (Tilford, Robbins, & Hobbs, 2001).

Well-being is defined by economists in terms of a welfare or utility function, whose determinants include the health of family members and the availability of time to pursue desired activities. The importance of nonfinancial aspects of ill health or disability on family members, sometimes referred to as "spillover" effects, has been documented in a growing literature (Brouwer, van Exel, & Tilford, 2009; Reichman, Corman, & Noonan, 2008). For example, research conducted using a representative sample of families of children of all ages with spina bifida identified through a state birth defects surveillance system has quantified the negative impact on the health of parental caregivers (Tilford et al., 2005) and their use of time, including sleep and social activities (Grosse, Flores, Ouyang, Robbins, & Tilford, 2009). This chapter focuses on financial impacts, both objective and subjective.

Having a child with a disability can affect family finances through out-of-pocket expenditures, changes in paid employment, and family composition. The potential influence of child disability on economic well-being operating through family composition is often not recognized. It is well established that children living in single-parent families are much more likely to experience economic disadvantage, and research suggests that child ill health can reduce the likelihood of a child living in a two-parent family (Reichman, Corman, & Noonan, 2004). There is inconclusive evidence whether having a child with a disabling condition such as spina bifida is associated with parents' relationship status (Grosse et al., 2009). On the other hand, there is evidence that the probability of parental divorce is reduced for children with Down syndrome relative to other congenital conditions and to children in general (Urbano & Hodapp, 2007). The remainder of this section takes family composition as a given.

Greater demands for caregiving may lead to reduced time available for paid employment, which may be offset in part or in full by the increased need for income to meet expenses. The net effect on parental employment and earnings is theoretically indeterminate (Emerson, 2007; Salkever, 1982). In general, though, the expectation is that parental employment is reduced. This can occur if either one parent leaves the labor force altogether or one or both parents reduce hours of paid employment (Parish, Seltzer, Greenberg, & Floyd, 2004). Reduction in employment due to child disability is not necessarily voluntary, particularly in single-parent households. Employment effects may vary with the degree of the individual child's needs and the child's age. One longitudinal study of a cohort of 103 two-parent families of children with intellectual disability followed from age 3 to age 11 found that at age 3 many mothers had stopped work, reduced their hours of work, or changed work to obtain a more flexible work schedule to meet their child's needs (Gallimore, Coots, Weisner, Garnier, & Guthrie, 1996). These differences were attenuated and not statistically significant at age 7 or 11.

In addition to employment status and hours of work, parents of children with disabilities may experience lower earnings as a result of decreased attachment to the labor market. Parents of children with disabilities are often reported to take lower paying jobs that are less intensive or permit greater flexibility in scheduling or they may pass up opportunities for promotion (Freedman, Litchfield, & Warfield, 1995). Periodic absences from the work force can lead to permanently lower earnings trajectories. Therefore, differences in the quantity of employment should be considered as conservative estimates of the impact on parental earnings.

In order to derive valid estimates of family impacts of disability, representative population samples of cases and unaffected children are needed. A systematic review identified 17 studies published from 1989 through 2005 that addressed the economic impacts on families of having a child with a disability (Anderson, Dumont, Jacobs, & Azzaria, 2007). Most of those studies employed convenience samples of case families recruited through parent support groups, clinics, or assistance programs. Also, only 9 of the 17 studies included a comparison group of families with nondisabled children, which is needed to calculate the incremental or attributable financial impact of having a child with a disability. Findings summarized by Anderson et al. (2007) were diverse. The estimated annual out-of-pocket cost of caring for a child with a disability ranged from $108 to $8742 per year, and the caregiver time cost was reported to vary from 4 to 84 h per week. Only one study summarized by Anderson et al. (2007), however, utilized a representative, population-based sample of families of children both with and without disabilities (Newacheck, Inkelas, & Kim, 2004).

3.1. Parental employment and earnings

This section, summarizes evidence on the opportunity cost to families of time spent in unpaid caregiving services in terms of foregone paid employment. A full measure of opportunity cost could include other time uses, including volunteer service, leisure, social participation, and self-care, notably sleep (Tilford et al., 2001). In addition to quantitative analyses, qualitative research with parents of children or adults with developmental disabilities provides insights into employment barriers and stresses (Shearn & Todd, 2000).

First, a selected number of studies using convenience samples of families of children with disabilities, with a particular focus on Down syndrome, are reviewed. An inherent limitation of convenience samples is that one cannot necessarily generalize to families outside the samples. Also, findings from convenience samples are frequently contradictory and should be discounted. Next, we review data from studies that have analyzed parental employment for representative samples of families. Some studies specifically sampled families with children who had a disability or a chronic health condition, and others analyzed general household surveys.

3.1.1. Convenience samples

Studies that have analyzed data on convenience sample of parents of children with Down syndrome or other disabilities have found mixed evidence on employment effects relative to parents of unaffected children. One frequently cited study found an effect on hours of work but not on the probability of being employed. Barnett and Boyce (1995) interviewed 237 parents of children with Down syndrome recruited through parent support groups and public schools and administered a time use survey that had previously been administered to a national sample. The investigators found that mothers of children with Down syndrome under age 17 were not significantly less likely to be in paid employment but averaged seven fewer hours per week in paid employment. Similarly, Landis (1992) reported that 65 mothers of young children with disabilities receiving early intervention services were not significantly less likely to be in paid employment but were much less likely to be employed full time relative to all mothers based on census data for the same state.

Among other convenience sample studies, one found a reduced probability of maternal employment, whereas others did not. Roach, Orsmond, and Barratt (1999) recruited 41 two-parent families of young children with Down syndrome in an academic research study with 29 socioeconomically matched families with typically developing children; the majority of parents in both groups had college degrees. The Down syndrome mothers were significantly less likely to be employed, 56.1% vs. 76.0%. By contrast, Crowe (1993) found that among three groups of mothers—45 with children with Down syndrome, 45 with children with multiple disabilities, and 45 with typically developing children aged 6 months to 5 years—there were no significant differences in employment. Also, average weekly hours of paid employment were highest for the Down syndrome group 5.9, compared with 2.3 for the multiple disabilities group and 3.4 for the matched controls. Likewise, Crowe and Florez (2006) analyzed data for a group of 30 mothers of children with developmental disabilities and 30 matched mothers of typically developing children aged 3–14 years. Mean weekly hours of paid employment were higher for the disability group, 27.4 vs. 21.5 for the mothers of typically developing children. Finally, Warfield (2001) interviewed a sample of 122 mostly middle-class mothers of 5-year-old children enrolled in an early intervention study, of whom 62–70% were employed for pay. Mothers of children with Down syndrome were more likely to be employed full time, 46.2%, than were either mothers of children with motor impairments, 38.5%, or those with developmental delay, 15.4%.

A case-only study design can elicit information from parents about perceptions or experience of role incompatibility between child care and paid work. For example, one US study recruited 166 mothers of toddlers aged 12–15 months receiving early intervention services and collected information about work plans (Booth & Kelly, 1999). About 45% of mothers reported that their child's condition affected their work plans to some extent, which varied based on the diagnosis. Mothers of children with Down syndrome were about two-thirds as likely as mothers of children with developmental delay of unknown etiology or other diagnoses to report altered work plans. A UK study that enrolled a convenience sample of 16 families of children with disabilities aged 3–17 years found that in 12 (75%) families the mother reported being unable to work because of their child's condition (Curran, Sharples, White, & Knapp, 2001). A Canadian survey of 148 parents of children with fetal alcohol spectrum disorder (FASD) using the Health Services Utilization Inventory reported that short-term loss of work days among employed parents averaged 2% of annual earnings (Stade, Ungar, Stevens, Beyene, & Koren, 2006).

3.1.2. Household surveys—generic

Numerous published analyses of representative samples of households of children have examined the influence of child disability and maternal employment, and most have found differences in either the probability of employment or hours of work conditional on employment among at least a subset of households. Using the 1972 NHIS, Salkever (1982) found large, statistically significant negative differences in maternal employment among White two-parent households but not among single-parent or non-White households. There was a 20% reduction in maternal employment (a difference of 6 percentage points from a 29 percentage point sample mean) associated with having a child with a disability, and the magnitude of the difference in employment varied with the number and severity of conditions. No impact on hours of work conditional on employment was observed.

A similar analysis by Breslau, Salkever, and Staruch (1982) of a specially constructed dataset of children receiving specialty care for various conditions and a random sample of families of children in Cleveland, Ohio, reported similar findings. Specifically, there was a large negative effect of child disability [measured by activities of daily living (ADL)] on maternal employment among lower-income two-parent families, a smaller negative effect on middle-income families, and no negative effect on single-parent families. Unlike Salkever (1982), a negative effect on hours of work conditional on employment was also detected. In contrast to both studies, an analysis of data from the 1984 Survey of Income and Program Participation

(SIPP) found a significant negative association of child disability with the employment of single mothers but not that of married mothers (Wolfe & Hill, 1995).

More recent US survey data have generally confirmed negative cross-sectional associations of child disability with maternal employment. For example, an analysis of data from the 1994 NHIS Disability supplement reported that mothers of a child with a disability were 75% as likely to be employed (Kuhlthau & Perrin, 2001). Another analysis of the same dataset reported that school-aged children with a disability who lived in two-parent families had an adjusted odds ratio of not having two full-time employed parents of 1.27; those who lived in a single-parent household had an adjusted odds ratio of 1.66 of not having a full-time employed parent (Heck & Makuc, 2000).

Two analyses of SIPP data collected during the 1990s found that having a child with a disability was associated with reductions in employment among both married and single mothers (Porterfield, 2002; Powers, 2003). One of these studies found that among single mothers there was a significant negative effect of having a young child (ages 0–5) with disability on both part-time and full-time employment, but no effect of child disability at older ages (Porterfield, 2002). Among married women, having a young child with a disability was associated with a reduction in the probability of full-time work but no reduction in work overall. Also, there was an interaction with education, with little effect on the employment of highly educated mothers. The second study reported that having a child with a limitation in the ability to do regular school work because of a physical, learning, or mental health condition reduced the probability of employment by 6.0 percentage points for married women and by 11.0 percentage for female household heads (Powers, 2003); no difference by age of the child was reported.

An analysis of data from the Panel Study on Income Dynamics 1997 Child Supplement identified specific characteristics of children's health that adversely affected maternal employment, which varied by marital status (Gould, 2004). For single mothers, time-intensive illnesses were associated with fewer hours of work. For married mothers, it was severe conditions with unpredictable time components that were associated with both less probability of working and fewer hours of work if employed.

An analysis of 1999–2000 NHIS data examined employment characteristics among 4732 low-income single parents (Loprest & Davidoff, 2004). The data came from the core child questionnaire with information on one randomly sampled child (<18 years) in each household. Because only one child in a family was sampled, mothers of disabled children are included in the comparison group (Powers, 2001). Loprest and Davidoff used a screener to identify children with special needs and subdivided them into three types: those with chronic health conditions, increased use of services, and activity limitation. Activity limitation was based on responses to five questions, whether the child was "limited in any way," needed help with personal care, or had impairments in mobility, vision (blindness), or hearing (Davidoff, 2004). Loprest and Davidoff found that mothers of children who were classified as having an activity limitation had a 6 percentage point lower adjusted probability of being employed and those who were employed averaged 2.5 fewer h per week of paid work. By contrast, having a child with a chronic medical or physical condition alone was not significantly associated with variation in maternal employment. It should be noted that the prevalence of activity limitations among parents in this sample was about twice as high for parents of children with special needs, although Loprest and Davidoff controlled for parental characteristics in their regression models.

Powers (2001) analyzed data from the School Enrollment Supplement to the October 1992 Current Population Survey (CPS). She used reports of children's impairments to predict reported difficulty in learning and used predicted learning difficulties to predict maternal employment. The sample included roughly 9500 two-parent families and 2800 single-parent families with school-aged children. Overall, the probability of employment was reduced by 6.5 percentage points for married women and 10.0 percentage points among female heads; similar findings were also reported with SIPP data (see Powers, 2003). After controlling for maternal health and potential bias in the reporting of learning difficulties, the adjusted reductions were 3.9 percentage points and 7.5 percentage points, respectively (Powers, 2001).

The 1979 National Longitudinal Survey of Youth (NLSY) cohort, along with the Child and Youth Supplement data collected by the Bureau of Labor Statistics since 1986, represents an important data resource which has been used sparingly to examine parental employment effects of child health, although a number of studies have used it to examine the effects of maternal employment on child development (Blau & Grossberg, 1992). Norberg (1998) analyzed the 1994 wave of the NLSY to examine maternal employment patterns during the first 5 years after the birth of a singleton infant relative to the presence of child health problems at birth; the sample consisted of 6604 children born to 3785 mothers between 1980 and 1994. A single "high risk" category was created for infants who had intrauterine growth retardation, a congenital defect diagnosed through prenatal testing (amniocentesis or ultrasound), or an extended birth hospitalization. The majority of mothers returned to work within the first year of birth, but return to work was delayed for mothers of high-risk infants. Controlling for the mother's work status prior to birth, the probability of being employed during the first 5 years after birth was 55% lower for mothers of high-risk infants.

Porterfield and Tracey (2003) analyzed NLSY data collected through 1998 on up to three births for women aged 19–40 years at delivery to examine changes in maternal employment and family income within the first 6 years after delivery across births. They compared families with a child with a disability or special health care need (e.g., asthma) and those with only unaffected children. Among single mothers, differences in employment, hours of work, and income were observed at 3 years but not at 6 years. By contrast, married women who had a child with a disability had significantly lower employment and hours of work and were more likely to have income below 200% of the federal poverty level at both 3 years and 6 years. In addition, they were significantly less likely to own their own home at 6 years after the birth of their first child. The investigators also analyzed pre-birth socioeconomic characteristics of the families and found no significant differences, suggesting that the causal effect was from child disability or ill health to lowered economic status.

Corman, Noonan, and Reichman (2005) analyzed data on a sample of almost 4000 low-income urban mothers from 20 cities who were followed up 12–18 months postpartum, the Fragile Families and Child Wellbeing Study. The sample was 78% ethnic minority and 74% unmarried; overall 54% were currently employed. The investigators found that having a child in poor health decreased the likelihood that a mother worked for pay by an average of 8 percentage points. In addition, it was associated with a reduction by more than 3 h per week of work among those who were employed. A subgroup analysis found that among high school graduates there was a 19 point reduction in employment but no reduction among women either with less education or with college education.

A study from Australia used data from a national 1997 Time Use Survey and compared 832 mothers of children without disability with 203 mothers of children with disability (Gordon, Rosenbloom, & Cuskelly, 2007). The probability of working for pay was slightly reduced for 151 women whose children had mild to moderate disability, 55.6% vs. 60.9%, but among 52 mothers of children with severe to profound limitations, it was sharply lower at 38.5%. In addition, mothers of children with disability were about half as likely to work full-time, whether the disability was mild to moderate, 14.6%, or severe to profound, 11.5%, compared with other mothers, 25.1%. A subgroup analysis found that differences in employment were restricted to mothers with partners; the employment of single (lone) parents was unaffected.

To summarize, findings from large household surveys consistently report that certain subgroups of mothers of children with disabilities are either less likely to work for pay or, conditional on employment, less likely to work full-time. Most analysts have interpreted these associations as evidence of causal effects of child ill health or disability, although the direction of causality is unclear. Also, there is evidence that it may be problematic to generalize across types of conditions. One study reported that limitations in maternal employment are specific to child disability, as characterized by activity limitations, and not chronic medical conditions in general (Loprest & Davidoff, 2004).

Some investigators report that differences in employment attributable to child disability or ill health are restricted to mothers in two-parent households (Breslau et al., 1982; Gordon et al., 2007; Salkever, 1982). Others have reported larger effects on employment of single parents (Heck & Makuc, 2000; Powers, 2001, 2003; Wolfe & Hill, 1995). Two studies reported that among single parents negative effects on employment were restricted to young children (Porterfield, 2002; Porterfield & Tracey, 2003), although another study found no such pattern (Powers, 2003).

3.1.3. Condition-specific analyses

A few condition-specific analyses of impacts on parental employment of having a child with a disability have been published using representative population-based samples. Several of these used registries of people with validated diagnoses to identify people with conditions, including two European studies specific to Down syndrome. One study from Sweden surveyed 85 families with young children (mean age 4.7 years) with Down syndrome and 89 families with children of the same ages who did not have an impairment (Hedov et al., 2002; Hedov et al., 2006). Approximately 90% of both groups of mothers worked outside the home, which reflects the availability of high-quality child care in Sweden. Despite equivalent probability of being employed outside the home, the mothers in the Down syndrome group were significantly less likely to work full-time. Overall, 22% of mothers of Down syndrome children worked full-time, compared with 45% of mothers of unaffected children. In addition, five Down syndrome mothers and one Down syndrome father took more than 100 paid sick days in 1 year, compared with none of the non-Down syndrome parents (Hedov et al., 2006). That does not include paid days off to care for a sick child; both Down syndrome mothers and fathers took three times as many paid days off to care for a sick child as did other parents.

In the United Kingdom, investigators recruited 181 families with a child born with Down syndrome during 1973–1980 in the Manchester Down Syndrome Cohort, and most were followed up when the children were 10–17 years old (Cunningham, 1996). During the early years of the study, mothers were given encouragement to engage in paid employment and were as likely to work as a comparison group. Subsequently, when the children were of school age, 40% of mothers reported that difficulties in scheduling had made work difficult, and the probability of employment had decreased relative to comparison mothers (Cunningham, 1996).

Although no published North American studies using representative samples of families with children with Down syndrome have examined parental employment, analyses for other conditions have been published. One study from Arkansas during 2001–2002 surveyed the primary parental caregivers of 98 children aged 2–17 years with spina bifida identified through a birth defects surveillance system, almost all of whom were mothers (Tilford, Grosse, Goodman, & Li, 2009). The investigators compared their employment patterns with a representative sample of 416 mothers in Arkansas from the 2001–2002 CPS. The largest difference was in the percentage who worked for pay in the past year, 54.1% vs. 76.7%; a smaller but still significant difference was observed in average number of weeks worked, 40.4 vs. 44.8. No difference in usual weekly hours of work was found. Regression models predicted an average reduction of 9.2 h per week. This varied by the severity of disability as proxied by the anatomic level of the spina bifida lesion, from 7.8 to 11.3 h per week. It also varied by the age of the child, from a predicted 13.3 h per week for infants to 6.2 h per week for 20 year-olds. The reduction primarily reflected lower employment probabilities rather than reduced hours among those who were employed. Tilford and colleagues also found that among those who were employed average hourly earnings were 25% lower. Another analysis of the same data reported effects on other use of time, including a marked reduction in caregiver sleep time by lesion level (Grosse et al., 2009).

A study from Canada collected data during 2001–2002 from a stratified random sample of 468 caregivers (95% natural parents) of children with cerebral palsy receiving rehabilitation services in the province of Ontario and compared responses with Ontario respondents in the Canadian National Longitudinal Survey of Children and Youth (Brehaut et al., 2004). A smaller proportion of subjects in the cerebral palsy sample reported working for pay compared with the population sample, 66.0% vs. 81.2%. Furthermore, among those that did work for pay, a slightly smaller proportion of the cerebral palsy sample reported working full-time, 67.5% vs. 73.2%.

Four recent publications reported data on employment patterns for representative US samples of parents of children with an autism spectrum disorder (ASD) as identified by the parents. First, an analysis of the National Household Education Survey (NHES)-After School Programs and Activities Survey 2005 assessed parental employment. Montes and Halterman (2006) found that mothers of children grades K-8 with ASD were 21% less likely to be employed than other mothers, 53% vs. 67%. Fathers of children with ASD were also less likely to be employed (82% vs. 93%) and more likely to work part-time. Montes and Halterman (2008a) calculated the mean loss of parental earnings to be $6000 per year for each child with ASD. They also reported that children with ASD were 38% less likely to live in a higher-income household, controlling for parental age, parental education, race/ethnicity, and other determinants of income. Likewise, children with other disabilities were 32% less likely to live in a higher-income household after adjustment for confounding. On the other hand, the reduction in earned income was much greater for the families with a child with ASD, 14%, compared with a 2% loss of income for families of children with other disabilities.

An analysis of data from the National Survey of Children's Health compared socioeconomic status and family income for children with ASD and other developmental disorders (Montes & Halterman, 2008b). Unlike their earlier study (Montes & Halterman, 2008a), Montes and Halterman (2008b) found that families with a child with ASD did not appear to differ in family income from families of typically developing children whereas families with children with other developmental disorders were substantially less likely to have high incomes. On the other hand, parents of children with ASD were more than seven times as likely as parents of typically developing children to have had to alter employment in the previous year because of child care needs.

A recent study examined parental reports of financial problems or reduced parental employment due to the child's condition in the 2005–2006 National Survey of Children with Special Health Care Needs (NS-CSHCN)—examined data on 2088 children aged 3–17 years with ASD, 9534 other children with "emotional, developmental, or behavioral problems," and 26,751 other children with "special health care needs," including health conditions such as asthma (Kogan et al., 2008). The majority (57.1%) of the ASD sample reported that a family member had reduced or stopped employment because of their child's condition; the equivalent percentages for the group with non-ASD developmental or mental health issues was 36.3% and for the children with other health issues it was still lower, 17.4%. Another analysis of the same dataset reported that the adjusted odds ratios for work loss by one or more family members related to the child's health care needs was a direct function of the child's disability: 2.0 for children with very little limitation, 3.9 for children with some limitations, and 7.9 for children with a great deal of limitation (Okumura, Van Cleave, Gnanasekaran, & Houtrow, 2009).

To summarize, two North American studies have reported that the primary parental caregiver of children with either spina bifida (Tilford et al., 2009) or cerebral palsy (Brehaut et al., 2004) is significantly less likely to be employed for pay but not significantly less likely to work full-time conditional on employment, whereas a Swedish study reported the opposite pattern for parents of children with Down syndrome (Hedov et al., 2002, 2006). The difference in findings across studies likely reflects structural differences across countries in the availability of affordable child care and flexibility in paid leave.

US samples of parents of children with autism or related disorders (ASD) typically report lower employment probabilities on average than parents of unaffected children as well as parents of children with other developmental disabilities (Kogan et al., 2008; Montes & Halterman, 2008a, b). More broadly, it is reported by Okumura et al. (2009) that barriers to parental employment and reported work loss are a direct function of the severity of a child's disabilities. However, the validity of the parent-reported diagnoses in the studies with ASD data is uncertain. As noted above, there is conflicting information about the validity of parental reports for specific pediatric conditions (Miller et al., 2001; Rasmussen et al., 1990). It is important to assess the diagnostic validity of parent reports of ASD and other disabling conditions in household surveys.

3.1.4. Employment effects across the lifespan

Few studies have examined the financial and employment effects on families caring for adult offspring with disabilities. One cross-sectional study from Australia compared a convenience sample of 25 families of adults aged 17–21 years who had both intellectual disability and either a physical or behavioral disability with another convenience sample of 25 families of unaffected adult children of the same ages (Einam & Cuskelly, 2002). Among mothers, the probability of paid employment was 52% among the former and 76% among the latter. The difference in full-time employment was even greater; 8 and 28% of mothers in the two groups, respectively, worked more than 30 h per week. However, a US cross-sectional study found that most mothers of adolescents or young adults (ages 10–23 years) with selected conditions (22 with Fragile X syndrome, 39 with Down syndrome, and 174 with ASD) were employed (68.2, 76.9, and 70.7%, respectively) (Abbeduto et al., 2004). Mean family incomes were also comparable across the three groups.

A cross-sectional study from Sweden involving a convenience sample of 17 young adults with ASD, aged 19–39 years, found that six reported receiving informal caregiving assistance (Järbrink, McCrone, Fombonne, Zandén, & Knapp, 2007). Six parents likewise reported providing an average of 11 h per week of caregiving services, but only two said that this had affected the number of hours of paid work to an unknown extent. It was not possible to quantify the number of hours of paid employment lost, but this appeared small in magnitude. By contrast, Järbrink (2007) reported that parental loss of paid work for children with ASD amounted to $5400 per child per year.

Only one longitudinal study to date has used cohort data to assess the employment effects of developmental disability across the lifespan. The Wisconsin Longitudinal Study (WLS), a cohort of roughly 10,000 largely White Wisconsin high school graduates from 1957, most of whom were re-interviewed in 1975 and 1992, provides unique information from a representative, population sample on the long-term impacts of child disability on parents (Seltzer, Greenberg, Floyd, Pettee, & Hong, 2001). The WLS also includes data derived from interviews of a set of siblings of the original respondents that were conducted during 1957, 1977, and 1994. The investigators identified 165 parents of a child with a developmental disability, most of whom had intellectual disability, and 53 parents of an adult child with an adult-onset severe mental health problem, as identified during the last survey round. These families were matched with a stratified random sample of 218 parents from the same samples who had only unaffected children.

The WLS data document a substantial employment and financial impact of having a child with a disability which varied in magnitude with the life stage. When the mothers were approximately 36 years of age, those who had a child with a developmental disability worked significantly fewer weeks, 27% less, than mothers in either of the other two groups (Seltzer et al., 2001). In the last survey round, when parents were in their early 50s, there was no longer a significant reduction in the probability of being employed.

The WLS data were reanalyzed by Parish et al. (2004). After control for confounding almost no difference in the probability of being employed was reported overall, but the mothers of children with developmental disabilities had lower labor force attachment and earnings. Mean earnings for this group were almost 50% lower when the mother was 36 years of age. The negative effect on maternal earnings diminished as disabled children became adults but did not entirely disappear. When the women were in their early 50s, the gap in earnings had shrunk by more than half, but was still sizeable. Also, parents of children with developmental disability during the last survey round had 27% lower household savings on average. This last finding is evidence of a lasting negative economic effect on parents of having a child with a developmental disability.

3.2. Out-of-pocket expenditures and financial burden

Families of children with disabilities or special health care needs incur greater out-of-pocket expenditures for medical and other services for their children and have perceptions of greater financial burden or stress in comparison with other parents (Parish & Cloud, 2006). A methodological challenge is deciding which measures of financial burden to use. Attitudinal and objective economic measures of financial burden, although correlated, classify different families as experiencing a burden (Oswald et al., 2005). Attitudinal measures of inadequate insurance and income relative to medical needs include questions such as whether respondents believe that insurance was insufficient to meet perceived needs for medical care. Economic indicators include out-of-pocket medical expenditures as a percentage of family income and whether medical care was delayed because of lack of money. In one study, similar percentages of children with special health care needs were underinsured by both definitions, but only half of those children had parents who met both sets of criteria (Oswald et al., 2005). Typically, researchers using the economic approach classify families spending more than 5% or 10% of their income on health care as being underinsured (Blewett, Ward, & Beebe, 2006).

Out-of-pocket medical spending per child as a percentage of family income has been used as an indicator of both underinsurance and financial burden. Often, when total out-of-pocket spending for the family is used as the denominator, the ratio is referred to as an indicator of underinsurance (Blewett et al., 2006), although others interpret it as a measure of "financial insecurity" or "burdensome health care costs" (Merlis, 2002). Thus, for example, in 1996 one-seventh of families (14%) with incomes below the federal poverty line spent more than 10% of their income on health care, compared with 1% of families with incomes at least 400% of the poverty level (Merlis, 2002). When analysts use spending on a particular child with a health condition as the denominator, it is generally used as a measure of the financial burden of the child's condition (Newacheck & Halfon, 1986). Absolute out-of-pocket medical expenditures rise with family income but decrease in relative terms as income rises, regardless of whether the family has a child with a chronic condition or disability (Galbraith, Wong, Kim, & Newacheck, 2005).

Families with children with disabilities or special needs report higher absolute out-of-pocket medical expenditures relative to other families. Using 1999–2000 MEPS data, Newacheck et al. (2004) reported that children with disabilities incurred average total medical expenditures (excluding dental and vision) 5.6 times higher than other children. Children with disabilities were more likely to be covered by health insurance, and most of those medical expenditures were reimbursed by public or private insurers. Out-of-pocket expenditures incurred by families were about 50% higher in absolute terms for children with disabilities relative to unaffected children but lower as a percentage of medical expenditures, 8.3% vs. 18.2%. Newacheck and Kim (2005) reported similar patterns for children with special health care needs. In other words, health insurance moderated the financial impact on families and reduced but did not eliminate the disparity in financial burdens across families. It should be noted that a small minority of families accounted for the bulk of out-of-pocket expenditures associated with child disability; 10% of families whose annual expenses totaled $644 or more accounted for 84.8% of all such expenditures (Newacheck et al., 2004).

Another measure of financial burden is whether out-of-pocket expenditures exceed a specified percentage of family income. It is not uncommon for families of children with serious health conditions to spend more than 10% of their income on their child's health care needs. For example, a sample of 151 lower-middle income families in Minnesota who had a child with an expensive and disabling condition, the majority of whom had spina bifida, cerebral palsy, or cystic fibrosis, and who applied for a state program that paid for medical needs not covered by insurers reported spending on average 12.5% of their income for medical services for their child (Leonard, Brust, & Sapienza, 1992).

Newacheck and Kim (2005) used 2000 MEPS data and reported that lower-income families (<200% of federal poverty level) were about 11 times as likely as higher-income families (> 400% of federal poverty level) to have out-of-pocket expenditures that exceeded 5% of family income. Other researchers have used MEPS data to look at overall family out-of-pocket medical expenditures, including the family's share of health insurance premiums, as a percent of family income. Yu, Dick, and Szilagyi (2008) reported that among families of children with special health care needs, the share of families with out-of-pocket expenditures exceeding 10% of family income increased from 15.4 to 21.7% between 2001 and 2004, and the share with expenses over 20% of income doubled from 4.6 to 9.2%.

Children with Down syndrome have higher medical expenditures than do children with many other conditions, and therefore out-of-pocket medical expenditures are also higher. For children with disabilities in general total medical expenditures are five to six times higher than those for other children (Newacheck et al., 2004). An analysis of health insurance claims data for privately insured children aged 0–4 years found mean medical care expenditures during 2004 to be 12 times as high for children with Down syndrome compared with other children (Boulet, Molinari, Grosse, Honein, & Correa-Villaseñor, 2008); expenditures were particularly elevated during the first 2 years of life among the one-half of children with Down syndrome who had congenital heart defects. The analysts did not report out-of-pocket expenditures for children with Down syndrome, but other analyses of the same claims dataset for muscular dystrophy and spina bifida reported that out-of-pocket expenditures accounted for 9% of medical expenditures (Ouyang, Grosse, Armour, & Waitzman, 2007; Ouyang, Grosse, & Kenneson, 2008). This is similar to the out-of-pocket share reported for all children with disabilities in MEPS data (Newacheck et al., 2004). On this basis, one can extrapolate that the median out-of-pocket medical expenditure for privately insured children with Down syndrome was approximately $1000 in 2004 dollars. Of course, half of families incurred higher out-of-pocket expenditures, some of them many times higher.

Although medical spending is easily quantified, it may constitute a small share of all spending by families on children with disabilities or special needs. Medical expenses typically make up only a small portion of overall spending by families caring for children with special needs (Meyers, Lukemeyer, & Smeeding, 1998). Non-medical expenses include transportation to doctors and therapists, modifications to houses, specialized child care, and special food, clothing, and other items. Spending on developmental or behavioral therapies is often classified as non-medical and excluded from reimbursement by insurers. Therefore, analyses that are restricted to out-of-pocket medical expenses are likely to substantially understate the degree of financial burden on families with special needs children (Amendah, Grosse, Peacock, & Mandell, 2011; Ganz, 2006).

3.3. Subjective financial burden

Parents' perceptions of the financial impact of having a child with disability or special health care needs have been measured in a number of surveys. For example, a prospective study completed at age of 8 years of a cohort of 219 surviving children with extremely low birthweight born 1992–1995 and 176 children with normal birthweight found significant differences in reported financial impact and caregiver burden using the Impact on Family Scale (Drotar et al., 2006). Specifically, the family impacts were explained by the presence of chronic health conditions, functional limitations, and neurodevelopmental disabilities. In addition, family impacts were greater in families with lower socioeconomic status.

The NS-CSHCN surveys collect information on reported financial problems. In the 2001 survey, approximately 20% of parents of children with special health care needs reported that their child's condition had caused some financial problems (Kogan, Newacheck, Honberg, & Strickland, 2005; Kuhlthau, Hill, Yucel, & Perrin, 2005). The same overall frequency of financial problems was reported in the 2005–2006 NS-CSHCN survey (Kogan et al., 2008). The reported frequency of financial problems was directly linked to the severity of the condition: 38.7% for with ASD, 30.0% for children with other emotional, developmental, or behavioral problems, and 13.7% for other children with special health care needs (Kogan et al., 2008).

The 2005–2006 NS-CSHCN contains several specific measures of financial burden, some of which have been used as indicators of underinsurance. For example, the percent of children who were reported to not always be able to be seen by needed providers because of inadequate insurance was 9.3% for children with special health care needs and 6.2% for the referent group (Honberg, Kogan, Allen, Strickland, & Newacheck, 2009). This measure was elevated only among children with special health care needs who had activity limitations: 10.5% for those with some to moderate limitations and 14.8% among those with serious limitations versus 4.9% among those with no disabling limitation (Honberg et al., 2009). The percent reporting that they needed additional income to cover the child's medical expenditures was 34.9% for families of children with ASD, 25.5% for families of children with other emotional, developmental, or behavioral problems, and 12.6% for other children with special health care needs (Kogan et al., 2008).

3.4. Public benefits and family financial burden

Public benefits can potentially offset the financial burden to families of having a child with Down syndrome or a similar condition. In the past, low-income families in the United States with children could qualify for welfare benefits on a long-term basis under the Aid to Families with Dependent Children (AFDC) program, although this was often transitional to employment. Child disability was found to influence both the probability of transitioning to employment and remaining employed. Acs and Loprest (1999) analyzed 1990 SIPP data and found that mothers with children with disability were significantly less likely to transition from AFDC to employment. Lukemeyer, Meyers, and Smeeding (2000) analyzed a representative sample of California families receiving welfare under the AFDC program in 1993. The percentage of mothers who reported in a second interview during 1995 that they had been employed in the previous month was 39% overall, 29% among those with a child with a disability, and 19% among those with a child with a severe disability. After adjusting for covariates, severe limitations were associated with a 15 percentage point lower probability of employment and, among those employed, a reduction in hours worked by 15 h in the last month. An analysis of NLSY data reported that former welfare recipients were one-third more likely to experience job loss if they had a child with a disability (Earle & Heymann, 2002). Most low-income mothers with a child with a chronic health condition report experiencing either loss of work days or of employment due to their child's condition, regardless of whether they had ever received welfare (Smith et al., 2002).

One of the most important public benefits for families with children with a disability is public health insurance. This includes both Medicaid and the Children's Health Insurance Program (CHIP, formerly known as SCHIP), for families with relatively low incomes but not incomes low enough to qualify for Medicaid. An analysis of 1998 NHIS data found that low-income children with chronic illnesses who were not enrolled in Temporary Assistance for Needy Families (TANF) were three times as likely to lack health insurance (Wise, Wampler, Chavkin, & Romero, 2002).

For children with special health care needs, eligibility for state Medicaid or CHIP coverage has been shown to influence the financial burden experienced by moderate-income families (Parish, Shattuck, & Rose, 2009). A higher-income threshold for eligibility means that more families are eligible. Comparing states in which Medicaid or CHIP eligibility differed by one multiple of the federal poverty level, families with children with special health care needs living in states with the higher Medicaid or CHIP eligibility thresholds were 77% or 68% as likely to have a financial burden that exceeded 3% of family income.

A study of low-income families with children in California during 1995 found that a sizeable minority of families had appreciable out-of-pocket expenses related to child conditions, not taking into account child care expenses (Lukemeyer et al., 2000; Meyers et al., 1998). Overall, 38% of families had out-of-pocket expenses, and among those, 43% (or 16% of the sample) spent more than $100 per month. Overall, only 23% of special expenses were medical. The authors calculated that subtracting special expenses from income would lead to an additional 9% of families being reclassified as being in severe poverty, with income less than 75% of the federal poverty level. Those families whose children were enrolled in Medicaid had significantly lower out-of-pocket expenses than comparable families whose children were either uninsured or covered by private health insurance.

For middle-class families of children with Down syndrome whose incomes are too high to qualify for Medicaid or CHIP, state Medicaid waivers can be an important means of ensuring access to needed services and reducing financial burden to the family. Waivers can allow families to enroll their child in Medicaid and have their medical care or developmental services reimbursed. This can serve as a secondary insurance to help cover expenses not covered by primary private insurance. The best known is the Deeming Waiver, formerly known as the Katie Beckett Waiver. Many children with Down syndrome are on such waivers, which can substantially reduce the financial burden experienced by their parents.

The most important cash benefit for low-income families with a child with Down syndrome is Supplemental Security Income (SSI) payments made by the Social Security Administration (SSA) to caregivers of children younger than age 18 who have disabilities characterized by "marked and severe functional limitations" for at least 12 months. SSI eligibility is based on either a diagnosis such as Down syndrome or the assessment of limitations, but the family must also meet limits on income and assets. Approximately 2% of US adolescents received SSI payments during 2007 (Social Security Administration, 2008). The average monthly SSI payment in December 2007 was $468. In general, a person who qualifies for SSI also qualifies for Medicaid.

Data on SSI beneficiaries are available from the 2001–2002 National Survey of SSI Children and Families (NSCF), a nationally representative survey of children (aged 17 and under) and young adults (aged 18–23) receiving SSI at the end of 2000 or who previously received or applied for SSI payments and were not currently institutionalized. Approximately 50% in each age group were either Black or multiracial and 64% were male. A mental disability was reported by 56% of children aged 6–12 years and 59% of adolescents, but no specific medical diagnoses were reported in the SSA tabulations. Half of all children receiving SSI payments lived in a family with no earner, and only one of six lived in a family earning more than $2000 per month during 2001 (Rupp et al., 2005–2006). On average, SSI payments accounted for 50% of family income. Most have public health insurance that covers all or almost all health care needs. More than two-thirds of families reported no out-of-pocket medical expenses for the child's health care in the previous year, and among those who did, median expenses were $200.

The California survey of AFDC families showed a strongly protective effect of SSI on the income adequacy of low-income families with eligible children. Among families with a severely disabled child, the percentage with income below 75% of the federal poverty level was 68.9% among those in which no child received SSI benefits (about half of the total) and 6.6% for families in which at least one child received SSI benefits (Lukemeyer et al., 2000; Meyers et al., 1998). The latter families were economically better off relative to families in the sample who had either a child with mild-to-moderate disability or no child with a disability, for whom 62.7 and 62.3% had equivalently low family incomes. Receipt of SSI benefits can also reduce the financial pressure on a single parent to work and is reported to be associated with significantly reduced probability of paid employment and hours of work among low-income single parents (Loprest & Davidoff, 2004).

To summarize, health insurance and transfer programs can help protect vulnerable families of children with severe disabilities from financial stress. Public health insurance is particularly beneficial because of low out-of-pocket payments and coverage for developmental services that are often not covered by private health plans. Consequently, families whose children are eligible for Medicaid or CHIP, based on either income or disability waivers, are less likely to incur high out-of-pocket expenditures as a percentage of income. The most protective transfer program is SSI, which provides cash payments to lower-income families to help cover various expenses associated with caring for a child with a severe disability.

4. Conclusions

Families with a child with Down syndrome, like those with children who have other serious disabilities and chronic health conditions, are at risk of experiencing financial stress as a result of parental caregiving demands and the need for money to pay for services not covered by insurance or public programs. Often, caregiving demands lead to lower frequency or intensity of paid employment among mothers, although this may be less likely among more highly educated mothers and those living in families with higher incomes. In particular, mothers of the most severely affected children with multiple disabilities or requiring intensive medical supervision are the least likely to be engaged in full-time employment. The study findings summarized in this chapter are quite heterogeneous. Some investigators have reported differences in employment probabilities but not hours of work among those who are employed, others have reported differences in hours but not in labor force participation, and many have reported impacts on both. Some studies have reported larger impacts on maternal employment in two-parent families and others in single-parent families. Although it is difficult to generalize about the magnitude of lost earnings for parents of children with disabilities, the majority of studies have found important effects. Mothers of younger school-age children with developmental disabilities in particular are typically reported to have 15–50% lower probability of employment than mothers of other children of the same ages.

Measures of financial burden and underinsurance show that families of children with special needs or disabilities in the United States are at elevated risk of financial hardship. This is particularly true for lower-income families, since family wealth and income can buffer the economic impact on the family of ill health and disability. Public health insurance is associated with lower measures of underinsurance and financial burden, holding income constant. SSI is particularly helpful for low-income families that qualify.

The degree of economic burden experienced by Down syndrome families may be somewhat less than for those of children with disabilities because they often have greater material resources and social advantages relative to other families who have children with special needs, which may account for the so-called Down syndrome advantage (Cahill & Glidden, 1996). Few studies, though, have compared the financial impacts on families of having a child with Down syndrome relative to those with other special needs. Also, studies have not quantified the financial impact on American families who chose to enroll a child with Down syndrome in intensive (and expensive) behavioral therapies not reimbursed by health insurers.

A meeting held in November 2007 sought to frame a public health research agenda for Down syndrome (Rasmussen et al., 2008). The non-federal participants identified roughly 20 priorities for research. One mentioned health insurance and developmental or educational services (p. 3004): "More information is also needed on the effect of services and supports, such as health insurance, day care, education, and developmental services, on the quality of life (e.g., well-being, functioning, and finances) of families and persons with DS." The economic impact of Down syndrome on families was not mentioned as a consideration, nor was there consideration of potential policies to mitigate those economic impacts. Despite an impressive amount of epidemiologic research on birth defects, relatively little is known, other than one recently published study, about the economic characteristics of American families who have children with Down syndrome (Schieve et al., 2009), and virtually nothing is known about their out-of-pocket spending on services, particularly therapies not covered by health insurance.

Acknowledgments

Cynthia Hinton, Cynthia Moore, Lijing Ouyang, Patricia Pastor, Sonja Rasmussen, Laura Schieve, Mike Soucie, and Mick Tilford all provided helpful comments. Full responsibility for any errors rests with the author.

Disclaimer: The findings and conclusions in this chapter are those of the authors and do not necessarily represent the official position of the Centers for Disease Control and Prevention.

REFERENCES

Down syndrome epidemiology

Besser, L. M., Shin, M., Kucik, J. E., & Correa, A. (2007). Prevalence of Down syndrome among children and adolescents in metropolitan Atlanta. *Birth Defects Research (Part A), 79*, 765–774.

Bishop, J., Huether, C. A., Torfs, C., Lorey, F., & Deddens, J. (1997). Epidemiologic study of Down syndrome in a racially diverse California population, 1989–1991. *American Journal of Epidemiology, 145*, 134–147.

Cahill, B. M., & Glidden, L. M. (1996). Influence of child diagnosis on family and parental functioning: Down syndrome versus other disabilities. *American Journal of Mental Retardation, 101*, 149–160.

Canfield, M. A., Honein, M. A., Yuskiv, N., Xing, J., Mai, C. T., Collins, J. S., et al. (2006). National estimates and race/ethnic-specific variation of selected birth defects in the United States, 1999–2001. *Birth Defects Research (Part A), 76*, 747–756.

Carr, J., & Hewett, S. (1982). Children with Down syndrome growing up. *Association of Child Psychology and Psychiatry News, 4*, 10–13.

Corrice, A. M., & Glidden, L. M. (2009). The Down syndrome advantage: Fact or fiction? *American Journal of Intellectual and Developmental Disability, 114*, 254–268.

Croen, L. A., Grether, J. K., & Selvin, S. (2001). The epidemiology of mental retardation of unknown cause. *Pediatrics, 107*, E86.

Cunningham, C. C. (1996). Families of children with Down syndrome. *Down Syndrome Research and Practice, 4*, 87–95.

Decouflé, P., Boyle, C. A., Paulozzi, L. J., & Lary, J. M. (2001). Increased risk for developmental disabilities in children who have major birth defects: A population-based study.*Pediatrics, 108*, 728–734.

Doria-Rose, V. P., Kim, H. S., Augustine, E. T., & Edwards, K. L. (2003). Parity and the risk of Down's syndrome. *American Journal of Epidemiology, 158*, 503–508.

Drews, C. D., Yeargin-Allsopp, M., Decouflé, P., & Murphy, C. C. (1995). Variation in the influence of selected sociodemographic risk factors for mental retardation. *American Journal of Public Health, 85*, 329–334.

Dzurova, D., & Pikhart, H. (2005). Down syndrome, paternal age and education: Comparison of California and the Czech Republic. *BMC Public Health, 5*, 69.

Ericson, A., Eriksson, M., & Zetterstrom, R. (1984). The incidence of congenital malformations in various socio-occupational groups in Sweden. *Acta Paediatrica Scandinavica, 73*, 664–666.

Forrester, M. B., & Merz, R. D. (2002). Epidemiology of Down syndrome (Trisomy 21), Hawaii, 1986–97. *Teratology, 65*, 207–212.

Freeman, S. B., Bean, L. H., Allen, E. G., Tinker, S. W., Locke, A. E., Druschel, C., et al. (2008). Ethnicity, sex, and the incidence of congenital heart defects: A report from the National Down Syndrome Project. *Genetics in Medicine, 10*, 173–180.

Frohnert, B. K., Lussky, R. C., Alms, M. A., Mendelsohn, N. J., Symonik, D. M., & Falken, M. C. (2005). Validity of hospital discharge data for identifying infants with cardiac defects. *Journal of Perinatology, 25*, 737–742.

Fujiura, G. T. (1998). Demography of family households. *American Journal on Mental Retardation, 103*, 225–235.

Gath, A., & Gumley, D. (1986). Family background of children with Down's syndrome and of children with a similar degree of mental retardation. *British Journal of Psychiatry, 149*, 161–171.

Hodapp, R. M., Ly, T. M., Fidler, D. J., & Ricci, L. A. (2001). Less stress, more rewarding: Parenting children with Down syndrome. *Parenting: Science and Practice, 1*, 317–337.

Hodapp, R. M., & Urbano, R. C. (2008). Demographics of African-American vs. European-heritage mothers of newborns with Down syndrome. *Journal of Policy and Practice in Intellectual Disability, 5*, 187–193.

Hodapp, R. M., & Urbano, R. C. (2009). Using large-scale databases to examine families of children with intellectual and developmental disabilities. In *International review of research in mental retardation* (vol. 37, pp. 131–177). Elsevier.

Hodapp, R. M., Urbano, R. C., & Rosenbloom, S. T. (2008). Mothers of newborns with Down syndrome: Demographic characteristics. Unpublished paper. Nashville, TN: Vanderbilt University.

Hook, E. B., Carothers, A. D., & Hecht, C. A. (1999). Elevated maternal age-specific rates of Down syndrome liveborn offspring of women of Mexican and Central American origin in California. *Prenatal Diagnosis, 19*, 245–251.

Huether, C. A., Ivanovich, J., Goodwin, B. S., Krivchenia, E. L., Hertzberg, V. S., Edmonds, L. D., et al. (1998). Maternal age specific risk rate estimates for Down syndrome among live births in whites and other races from Ohio and metropolitan Atlanta, 1970–1989. *Journal of Medical Genetics, 35*, 482–490.

Khoshnood, B., De Vigan, C., Vodovar, V., Bréart, G., Goffinet, F., & Blondel, B. (2006). Advances in medical technology and creation of disparities: The case of Down syndrome. *American Journal of Public Health, 96*, 2139–2144.

Khoshnood, B., Pryde, P., Blondel, B., & Lee, K. S. (2003). Socioeconomic and state-level differences in prenatal diagnosis and live birth prevalence of Down's syndrome in the United States. *Revue d'Epidemiologie et Sante Publique, 51*, 617–627.

Knox, E. G., & Lancashire, R. J. (1991). *Frequencies and social variations. Epidemiology of congenital malformations*. London: HMSO.

Kuppermann, M., Learman, L. A., Gates, E., Gregorich, S. E., Nease, R. F. Jr., Lewis, J., et al. (2006). Beyond race or ethnicity and socioeconomic status: Predictors of prenatal testing for Down syndrome. *Obstetrics and Gynecology, 107*, 1087–1097.

Lopez, P. M., Stone, D., & Gilmour, H. (1995). Epidemiology of Down's syndrome in a Scottish city. *Paediatric and Perinatal Epidemiology, 9*, 331–340.

Miller, J. E., Gaboda, D., & Davis, D. (2001). Early childhood chronic illness: Comparability of maternal reports and medical records. *Vital Health Statistics Series 2, Data evaluation and methods research, 131*, 1–10.

Most, D. E., Fidler, D. J., Booth-LaForce, C., & Kelly, J. (2006). Stress trajectories in mothers of young children with Down syndrome. *Journal of Intellectual Disability Research, 50*, 501–514.

Rasmussen, S. A., Mulinare, J., Khoury, M. J., & Maloney, E. K. (1990). Evaluation of birth defect histories obtained through maternal interviews). *American Journal of Human Genetics, 46*, 478–485.

Rasmussen, S. A., Whitehead, N., Collier, S. A., & Frías, J. L. (2008). Setting a public health research agenda for Down syndrome: Summary of a meeting sponsored by the

Centers for Disease Control and Prevention and the National Down Syndrome Society. *American Journal of Medical Genetics (Part A), 146A*, 2998–3010.

Rasmussen, S. A., Wong, L. Y., Correa, A., Gambrell, D., & Friedman, J. M. (2006). Survival in infants with Down syndrome, Metropolitan Atlanta, 1979–1998. *Journal of Pediatrics, 148*, 806–812.

Rosano, A., Del Bufalo, E., & Burgio, A. (2008). Status socio-economico e occorrenza di malformazioni congenite. *Epidemiologia e Prevenzione, 32*, 21–26.

Schieve, L. A., Boulet, S. L., Boyle, C., Rasmussen, S. A., & Schendel, D. (2009). Health of children 3 to 17 years of age with Down syndrome in the 1997–2005 National Health Interview Survey. *Pediatrics, 123*, e253–e260.

Seltzer, M. M., Krauss, M. W., & Tsunematsu, N. (1993). Adults with Down syndrome and their aging mothers: Diagnostic group differences. *American Journal of Mental Retardation, 97*, 496–508.

Shepperdson, B. (1985). Changes in the characteristics of families with Down's syndrome children. *Journal of Epidemiology and Community Health, 39*, 320–324.

Sherman, S. L., Allen, E. G., Bean, L. H., & Freeman, S. B. (2007). Epidemiology of Down syndrome. *Mental Retardation and Developmental Disabilities Research Reviews, 13*, 221–227.

Shin, M., Besser, L. M., Kucik, J. E., Lu, C., Siffel, C., & Correa, A. (2009). Prevalence of Down syndrome among children and adolescents in 10 regions of the United States. *Pediatrics, 124*, 1565–1571.

Siffel, C., Correa, A., Cragan, J., & Alverson, C. J. (2004). Prenatal diagnosis, pregnancy terminations and prevalence of Down syndrome in Atlanta. *Birth Defects Research (Part A), 70*, 565–571.

Torfs, C. P., & Christianson, R. E. (2003). Socioeconomic effects on the risk of having a recognized pregnancy with Down syndrome. *Birth Defects Research (Part A), 67*, 522–528.

Urbano, R.C, & Hodapp, R. M. (2007). Divorce in families of children with Down syndrome: A population-based study. *American Journal of Mental Retardation, 112*, 261–274.

Vrijheid, M., Dolk, H., Stone, D., Abramsky, L., Alberman, E., & Scott, J. E. (2000). Socioeconomic inequalities in risk of congenital anomaly. *Archives of Diseases of Childhood, 82*, 349–352.

Yang, Q., Rasmussen, S. A., & Friedman, J. M. (2002). Mortality associated with Down's syndrome in the USA from 1983 to 1997: A population-based study. *Lancet, 359*, 1019–1025.

Family economic impacts of child disability

Abbeduto, L., Seltzer, M. M., Shattuck, P., Krauss, M. W., Orsmond, G., & Murphy, M. M. (2004). Psychological well-being and coping in mothers of youths with autism, Down syndrome, or fragile X syndrome. *American Journal of Mental Retardation, 109*, 237–254.

Acs, G., & Loprest, P. (1999). The effect of disabilities on exits from AFDC. *Journal of Policy Analysis and Management, 18*, 28–49.

Amendah, D., Grosse, S. D., Peacock, G., & Mandell, D. S. (2011). The economic costs of autism: A review. In D. G. Amaral, G. Dawson, & D. H. Geschwind (Eds.) *Autism Spectrum Disorders*, in press. New York: Oxford University Press.

Anderson, D., Dumont, S., Jacobs, P., & Azzaria, L. (2007). The personal costs of caring for a child with a disability: A review of the literature. *Public Health Reports, 122*, 3–16.

Barnett, W. S., & Boyce, G. C. (1995). Effects of children with Down syndrome on parents' activities. *American Journal of Mental Retardation, 100*, 115–127.

Blau, F., & Grossberg, A. (1992). Maternal labor supply and children's cognitive development. *Review of Economics and Statistics, 74*, 474–481.

Blewett, L. A., Ward, A, & Beebe, T. J. (2006). How much health insurance is enough? Revisiting the concept of underinsurance. *Medical Care Research and Review, 63*, 663–700.

Booth, C. L., & Kelly, J. F. (1999). Child care and employment in relation to infants' disabilities and risk factors. *American Journal of Mental Retardation, 104*, 117–130.

Boulet, S. L., Molinari, N. A., Grosse, S. D., Honein, M. A., & Correa-Villaseñor, A. (2008). Health care expenditures for infants and young children with Down syndrome in a privately insured population. *Journal of Pediatrics, 153*, 241–246.

Brehaut, J. C., Kohen, D. E., Raina, P., Walter, S. D., Russell, D. J., Swinton, M., et al. (2004). The health of primary caregivers of children with cerebral palsy: How does it compare with that of other Canadian caregivers? *Pediatrics, 114*, e182–e191.

Breslau, N., Salkever, D., & Staruch, K. S. (1982). Women's labor force activity and responsibilities for disabled dependents: A study of families with disabled children. *Journal of Health and Social Behavior, 23*, 169–183.

Brouwer, W. B. F., van Exel, N. J. A., & Tilford, J. M. (2009). Incorporating caregiver and family effects in economic evaluations of child health. In W. Ungar (Ed.) *Economic Evaluation in Child Health* (pp. 55–76). New York: Oxford University Press.

Corman, H., Noonan, K., & Reichman, N. E. (2005). Mothers' labor supply in fragile families: The role of child health. *Eastern Economic Journal, 31*, 601–616.

Crowe, T. K. (1993). Time use of mothers with young children: The impact of a child's disability. *Developmental Medicine & Child Neurology, 35*, 621–630.

Crowe, T. K., & Florez, S. I. (2006). Time use of mothers with school-age children: A continuing impact of a child's disability. *American Journal of Occupational Therapy, 60*, 194–203.

Curran, A. L., Sharples, P. M., White, C., & Knapp, M. (2001). Time costs of caring for children with severe disabilities compared with caring for children without disabilities. *Developmental Medicine & Child Neurology, 43*, 529–533.

Davidoff, A. (2004). Identifying children with special health care needs in the National Health Interview Survey: A new resource for policy analysis. *Health Services Research, 39*, 53–71.

Drews, C. D., Yeargin-Allsopp, M., Decouflé, P., & Murphy, C. C. (1995). Variation in the influence of selected sociodemographic risk factors for mental retardation. *American Journal of Public Health, 85*, 329–334.

Drotar, D., Hack, M., Taylor, G., Schluchter, M., Andreias, L., & Klein, N. (2006). The impact of extremely low birth weight on the families of school-aged children. *Pediatrics, 117*, 2006–2013.

Earle, A., & Heymann, S. J. (2002). What causes job loss among former welfare recipients: The role of family health problems. *Journal of the American Medical Women's Association, 57*, 5–10.

Einam, M, & Cuskelly, M. (2002). Paid employment of mothers and fathers of an adult child with multiple disabilities. *Journal of Intellectual Disability Research, 46*, 158–167.

Emerson, E. (2007). Poverty and people with intellectual disabilities. *Mental Retardation and Developmental Disabilities Research Reviews, 13*, 107–113.

Freedman, R. I., Litchfield, L. C., & Warfield, M. E. (1995). Balancing work and family: Perspectives of parents of children with developmental disabilities. *Families in Society: The Journal of Contemporary Human Services, 76*, 507–514.

Galbraith, A. A., Wong, S. T., Kim, S. E., & Newacheck, P. W. (2005). Out-of-pocket financial burden for low-income families with children: Socioeconomic disparities and effects of insurance. *Health Services Research, 40*, 1722–1736.

Gallimore, R., Coots, J., Weisner, T., Garnier, H., & Guthrie, D. (1996). Family responses to children with early developmental delays. II: Accommodation intensity and activity in early and middle childhood. *American Journal of Mental Retardation, 101*, 215–232.

Ganz, M. L. (2006). The costs of autism. In S. Moldin, & J. Rubenstein (Eds.) *Understanding autism: From neuroscience to treatment* (pp. 476–502). Boca Raton, FL: Taylor and Francis Group.

Gordon, M., Rosenman, L., & Cuskelly, M. (2007). Constrained labour: Maternal employment when children have disabilities. *Journal of Applied Research in Intellectual Disabilities, 20*, 236–246.

Gould, E. (2004). Decomposing the effects of children's health on mother's labor supply: Is it time or money? *Health Economics, 13*, 525–541.
Grosse, S. D., Flores, A. L., Ouyang, L., Robbins, J. M., & Tilford, J. M. (2009). Impact of spina bifida on parental caregivers: Findings from a survey of Arkansas families. *Journal of Child and Family Studies, 18*, 574–581.
Heck, K. E., & Makuc, D. M. (2000). Parental employment and health insurance coverage among school-aged children with special health care needs. *American Journal of Public Health, 90*, 1856–1860.
Hedov, G., Anneren, G., & Wikblad, K. (2002). Swedish parents of children with Down's syndrome. *Scandinavian Journal of Caring Sciences, 16*, 424–430.
Hedov, G., Wikblad, K., & Anneren, G. (2006). Sickness absence in Swedish parents of children with Down's syndrome: Relation to self-perceived health, stress and sense of coherence. *Journal of Intellectual Disability Research, 50*, 546–552.
Honberg, L. E., Kogan, M. D., Allen, D., Strickland, B. B., & Newacheck, P. W. (2009). Progress in ensuring adequate health insurance for children with special health care needs. *Pediatrics, 124*, 1273–1280.
Järbrink, K. (2007). The economic consequences of autistic spectrum disorder among children in a Swedish municipality. *Autism, 11*, 453–463.
Järbrink, K., McCrone, P., Fombonne, E., Zandén, H., & Knapp, M. (2007). Cost-impact of young adults with high-functioning autistic spectrum disorder. *Research in Developmental Disabilities, 28*, 94–104.
Kogan, M. D., Newacheck, P. W., Honberg, L., & Strickland, B. (2005). Association between underinsurance and access to care among children with special health care needs in the United States. *Pediatrics, 116*, 1162–1169.
Kogan, M. D., Strickland, B. B., Blumberg, S. J., Singh, G. K., Perrin, J. M., & van Dyck, P. C. (2008). A national profile of the health care experiences and family impact of autism spectrum disorder among children in the United States, 2005–2006. *Pediatrics, 122*, e1149–e1158.
Kuhlthau, K. A., Hill, K. S., Yucel, R., & Perrin, J. M. (2005). Financial burden for families of children with special health care needs. *Maternal and Child Health Journal, 9*, 207–218.
Kuhlthau, K. A., & Perrin, J. M. (2001). Child health status and parental employment. *Archives of Pediatrics and Adolescent Medicine, 155*, 1346–1350.
Landis, L. J. (1992). Marital, employment and child care status of mothers with infants and toddlers with disabilities. *Topics in Early Childhood Special Education, 12*, 496–507.
Leonard, B., Brust, J. D., & Sapienza, J. (1992). Financial and time costs to parents of severely disabled children. *Public Health Reports, 107*, 302–312.
Loprest, P., & Davidoff, A. (2004). How children with special health care needs affect the employment decisions of low-income parents. *Maternal and Child Health Journal, 8*, 171–182.
Lukemeyer, A., Meyers, M., & Smeeding, T. (2000). Expensive children in poor families: Out-of-pocket expenditures for the care of disabled and chronically ill children in welfare families. *Journal of Marriage and the Family, 62*, 399–415.
Merlis, M. (2002). Family out-of-pocket spending for health services: A continuing source of financial insecurity. The Commonwealth Fund, publication number 509. Retrieved February 1, 2010, from http://www.commonwealthfund.org/~/media/Files/Publications/Fund%20Report/2002/Jun/Family%20Out%20of%20Pocket%20Spending%20for%20Health%20Services%20%20A%20Continuing%20Source%20of%20Financial%20Insecurity/merlis_oopspending_509%20pdf.pdf
Meyers, M., Lukemeyer, A., & Smeeding, T. (1998). The cost of caring: Childhood disability in poor families. *Social Service Review, 72*, 209–233.
Montes, G., & Halterman, J. (2006). Characteristics of school-age children with autism. *Journal of Developmental & Behavioral Pediatrics, 27*, 379–385.

Montes, G., & Halterman, J. S. (2008a). Association of childhood autism spectrum disorders and loss of family income. *Pediatrics*, *121*, e821–e826.

Montes, G., & Halterman, J. S. (2008b). Child care problems and employment among families with preschool-aged children with autism in the United States. *Pediatrics*, *122*, e202–208.

Newacheck, P. W., & Halfon, N. (1986). The financial burden of medical care expenses for children. *Medical Care*, *24*, 1110–1117.

Newacheck, P. W., Inkelas M, & Kim, S. E. (2004). Health services use and health care expenditures for children with disabilities. *Pediatrics*, *114*, 79–85.

Newacheck, P. W., & Kim, S. E. (2005). A national profile of health care utilization and expenditures for children with special health care needs. *Archives of Pediatric and Adolescent Medicine*, *159*, 10–17.

Norberg, K. (1998). The effects of daycare reconsidered. NBER Working Paper No. 6769. Cambridge, MA.

Okumura, M. J., Van Cleave, J., Gnanasekaran, S., & Houtrow, A. (2009). Understanding factors associated with work loss for families caring for CSHCN. *Pediatrics*, *124*, S392–S398.

Oswald, D. P., Bodurtha, J. N., Broadus, C. H., Willis, J. H., Tlusty, S. M., Bellin, M. H., et al. (2005). Defining underinsurance among children with special health care needs: A Virginia sample. *Maternal and Child Health Journal*, *9*, S67–S74.

Ouyang, L., Grosse, S. D., Armour, B. S., & Waitzman, N. J. (2007). Health care expenditures of children and adults with spina bifida in a privately insured U.S. population. *Birth Defects Research (Part A)*, *79*, 552–558.

Ouyang, L., Grosse, S. D., & Kenneson, A. (2008). Health care utilization and expenditures for children and young adults with muscular dystrophy in a privately insured population. *Journal of Child Neurology*, *23*, 883–888.

Parish, S. L., & Cloud, J. M. (2006). Financial well-being of young children with disabilities and their families. *Social Work*, *51*, 223–232.

Parish, S. L., Seltzer, M. M., Greenberg, J. S., & Floyd, F. (2004). Economic implications of caregiving at midlife: Comparing parents with and without children who have developmental disabilities. *Mental Retardation*, *42*, 413–426.

Parish, S. L., Shattuck, P. T., & Rose, R. A. (2009). Financial burden of raising CSHCN: Association with state policy choices. *Pediatrics*, *124*, S435–S442.

Porterfield, S. L. (2002). Work choices of mothers in families with children with disabilities. *Journal of Marriage and the Family*, *64*, 972–981.

Porterfield, S.L., & Tracey, C. (2003). Disentangling the dynamics of family poverty and child disability: Does disability come first? Working Paper No. 03–01. Center for Social Development, Washington University, St. Louis, MO. Retrieved February 14, 2009, from http://csd.wustl.edu/Publications/Documents/WP03-01.pdf.

Powers, E. T. (2001). New estimates of the impact of child disability on maternal employment. *American Economic Review*, *91*, 135–139.

Powers, E. T. (2003). Children's health and maternal work activity: Estimates under alternative disability definitions. *Journal of Human Resources*, *38*, 522–556.

Reichman, N. E., Corman, H., & Noonan, K. (2004). Effects of child health on parents' relationship status. *Demography*, *41*, 569–584.

Reichman, N. E., Corman, H., & Noonan, K. (2008). Impact of child disability on the family. *Maternal and Child Health Journal*, *12*, 679–683.

Roach, M. A., Orsmond, G. I., & Barratt, M. S. (1999). Mothers and fathers of children with Down syndrome: Parental stress and involvement in childcare. *American Journal of Mental Retardation*, *104*, 422–436.

Rupp, K., Davies, P. S., Newcomb, C., Iams, H., Becker, C., Mulpuru, S., et al. (2005–2006). A profile of children with disabilities receiving SSI: Highlights from the National Survey of SSI Children and Families. *Social Security Bulletin*, *66*, 21–48.

Salkever, D. (1982). Children's health problems and maternal work status. *Journal of Human Resources*, *17*, 94–109.
Seltzer, M. M., Greenberg, J. S., Floyd, F. J., Pettee, Y., & Hong, J. (2001). Life course impacts of parenting a child with a disability. *American Journal of Mental Retardation*, *106*, 265–286.
Shearn, J., & Todd, S. (2000). Maternal employment and family responsibilities: The perspectives of mothers of children with intellectual disabilities. *Journal of Applied Research in Intellectual Disabilities*, *13*, 109–131.
Smith, L. A., Romero, D., Wood, P. R., Wampler, N. S., Chavkin, W., & Wise, P. H. (2002). Employment barriers among welfare recipients and applicants with chronically ill children. *American Journal of Public Health*, *92*, 1453–1457.
Social Security Administration. (2008). *SSI Annual Statistical Report, 2007*. Retrieved February 12, 2009, from http://www.ssa.gov/policy/docs/statcomps/ssi_asr/.
Stade, B., Ungar, W. J., Stevens, B., Beyene, J., & Koren, G. (2006). The burden of prenatal exposure to alcohol: Measurement of cost. *Journal of FAS International*, *4*, e5. Available from: http://www.motherisk.org/JFAS_documents/JFAS_6005_e5.pdf.
Tilford, J. M., Grosse, S. D., Goodman, A. C., & Li, K. (2009). Labor market productivity costs for caregivers of children with spina bifida: A population-based analysis. *Medical Decision Making*, *29*, 23–32.
Tilford, J. M., Grosse, S. D., Robbins, J. M., Pyne, J. M., Cleves, M. A., & Hobbs, C. A. (2005). Health state preference scores of children with spina bifida and their caregivers. *Quality of Life Research*, *14*, 1087–1098.
Tilford, J. M., Robbins, J. M., & Hobbs, C. A. (2001). Improving estimates of caregiver time cost and family impact associated with birth defects. *Teratology*, *64*, S37–S41.
Warfield, M. E. (2001). Employment, parenting, and well-being among mothers of children with disabilities. *Mental Retardation*, *39*, 297–309.
Wise, P. H., Wampler, N. S., Chavkin, W., & Romero, D. (2002). Chronic illness among poor children enrolled in the Temporary Assistance for Needy Families program. *American Journal of Public Health*, *92*, 1458–1461.
Wolfe, B. L., & Hill, S. C. (1995). The effect of health on the work effort of single mothers. *Journal of Human Resources*, *30*, 42–62.
Yu, H., Dick, A. W., & Szilagyi, P. G. (2008). Does public insurance provide better financial protection against rising health care costs for families of children with special health care needs? *Medical Care*, *46*, 1064–1070.

Other Issues

CHAPTER TEN

Health Research, the Needs of Persons with Down Syndrome and Their Families

Susan J. Buckley

Contents

Abstract

Advances in general medicine, in particular antibiotics and pediatric cardiac surgery, have dramatically increased survival and longevity for individuals with Down syndrome. Studies focused on identifying their specific healthcare needs have led to screening and preventative healthcare programmes. However, it is argued that reviews of the increased likelihood of a range of illnesses can be both frightening and not practically helpful to parents. Many children with Down syndrome are as healthy as their siblings. Individuals with Down syndrome vary widely on all family, health, and development characteristics and, as yet, the health data does not reflect these differences when discussing risk. Researchers are urged to think carefully before writing and presenting data, checking its validity in the real world, and recognizing parents will be in the audience. There is still a need to inform healthcare professionals of the potential of individuals with Down syndrome.

Department of Psychology, Down Syndrome Education International, University of Portsmouth, UK

International Review of Research in Mental Retardation, Volume 39
ISSN 0074-7750, DOI 10.1016/S0074-7750(10)39010-0

1. Health Research, the Needs of Individuals with Down Syndrome and Their Families

It is a privilege to be asked to contribute an overview to this special issue from the perspective of the parent of a daughter with Down syndrome, now 40 years of age, as well as a professional researcher and practitioner in the field. My experience as a clinical psychologist and researcher spans the period from before education was a right for children with Down syndrome in the USA or the UK and before early intervention services and community services developed. I spent the first years of my career working in large institutions where the quality of care and quality of life for residents was extremely poor. We have come a long way since the 1960s but we also still have a way to go. There is still plenty of room for improvement in early intervention and educational opportunities—my particular areas of expertise—even in the most developed countries of the world. Taking an international perspective, access to even basic healthcare and education is still not available to the majority of children born with Down syndrome.

2. The Contribution of Medicine

Advances in medical care have dramatically improved the quality of life and life span of most individuals with Down syndrome in the last 40 years in the developed countries. In fact, it could be argued that these advances have made the most significant difference to their lives and those of their families, over and above the changes in attitudes, early intervention, and educational opportunities. A number of the authors in this volume identify that survival rates have increased as has length of life and provide the detailed data to support these facts. The two most significant advances have been the advent of antibiotics and the development of pediatric cardiology—since the two most significant causes of death were respiratory illnesses and cardiac defects. These can now be treated successfully for the majority of children and adults.

There have been two main steps forward driven by medical practitioners and clinical research. The first has been due to the increased understanding and improvements in the ability to treat a wide range of illnesses throughout the population. In other words, children and adults with Down syndrome have benefitted enormously from general advances in healthcare for everyone. Effective treatments are usually the same for individuals with Down syndrome as they are for any other person in the population with the same or similar condition.

The second has been a growing interest in the specific range of healthcare needs that may be more common among individuals with Down syndrome. This allows physicians and families to be aware and alert for the symptoms of these conditions. Most importantly, it enables preventative care and early detection systems to be put in place. The development of specialist Down Syndrome Clinics in a number of countries has given the physicians working in these settings a wealth of experience of the particular healthcare and social needs of individuals with Down syndrome and their families. Treatments for individual conditions may be the same as when they occur in others, but the pattern of multiple health care and management needs which may arise benefit from a specialist overview. The Down Syndrome Medical Interest Groups (DSMIG) formed by these physicians with a special interest in Down syndrome have led to preventative healthcare guidelines being developed and accepted by the medical professions in a number of countries, with the USA DSMIG leading the way.

None of this information was available when my daughter was born in 1969 and she received no specialist healthcare, screening, or early intervention services. When babies with Down syndrome were born 40 years ago, cardiac defects were often missed or identified but not corrected, hearing losses and thyroid deficiencies went undetected. We were fortunate, as my daughter had no heart defects. She did have a chronic "runny nose" until the age of 5 years but was otherwise as healthy as her siblings. She has never been an inpatient in hospital and, until she reached 32 years of age, had no particular healthcare needs at all. (She developed arthritis in one of her hips at 32 but according to her expert consultant it has progressed more slowly and caused less pain than would be expected for a person without Down syndrome. Last year she developed inflammatory bowel syndrome which has responded extremely well to the same drug treatments as would be given to anyone else). This raises for me an important question—how do parents make sense of all the information on possible health conditions and risks?

3. Some Cautions

Most of the chapters in this volume provide extensive and detailed reviews of the available information on medical conditions that can occur for individuals with Down syndrome. They tend to focus on those that occur more frequently for this population when compared to those without Down syndrome. However, this data is very difficult to make sense of as a parent. The first observation is that much of the data is very imprecise. Estimates of the risk of a particular condition occurring vary widely from study to study. The reviews in this volume do not give details of the sample sizes or how representative of the population they are for the studies mentioned. In addition, a parent or healthcare practitioner needs to know how likely it is that a particular child will get a condition. I would argue the only way to express this meaningfully is that the risk is 1 in *x* children or adults (specifying by age and gender if at all possible). A percentage increase in risk is meaningless to a parent and can be needlessly very worrying. There is a need for authors of medical review chapters – often written for other medical practitioners—to think about interpreting the actual, practical significance of the statistics in their chapters for parents and other health professionals.

Authors in this volume rightly suggest that parents of new babies with Down syndrome need accurate information on their healthcare needs. I would agree but this is actually difficult to do without being unnecessarily frightening. No one with a newborn infant without Down syndrome is given a list of the chances their child may get any particular illness even though we could do this. Many infants and young children with Down syndrome are healthy and happy, some are very sick and this will often be obvious from birth, and others have illnesses of varying severity.

I recently attended an educational meeting in a local maternity hospital. The audience was a range of healthcare professionals, including obstetricians, midwives, pediatricians, and geneticists plus students from these specialties. The aim was to update and inform them on the lives of infants and children with Down syndrome and they heard from parents, from specialists in providing screening and counselling information, and from a community pediatrician. The community pediatrician provides healthcare for the children from birth through to 18 years of age. She is a caring and very competent doctor and a champion for children with Down syndrome. However, she presented a set of slides which listed all the possible illnesses for which a child with Down syndrome was at extra risk. It was extremely depressing and certainly I sat there thinking that for those listening it would only support the view that their lives are so blighted by health problems, may be termination programmes are justified. I also sat there thinking of the 120 pre-school children we see regularly at any one time in our early intervention service—happy and usually well children, smiling, communicating, walking, playing, socializing—much loved and bringing much joy to their families—and wondered how we could present the health and illness information in a more balanced, accurate, and real way.

Not every child with Down syndrome is sick. Not every child has multiple additional health problems, yet reading the medical chapters in this volume would really depress most parents, especially those with infants, as it is almost impossible for them to work out what is relevant for their child—what the real risk of their child having any of these conditions at all actually is, or more than one at any one time. May be even more importantly, families with a pre-natal diagnosis and considering whether they continue the pregnancy and all the professionals who give them information and counselling, need much better presentation of all this medical risk information.

This brings us to the value of databases and health records. We need to know how illnesses co-occur in order to evaluate the real health experiences and quality of life of individuals with Down syndrome. Many children and adults are largely happy and healthy in my experience. The most important issues for the majority are ensuring that they receive the same healthcare as for the rest of the population, that is, the usual vaccination and immunization programmes, screening and treatment for any vision and hearing impairments, and, in addition, screening for thyroid dysfunction.

Although infants and children with Down syndrome are at increased risk of a range of illnesses, if they are actually suffering from any of them, the first signs will be actual symptoms—usually the same symptoms as any other child would experience—and the treatments will typically be the same. This is equally true of adult ill health. If there are potentially different responses to treatment, the specialist consultant will usually be aware of this as is highlighted in the chapter on cancers.

4. The Responsibilities of Researchers

If we consider the issues for the older persons with Down syndrome, the story of dementia is salutary. The chapter on dementia in this volume gives a very accurate review of current knowledge and the facts show that only a minority of adults have dementia at the end of their lives. I have a powerful memory of sitting in a conference attended by professionals and parents and hearing a pathologist tell us that everyone, 100% of adults with Down syndrome, would get dementia, based on the study of a small number of brains. I looked at the faces of the parents with babies with Down syndrome in their arms and I felt very, very angry. I felt that if I had heard this talk when my baby was only weeks or months old I would have been in despair and this reflected the feelings of parents at the meeting when talking together later. I knew the presenter was wrong as I had cared for a number of elderly people with Down syndrome in their fifties who were fit and did not die of dementia.

I have to say that this is not the only time I have listened to researchers of different disciplines present their data with apparently little awareness of the effects it would have on parents in their audience. It happens far too often. In the dementia example, the information was wrong but the presenter had made assumptions from pathology which she had not even checked out by talking with those caring for adults with Down syndrome.

It was premature to discuss the possible real-life significance of her findings. In other examples, the information may be correct, but the way it is presented is insensitive and does not adequately draw out the real-life implications for either parents or practitioners in the audience who are trying to understand how it is relevant for their child or the children and families they serve. Quite often, the limitations of a research study and whether or not it has any ecological validity are not made clear. An example of this would be work on recognizing emotions from still-face pictures—in the real world there are multiple cues to help a person identify how someone is feeling, from tones of voice to body postures and the context of the situation; therefore, it is not justifiable to suggest people with Down syndrome are poor at emotion recognition from the results of a still-face experiment.

If we consider the dementia example further, it can be argued that knowing a person is at increased risk leads to the early detection and treatment of an illness. That may be true when we have precise diagnostic criteria. We do not have these for dementia and since the message got out over a decade ago that everyone with Down syndrome gets dementia, I have seen many examples of adults wrongly thought to have dementia when they were actually depressed or even just unhappy and disturbed by a move of home, loss of a loved one or friend, or loss of a job. I have also been concerned to read papers where researchers are suggesting the early effects of dementia and the inevitable cognitive decline for all with Down syndrome may explain their results for some individuals in late adolescence or early adult life.

In summary, the chapters in this book provide scientists and physicians with a great deal of useful knowledge on the medical conditions studied and on treatment approaches, but researchers and physicians need to consider how to share information with parents in a sensitive way that is relevant to their child, whether at a meeting in a clinic or at a presentation at a meeting or conference.

5. Exploring Health Patterns

Two of the chapters in this volume report a range of interesting findings on patterns of illness in the community and on the effects of disability on the employment and financial status of families. Here again, the authors provide comprehensive reviews of the available literature.

It is important for health services to be aware that babies with Down syndrome are more likely to be premature and of low birth weight. However, the significance of the mean being 37.7 rather than 38.8 weeks gestation may not really carry significant additional risk for most of the babies, whereas a mean of 34 weeks might. Similarly, for birth weight what matters is how many babies are so small for dates that it has implications for their survival or health. Babies and children with Down syndrome are smaller and lighter for most of their early childhood. We are back to being careful to consider the real-life implications of a statistically significant finding.

As the authors point out, some of the other trends reported for the effects of ethnic backgrounds on birth, illness rates, or longevity need to be very carefully considered in terms of the available attitudes and services in different communities, especially as the studies are not all consistent in their findings.

For example, in the UK, the availability of good-quality child care has improved greatly in the last decade and this has made it possible for both parents to work, as is the case in Scandinavian countries. The advice given when a baby is first diagnosed will influence parental behavior. When parents are encouraged not to change their life plans but to carry on as they had planned for a typical baby joining their family, outcomes can be different. The educational and financial status of the family, the attitudes, services, and financial supports in their community, the support of the extended family, and the individual characteristics of the child with Down syndrome will all affect outcomes for a particular child and family.

This highlights yet again the difficulty of understanding the implications for an individual family of the results of large-scale surveys. We actually need to know how the range of factors listed above and others really do increase or reduce the stresses of caring for a child with Down syndrome and the effects on health, wealth, and employment. The effects of poverty, pollution, and poor housing are likely to affect a child with Down syndrome and their families in the same direction that they do for other children and families.

6. Individual Differences

The demographic factors influencing children and families are probably easier to identify and to quantify than the differences in the individual characteristics of children with Down syndrome. Studies of all children with Down syndrome in comparison with children without Down syndrome are, of course, important as they alert us to possible differences but we need finer-grained analyses as there is great diversity in this population. The extent of a child's healthcare needs and the nature of them matter—a life-threatening illness has a very different impact to an acute but treatable one or even a chronic but treatable one. The personality and behavioral characteristics of young children with Down syndrome vary widely and have a significant impact on the stresses involved in child care. The learning and language abilities of the children also vary widely. Each child and adult is an individual with the same rights and needs as the rest of the population plus some additional ones. The "child first" and "person first" message still needs to be stressed.

I learned slowly that my daughter with Down syndrome was more alike than different from her brother and sister. This became steadily more apparent as she became a teenager, reached puberty, wanted to wear her jeans to school, sit with the boys in the bus, and listen to the same pop groups as everyone else her age. It became absolutely clear when she moved to independent supported living at 22 years of age and fell madly in love. She wanted what everyone else her age wanted, to get away from home, have a place that was her private space, make her own decisions (and learn from her mistakes), have a close, loving, caring, and sexual relationship, have a meaningful leisure life and a job. She has succeeded on all fronts—always with the necessary support.

One topic that needs more up-to-date research is sexuality. The main references quoted in this volume are dated in the 1980s. We do not actually have any good scientific data even on fertility and much less on sexuality and relationships. My daughter has competently managed contraception by taking the contraceptive pill and by being supported through a family planning service available to all women in her community. Indeed, when she met and fell in love with her partner and we negotiated sexuality, I remarked to family and friends that the family planning service was excellent and the first time she had received a mainstream, inclusive service in her life. My daughter's benefits from and experience of loving relationships has also taught me not to underestimate the emotional and social competence of adults with Down syndrome.

Another topic that needs more research is the diagnosis of autism in children and adults with Down syndrome. The dual diagnosis of Down syndrome and autism is being made more frequently but we need to know more about the tendency for this to happen for children with the most severe intellectual delays and also to be diagnosed even when the children are socially and emotionally engaged so do not have the core social deficit of autism.

7. Important Progress

I have raised a number of issues about the presentation of findings so that they can be interpreted as they might apply to a particular individual in a family or clinic setting. I have also appealed for more sophisticated studies which actually allow us to tease out the effects of different family environments and individual characteristics so that we can understand and possibly predict individual risks and needs better. However, as the chapters in this volume indicate, we have made huge advances in knowledge of the healthcare needs of children with Down syndrome.

The most positive outcome of what we know is the preventative programmes and screening that are now possible and the guidelines to medical care available and accepted in medical practice in the USA and elsewhere. The information on the increased risk of many conditions is important in alerting physicians to consider them when treating a patient with Down syndrome. It is equally important that physicians know that there are some significant conditions such as solid cancer tumors and some types of heart disease that are less common; therefore, screening for these should not necessarily be the same as it is in the general population—mammograms and cervical smears would be two examples that would be distressing and are not warranted (although the significance of the latter could change as more adult women with Down syndrome lead normal lives).

8. In Conclusion

Healthcare advances for individuals with Down syndrome have largely been the result of advances in knowledge of illnesses and effective treatments for the whole population. There is still a need to ensure that children and, in particular, adults with Down syndrome actually access healthcare when they need it and that they receive care that is of the same quality as that offered to other non-disabled people in their communities. They will not be able to ask the same questions nor always be able to provide information in the same way, and informed support and advocacy is essential. Care staff in supported living settings need to be well informed and healthcare plans in place and monitored for all individuals.

There is also still a need to educate the medical profession in the healthcare needs of children and adults with Down syndrome. The advent of the internet should make this easy and there are now examples of the way this can be used effectively to educate health professionals (see Brighter Tomorrows 2010; Canister Books 2010; Skotko 2010). However, in my experience, the biggest need is still to educate health professionals about the potential of people with Down syndrome. Still too many parents complain of meeting professionals who are ill-informed, with low expectations, and generally negative views about the potential of children and adults with Down syndrome to lead happy and productive lives and bring life-long joy to their families.

RESOURCES

Skotko, B (2010). Online course for health professionals. http://brianskotko.com/
Brighter tomorrows http://brighter-tomorrows.org/
Canister books http://canisterbooks.com/diagnosisbook.php

Afterword

The past fifty years have produced landmark changes in the lives of people with Down syndrome and their families. It has been quite remarkable to observe, and be part of, the social, educational, and attitudinal progress that we recognize today. Since the early post–World War II period when more and more families began to refuse institutionalization, giant strides have been taken in creating supports for individuals and families and in creating more inclusive and welcoming communities.

Longevity studies reveal that, although disparities exist among racial groups, individuals with Down syndrome are living much longer lives—indeed many are living into their sixties. During these longer lives, they are benefitting from better pedagogy utilized by educators to include them in regular classrooms and to adapt curriculum for them according to principles of universal design for learning (UDL). Individuals with Down syndrome are also benefitting from more intensive skill development to seek and obtain employment, earn wages, accumulate assets, and live independently or semi-independently.

It is hard to overstate the timeliness and the importance of this special volume on health care issues in Down syndrome. By any objective measure, the progress we have witnessed in health care offered to children and adults with Down syndrome is a pivotal advance, if not the pivotal advance underpinning the successes of persons with Down syndrome we learn about whether from the National Down Syndrome Society's (NDSS) *My Great Story* public awareness campaign or from our own observations as we watch lives being lived in communities all around us.

Yet we know less than we think we know about persons with Down syndrome and certainly far less than there is to know and to apply. The distinguished researchers who authored this impressive volume about health care have greatly expanded the existing body of knowledge about the health of people with Down syndrome. In a scholarly and in depth manner these authors have covered the major health issues facing individuals with Down syndrome across the lifespan. Persons with Down syndrome can have a wide range of health problems, including congenital heart defects, obstructed digestive systems, thyroid conditions, ear and hearing problems, increased susceptibility to infection, sleep apnea, and respiratory problems. Individuals with Down syndrome also are at a higher risk of developing Alzheimer's disease.

Most significantly, this volume appears at a moment in time when the leadership of new champions in Congress and the increased political sophistication of the Down syndrome movement have wrought greater federal and state government focus on Down syndrome research and health care. In the Fiscal Year 2006 Senate Labor, Health and Human Services Appropriations bill, report language was included which called for the Director of the National Institutes of Health (NIH) to establish an NIH Down Syndrome Research Task Force to develop a strategic plan for research. This blueprint, and one subsequently published by the Centers for Disease Control and Prevention (CDC), a sister federal agency of NIH, emphasize the need for research on medical, cognitive, health and behavioral conditions affecting people with Down syndrome.

At a time when the NIH and CDC strategic plans offer roadmaps for basic research and longitudinal Down syndrome population surveillance, the special volume, and the new and newly accumulated knowledge it provides, will help individuals with Down syndrome and their families, researchers and clinicians reach benchmarks in the roadmaps more quickly.

The publication of this compilation on Down syndrome converges with other major developments in the policy arena that merit explanation.

In 2008, Congress passed the *Prenatally and Postnatally Diagnosed Conditions Awareness Act*. This landmark, bipartisan legislation will ensure that women who receive a positive prenatal or postnatal diagnosis of Down syndrome and other chromosomal disorders, and the physicians who serve them, have available up-to-date, scientific information about the disorder, including life expectancy, clinical course, health conditions associated with the syndrome, intellectual and functional development, and prenatal and postnatal treatment options. The law authorizes the development and distribution of accurate, evidenced-based information about Down syndrome through a variety of means—the publication and distribution of printed materials, the creation of hotlines, websites and informational clearinghouses. The intent of the law is also to foster the development of a coherent process for delivering accurate information about the diagnosis to medical and other health professionals to avoid any conflicting, inaccurate or incomplete information being given to women and their partners.

The passage of this Act only intensifies the need for carefully researched and collected information about health care issues related to Down syndrome and guidance regarding treatment options and management.

Another significant policy development occurred at the end of 2009 when *The Trisomy 21 Translational Research Parity Act* was introduced in Congress. The bill seeks to incorporate Down syndrome as an area of permissible research and surveillance at the NIH and the CDC. Additionally, it will create Down Syndrome Translational Research Centers of Excellence to conduct and support basic, clinical, and translational research, but research that is truly patient-oriented. The Centers of Excellence would be designed to foster partnerships between academic institutions and clinics to conduct translational research and help develop interventions, treatments, and therapeutics for Down syndrome.

The legislation would also establish a Down Syndrome Coordinating Committee to coordinate activities across the institutes of NIH and other federal programs as well as establish a National Down Syndrome Patient Registry and Biobank. By creating a common data entry and management system for Down syndrome patient data collection and analysis, the registry and biobank would greatly enhance opportunities for translational research and for improved clinical care for patients with Down syndrome.

As Dr. Elias Zerhouni MD, former director of NIH stated, "We are now poised to capitalize on . . . advances and improve the health of people with Down syndrome." The developments described above, including the release of the special volume on Down syndrome indeed indicate that we are launched into a period of significant and exciting discovery. The time has never been so promising for using emerging knowledge to give people with Down syndrome the brighter future we collectively envision.

Madeline Will
National Down Syndrome Society
Vice President of Public Policy
Director, National Policy Center

Index

Note: The letters 'f' and 't' following the locators refers to figures and tables cited in the text.

B

E

F

U

V

W

X

Contents of Previous Volumes

Volume 7

Volume 8

Volume 9

Volume 10

Volume 11

Volume 12

Volume 13

Volume 14

Volume 15

Volume 16

Volume 17

Volume 18

Volume 19

Volume 20

Volume 21

Volume 22

Volume 23

Volume 24

Volume 25

Volume 26

Volume 27

Volume 28

Volume 29

Volume 30

Volume 31

Volume 32

Volume 33

Volume 34

Volume 35

Volume 36

Volume 37

Volume 38